MEDICAL APPLICATIONS
OF
CLINICAL NUTRITION

Keats Titles of Relevant Interest

Brain Allergies by William H. Philpott, M.D. and Dwight K. Kalita, Ph.D.

Diet and Disease by E. Cheraskin, M.D., D.M.D.;
  W.M. Ringsdorf, D.M.D.; and J.W. Clark, D.D.S.

Diverticular Disease of the Colon by Neil Painter, M.D.

Mental and Elemental Nutrients by Carl C. Pfeiffer, Ph.D., M.D.

Minerals and Your Health by Len Mervyn, Ph.D.

Nutrients to Age Without Senility by Abram Hoffer, Ph.D., M.D. and
  Morton Walker, D.P.M.

Orthomolecular Nutrition by Abram Hoffer, Ph.D., M.D., and
  Morton Walker, D.P.M.

Physician's Handbook on Orthomolecular Medicine, edited by
  Roger J. Williams, Ph.D. and Dwight K. Kalita, Ph.D.

The Poisons Around Us by Henry A. Schroeder, M.D.

Predictive Medicine by E. Cheraskin, M.D. and W. M. Ringsdorf, D.M.D.

The Saccharine Disease by T.L. Cleave, M.D.

Selenium as Food and Medicine by Richard A. Passwater, Ph.D.

Trace Elements, Hair Analysis and Nutrition by Richard A. Passwater, Ph.D.
  and Elmer M. Cranton, M.D.

Victory Over Diabetes: A Bio-Ecologic Triumph by
  William H. Philpott, M.D., and Dwight K. Kalita, Ph.D.

MEDICAL APPLICATIONS OF CLINICAL NUTRITION

Edited by
JEFFREY BLAND, PH.D.
University of Puget Sound

Introduction by Norman Shealy, M.D.

with contributions by
Donald R. Davis, Ph.D.; William D. McArdle, Ph.D., and
John R. Magel, Ph.D.; Sheldon Reiser, Ph.D.;
Herbert K. Naito, Ph.D., and Henry F. Hoff, Ph.D.;
Abram Hoffer, M.D., Ph.D.; Raymond J. Shamberger, Ph.D.;
Denis Burkitt, M.D.; Scott Rigden, M.D.
and Jeffrey Bland, Ph.D.

Keats Publishing ✹ New Canaan, Connecticut

Library of Congress Cataloging in Publication Data
  Main entry under title:

  Medical applications of clinical nutrition.

  Includes bibliographical references and index.
    1. Nutrition disorders.   2. Diet therapy.   3. Nutriton.
I. Bland, Jeffrey, 1946–   . II. Davis, Donald, 1941–
[DNLM: 1. Diet therapy.   2. Nutrition.   3. Nutrition disorders.
WB 400 M489]
RC620.M38 1983   616.3'9   82-84365
ISBN 0-87983-327-0

MEDICAL APPLICATIONS OF CLINICAL NUTRITION

Printed in the United States of America

Keats Publishing, Inc.
27 Pine Street, New Canaan, Connecticut 06840

Dedication

The field of clinical nutrition is rapidly changing as a result of the vision of observant clinicians and innovative laboratory researchers. This book was written to reflect the vitality and excitement in the field of clinical nutrition as it applies to health care, and is dedicated to the many investigators and clinicians who have contributed in their own ways to the progress in this field.

CONTENTS

ACKNOWLEDGEMENTS

This book has been born out of several years of discussion among the various authors concerning the need for an overview of modern clinical nutrition as it applies to health care. After a number of drafts and editorial alterations, An and Nathan Keats of Keats Publishing were supportive of the publication of this manuscript to make this information available to the health practitioner. It is to them that a great amount of thanks go for the final publishing force necessary to make this book a reality.

The authors also thank Mr. Kenneth Anderson for his fine editorial and copy work done on the manuscript; and a special note of thanks goes to my secretarial staff, Ms. Mary Ludlow and Phyllis Hamilton for their fine work in integrating the various chapters and getting the book to flow together.

Finally, credit for the germ seed of the idea of this book should go to Drs. Norman Shealy and Elmer Cranton of the American Holistic Medical Association.

Jeffrey Bland, Ph.D.
Tacoma, Washington
April, 1983

ABOUT THE CONTRIBUTORS

Jeffrey Bland, Ph.D.

Dr. Bland is an associate professor of chemistry, specializing in nutritional biochemistry at the University of Puget Sound in Tacoma, Washington and is director of the Bellevue-Redmond Medical Laboratory. He serves as president of the Northwest Academy of Preventive Medicine and is actively working in research and writing in the area of early recognition of nutritional inadequacy. His Ph.D. in biochemistry was taken at the University of Oregon and he has been involved as a postdoctoral fellow in clinical chemistry.

Donald R. Davis, Ph.D.

Dr. Davis is a senior research associate at Clayton Biochemical Institute at the University of Texas at Austin and has written widely in the area of biochemical individuality and its relationship to nutritional needs. He is a former professor of chemistry at the University of California, Irvine, and has his doctorate in organic chemistry. For the past eight years his speciality has been in the area of nutritional biochemistry and establishing the diversity of biochemical individuality.

William D. McArdle Ph.D. and John R. Magel, Ph.D.

Drs. McArdle and Magel are professors at Queens College of City University of New York in physiology. Dr. McArdle was an author of the important book entitled *Nutrition, Weight Control and Exercise* and he and Dr. Magel have been working together in research relating to fitness, weight management and metabolic control.

Sheldon Reiser, Ph.D.

Dr. Reiser is a senior research scientist at the United States Department of Agriculture, Beltsville, Maryland station, on carbohydrate research. He has contributed greatly to the appreciation of physiological differences in metabolism between starch and sugar. His research group has been one of the most active groups in the world in establishing those differences.

Herbert K. Naito, Ph.D. and Henry F. Hoff, Ph.D.

Drs. Naito and Hoff are both scientists at the Cleveland Clinic Foundation, Cleveland, Ohio and have been engaged in extensive research into the process of atherogenesis. Their studies on the relationship of serum lipid disorders and atherosclerosis have been very important in delineating both the mechanism of atherogenesis and the dietary relationship thereof.

Abram Hoffer, M.D., Ph.D.

Dr. Hoffer has been a primary investigator for thirty years in the area of nutrition and behavior. He has been instrumental in establishing a molecular explanation for behavior disorders at the brain biochemical level and along with Dr. Humphry Osmond has proposed and provided experimental evidence for a brain biochemical mechanism for schizophrenia which is responsive to megavitamin therapies. Although their proposal still remains controversial, the impact that it has made on the psychiatric field has been tremendous and resulted in worldwide interest in biological and biochemical mechanisms of mental dysfunction.

Raymond J. Shamberger, Ph.D.

Dr. Shamberger works at the Cleveland Clinic Foundation as a senior research scientist, has been actively involved in research and publication in the area of trace element nutrition and the relationship of vitamin undernutriture to chronic physiological dysfunction. His work in selenium nutrition allowed for the recognition of the relationship of selenium deficiency to increased risk to cardiovascular disease and certain cancers.

Denis Burkitt, M.D.

Dr. Burkitt has worked as a public health service physician in South Africa for more than forty years and was, with Dr. T. L. Cleave, among the first individuals to recognize the extremely important relationship between low dietary fiber intake and increased risk to gastrointestinal diseases. His pioneering work in this area has been instrumental in initiating considerable research around the world in the role that dietary fiber plays in proper gastrointestinal function and which constituents of fiber are responsible for this action.

Scott Rigden, M.D.

Dr. Rigden is a family physician in Illinois who has integrated nutrition into the general practice of medicine at the family practice level effectively and has developed a number of teaching and training tools to help his patients recognize the importance of and integrate the concepts of improved nutrition in their daily lives. He has been an active member of the American Holistic Medical Association and has written a guide for physicians in the implementation of nutrition in their practices.

PREFACE

THE PAST TEN YEARS has seen a virtual explosion in information as it relates to the impact that nutrition—both prophylactic and therapeutic—has on human health and disease. The rate at which this information is accumulating is somewhat overwhelming to the average clinician, and sometimes it is difficult for medical practitioners who want to apply clinical nutrition to their daily practice to find approaches to implement these new concepts.

It was with this problem in mind that *Medical Applications of Clinical Nutrition* was born. Its various authors were asked specifically to relate areas of their own expertise in the nutritional science field to the needs of the average health practitioner and to bring to the clinician new therapeutic modalities for both the prevention and the management of various degenerative diseases through altered nutrition.

It is certainly not fair to suggest that all major killer diseases are caused by suboptimal nutrition, but there is an overwhelming amount of information now indicating that the progression and origin of many, if not all, of these diseases may be related to the malnutrition of overconsumptive undernutrition. The average American diet has been implicated as contributing to this form of borderline malnutrition of too much of too little.

Recent studies, such as the Health and Nutrition Examination Survey and the Dietary Goals of the United States, indicate that dietary changes decreased risk to morbidity—and potentially, mortality—from many of the degenerative diseases.

This book has focused on those well-documented areas of nutritional intervention which decrease the risk of many of the major killer diseases and it has put these approaches at a level that can be applied by practicing clinicians without the necessity of becoming specialists in the nutritional sciences.

It is hoped that this book will stimulate further discussion, inquiry and interest in the field of clinical nutrition as it applies to medical problems. Often, medical practitioners are put off by nutrition because of its very qualitative, nonscientific, historical legacies. We hope that this book will make it clear that modern nutrition has become a true science and is as applicable to health care as any of the other subspecialties of medicine.

This book has concentrated primarily on nutrition as it relates to prevention and management of many of the major diseases such as coronary heart disease, cerebrovascular problems, maturity-onset diabetes or gastrointestinal dysfunctions, rather than on iatrogenic nutritional problems such as hospital-induced malnutrition, postsurgical malnutrition, or specialty problems such as total parenteral nutrition.

After an introduction to the topic of clinical nutrition and its application to the medical sciences with emphasis on identification of early warning risk factors to nutritional inadequacy, Dr. Donald Davis discusses the important concept of biochemical diversity and its relationship to establishing nutritional needs. He points out that nutrition is for real people, and that statistical humans are of little interest in the field of clinical nutrition.

This leads to a detailed discussion of how to assess the individual patient for the potentiality of overconsumptive undernutrition, and then Drs. McArdle and Magel discuss the most prevalent nutritional problem exemplifying this type of malnutrition, that of weight management and its relationship to diet and exercise.

Dr. Reiser then addresses the very difficult topic of the physiological differences between starch and sugar. His excellent research enables him to indicate why some individuals are sucrose sensitive, as excessive levels of simple carbohydrate in their diet may contribute to increased risk to certain diet-related diseases.

Doctors Naito and Hoff then discuss diet and its relationship to pathogenesis of the blood vessel wall and arterio- and atherosclerosis. The diet/heart disease controversy is still raging vigorously and this lucidly written chapter helps to identify some of the facts that we do know with security concerning fats and other agents in the diet which may contribute to increased risk to the atherosclerotic process.

Dr. Hoffer then addresses a topic which only in the last five to ten years has received great attention in the nutritional literature, that of the relationship of diet to behavior. Drawing on his years of experience that Dr. Hoffer has had as a psychiatrist, he is able to pull together both clinical information and research data which supports the important role that proper diet plays in optimizing behavior and also the relationship of certain personality/behavior disorders to nutritional variance.

Dr. Raymond Shamberger next undertakes the important area of vitamin and mineral undernutriture and the relationship to clinical symptomatologies. There is still continuing debate as to whether vitamins and minerals in supplemental doses are beneficial for individuals who eat the standard American diet, and Dr.

Shamberger's discussion of this topic provides better information in the resolution of this debate.

Dr. Burkitt then discusses the role that dietary fiber plays in intestinal function and absorptive processes and traces both historically and from more recent experimental studies the important distinctions among different types of fiber and the roles that each may play in human digestive function.

Finally, Dr. Rigden ties all of this information together, writing about how clinical nutrition can apply to the practice of general medicine and be integrated into the day-by-day routine. Specific emphasis on behavior modification for patients and techiques for patient education in the nutrition area are stressed in Dr. Rigden's chapter.

Taken as a whole, this book can allow the clinician to recognize how to assess the patient's nutritional status and then to apply either preventive or therapeutic nutrition where it is required by modifying both macronutrient and micronutrient intake.

It is to be hoped that delivery of this information by improving the eating habits and life-style of the patient will be facilitated through this book by two mechanisms: better doctor education and the introduction of the physician to methods of patient behavior modification.

J.B.

INTRODUCTION

THERE WAS A TIME, in the days of Hippocrates, when nutrition was considered an extremely important part of medical care; and it is of some interest that Sir William Osler, often called the Father of American Medicine, wrote extensively on problems of poor nutrition and the "abominable" confections that people were eating in this country.

During an otherwise excellent medical school training at Duke University, a year of general surgical residency at Barnes Hospital—Washington University, and five years of neurosurgical training at Massachusetts General Hospital, I received no instruction in nutrition other than some information about diets for various illnesses including such things as the Sippy diet for peptic ulcer (since proven to be ineffective) and some information about diets for diabetes or for weight loss. The quality of nutrition was never discussed. Even today, only a few medical schools have any courses at all in nutrition and most of these are very inadequate. Even more appalling is the poor quality of nutrition fed at most hospitals in this country. There are several studies indicating patients may leave the hospital being nutritionally malnourished.

Because of this almost total deficit in medical training, most physicians continue to feel that patients need "only to eat a balanced diet"—whatever that means. Most physicians could hardly know since they haven't really been taught that. The Surgeon General has emphasized that Americans eat too much fat, salt and sugar.

How right that is! Many Americans consume approximately 18 percent of their calories as refined sugar which has no vitamins or minerals necessary for its metabolism. They consume another 18 percent of their calories in the form of refined, enriched white flour which is nutritionally deficient in approximately twenty-eight essential nutrients, especially vitamin B6, the most commonly deficient B vitamin in the diet of the American people. B6 deficiency has been highly associated with coronary artery disease and carpal tunnel syndrome, among other illnesses.

The outstanding work of Burkitt, Cleave and many others on the adverse effects of refined flour and sugar upon health have been largely ignored both in this country and abroad. In my own practice, 60 percent of patients who have been tested with blood levels of B vitamins have been found to be deficient in one or another of the B vitamins.

One of the great crises facing America today is the marked increase in the cost of medical care. It is quite likely that general health could be improved very significantly if people only ate better. A tremendous beginning for educating physicians has been made.

I have been fortunate to be privy to some of the earlier parts of *The Medical Applications of Clinical Nutrition* and consider this one of the most important books ever published. Jeffrey Bland, its general editor, has put his extensive knowledge of nutrition to excellent use.

In my opinion, every physician in this country should own and read this book. It could do more for health care than all the drugs and all the surgery in the country if doctors would only heed the important information contained herein. Intelligent physicians will take advantage of the many pearls provided by Jeffrey Bland and the other professionals who have contributed, and if physicians are as intelligent as I believe they are, the health of all Americans will surely benefit.

C. Norman Shealy, M.D., Ph.D.
Springfield, Missouri

PART I

THE NUTRITION-DISEASE LINK

1

THE POTENTIAL FUTURE
OF NUTRITIONAL MEDICINE

———————— ◄•► ————————

JEFFREY BLAND, PH.D.

NUTRITION has become an increasingly popular topic in the fields of health care over the past few years. This increased interest has led to the more frequent recognition of the malnutrition related to overconsumption/undernutrition. This form of malnutrition, which is not characterized by diseases of frank deficiency (kwashiorkor, marasmus, beri-beri, scurvy, pellagra or rickets), but rather by increased risk to many of the degenerative diseases such as coronary heart disease, maturity onset diabetes and conditions associated with obesity, as well as syndromes that were previously characterized as being psychogenic in origin (depression, lassitude, fatigue, malaise, neuroses and the preclinical signs of anemia) has been occupying more and more time in the training of clinicians. The recognition and management of these dietary-related health problems are at the frontier of modern clinical nutrition. Patients are coming to their physicians with questions concerning the significance of cholesterol, sugar in the American diet, vegetarianism, megavitamin therapy, the use of nutritional supplements and many other nutritional controversies.[1] Where do physicians derive their nutrition information to respond to these questions? One need only go back and trace the history of nutrition education to fully appreciate the present position that the physician finds him or herself in when attempting to field these questions and to integrate nutritional concepts in the practice.

The history of clinical nutrition can be divided into four distinct eras: the first began in the nineteenth century and extended into the early twentieth century when it was recognized for the first time that food contained constituents which were essential for human function and that different foods provided different amounts

5

of these essential agents. Near the end of this era David Cuthbertson reported his studies of mineral and nitrogen metabolism in patients, demonstrating that rapid weight loss was associated with negative nitrogen balance and could only be rectified by providing adequate dietary protein associated with certain foods.

The second era was initiated in the early decades of the twentieth century and might be called "the vitamin period." Vitamins came to be recognized in foods and deficiency syndromes were described. Famous names associated with this era include Eijkman, Funk, Szent-Györgyi, King, McCollum and Davis, Osborne and Mendel, Wolbach and Goldberger.[2]

As vitamins became recognized as essential food constituents necessary for health, it became tempting to suggest that every disease and condition for which there had been no previous effective treatment might be responsive to vitamin therapy. At that point in time, medical schools started to become more interested in having their curricula integrate nutritional concepts into the basic sciences. Much of the focus of this education was on the recognition of vitamin deficiency symptoms. Herein lay the beginnings of what ultimately turned from ignorance to denial of the value of nutritional therapies in medicine. Reckless claims were made for effects of vitamins that were far beyond what could be actually achieved from the use of these essential nutrients.

In the third era of nutritional history in the early 1950s to mid 1960s, vitamin therapy began to fall into disrepute. Concommitant with this, nutrition education in medical schools also became less popular. It was just a decade before this that many drug companies had found their vitamin sales skyrocketing and were quick to supply practicing physicians with generous samples of vitamins and literature extolling the virtue of supplementation for a variety of health-related conditions. Expectations as to the success of vitamins in disease control were exaggerated. As we now know in retrospect, vitamin and mineral therapies are much less effective when applied to health-crisis conditions than when applied to long-term problems of undernutrition which lead to chronic health problems. Although many practitioners had hoped that vitamin therapy would be similar in its impact to that of antibiotic therapy, the effects upon human physiology of vitamins versus antibiotics were vastly different; therefore, disillusionment concerning the usefulness of nutritional therapy resulted. Associated with this disillusionment, nutrition as a topic of discussion became an unpopular subject in medical school curricula, and over the next period of time medical schools that once had nutrition courses in their curricula dropped these required courses, hoping that the brief discussion of nutrition in courses such as biochemistry would be adequate.

As this educational vacuum developed, due to the reduced emphasis on nutrition in medical institutions, it was filled by lay nutritionists and individuals who purported to have miracle cures using nutritional remedies. As a result, the past ten to fifteen years have seen a reputation surrounding nutrition grow as a "soft science" with little relevance to clinical medicine as long as a person is consuming foods from the four food groups.

The stigma surrounding nutrition education in medical schools may have been further stimulated by the difference in academic lineage between the origin of health scientists and nutritionists. Traditionally, health scientists have been schooled in universities, which have a pure research bias in their pedagogy, whereas nutrition has grown up in the land-grant state colleges, closely tied to dietetics, home economics, agriculture and animal husbandry. The more utilitarian education that was traditionally offered by the land-grant college may have resulted in a rejection by the "pure scientists" educating the health scientists at the university. It should also be pointed out that a sex bias is likely involved as well. Traditionally, nutrition was the responsibility of the homemaker (a woman) and health care of the doctor (a man). The woman who wanted to be a professional nutritionist or dietician went to the land-grant college, whereas the man wanting to be a doctor went to the university. This distinction has contributed to the reputation that nutrition is soft science (and by association, poor science) and cannot be adequately integrated into a program of scientific medicine. It only recently has come to light that many of the major diseases may have part of their origin related to suboptimal nutrition.

Due to the recognition of the relationship of disease to the malnutrition of overconsumption/undernutrition, there has been a winning back of the sympathies of many health practitioners as to the importance of nutrition in terms of reflection upon the total diet and the impact of diet on specific individuals in the prevention of nutrient-related syndromes. This signals the fourth period of nutrition evolution in the past five years, which has witnessed the reintroduction of nutrition courses within the curricula of many schools training health practitioners and a new heightened emphasis on nutritional biochemistry and the role that nutrition can play in a total preventive health-care program. The emphasis of these programs is not only to train health practitioners didactically about the relationships that nutrition has to health, but in a broader sense to expose them clinically on the wards to the actual application of nutritional therapies to ambulatory or hospitalized patients.

Symposia have recently been held which discuss specifically the problems of how to effectively teach and train health practitioners in nutrition in a medical school setting,[3] and have led to the conclusion that considerable curricular redesign is necessary to transmit effectively the new information in the area of clinical nutrition to health practitioners.

A survey of practicing physicians and second-year medical students by Richard Podell has suggested that medical students and physicians learn about nutrition haphazardly and are highly dependent for their knowledge on nonprofessional literature.[4]

It was also found that there was a considerable difference in health practitioners from individual to individual, between their actual knowledge of nutrition and their belief in their knowledge of nutrition. A study by D. E. Dugdale and colleagues found that all groups of health practitioners had a high level of "perceived knowledge" of nutrition, but that the accuracy of the knowledge on objective questionnaires was surprisingly low, indicating that better quality control in the area of nutritional knowledge and better information transfer are essential in this field.[5]

Robert Olson has defined clinical nutrition as an interface between human ecology and internal medicine, with nutrition defined as the science of food and its relationship to health.[6] This broader definition of nutrition opens the door for a more intense look by health practitioners at what the contemporary nutrition information, accumulated over the past ten years, has to say about helping people keep healthy. The forty-five or more essential nutrients, necessary in the diets of humans to promote optimal physiological function, represent the most comprehensive list of essential dietary constituents of any organism in the phylogenetic tree. Human beings are more dependent upon their food supply system than any other organism, plant or animal, for optimal function. The red bread mold, *Neurospora crassa*, can manufacture all of its own vitamins, essential amino acids, and essential fatty acids from a few mineral salts, some water, light and a warm place to live, whereas humans require these agents to be manufactured by other plants or animals for their use. This dependency of humans upon essential nutrients makes them more vulnerable to nutritional inadequacies and to chronic nutritional deficiency syndromes. The recognition of this concept is exposing the vulnerability of humans to malnutrition and is revealing how undernutrition can result in chronic states of dysfunction.

It has been suggested by some investigators that possibly many of the degenerative diseases have twenty- to thirty-year latency periods from the time of their inception until the full-blown clinical symptomatology of that disease profile exists, and that these progressions may result in part from suboptimal nutrition. If this is so, then the impact of people's nutritional support upon their metabolism is controlled by their unique genetic lineage. It might be considered that the expression of these diseases is in part related to a conditional lethal mutation. Everyone carries genetic characteristics which could contribute to disease and ultimately death, but this may be prevented by optimal adjustment of the environment to prevent the expression of this characteristic. The adverse effects of this mutation is conditioned by the diet, life style and environment of the individual. This might explain why certain diets might be associated with a statistical increased risk of degenerative disease, but might not produce that disease in all people consuming that diet. The impact of a specific diet upon a unique individual will be determined by the genetics of that individual, and the conditional lethal mutant sensitivity of one individual may not be mirrored by another.

A number of nutritionally related diseases are known to be related to conditional lethal mutations. A partial list of these is seen in Table 1. Adjusting the diet of infants born with phenylketonuria, methylmalonic aciduria, or cystathioninuria to account for their unique genetic needs will allow prevention of the disease state that would result if this relationship were not recognized. It is argued that the diet-disease links proposed the past ten years are related to genetic sensitivity to certain dietary habits which express themselves as a disease after a multi-year latency period (e.g., atherosclerosis and a high fat diet). This model would account for why some individuals may become diseased following a certain dietary pattern and others with differing genetic sensitivity may not. From these arguments it follows that many diseases not now recognized as such may be conditional lethal mutations, where the modifiers are agents within the environment, such as diet.

Even in the face of these unique genetic determinants, it can be established that there are certain basic dietary considerations which will minimize the risk to nutrient-related health difficulties for most individuals and that community-based nutrition improvement programs should focus upon health improvement by delivery of this improved preventive nutrition. Such concepts as a diet lower in total dietary fat with higher levels of dietary fiber, and a diet with a density of micronutrients, as the vitamins and minerals, higher than in the average American diet, appear from most studies to be in the best interest of improved health and the prevention of degenerative disease.

TABLE 1.1
Representative Nutrient Responsive Conditional Lethal Diseases

phenylketonuria
maple syrup urine syndrome
juvenile-onset diabetes
methylmalonic aciduria
cystathioninuria
ornithinemia
homocystinuria
pyruvic decarboxylase deficiency
xanthurenic aciduria

Undernutrition Needs New Methods of Evaluation

As William Connor has pointed out, at first glance the notion that preventive nutrition needs further discussion seems superfluous, in that we have witnessed a spectrum of diseases emerging over the past fifty years which may be related to a relatively recent new type of malnutrition: that of overconsumption/undernutrition.[7] Inspection of Table 1.2 will illustrate the diseases of overconsumption and the relationship to specific nutritional excesses.

TABLE 1.2
Diseases of Overconsumption and The Suggested Nutrient Excesses

Atherosclerosis, coronary heart disease and stroke	Cholesterol, saturated fat, and calories
Hypertension	Salt and calories
Obesity	Calories
Diabetes mellitus	Calories
Cholesterol gallstones	Cholesterol and fat
Cancer of the breast	Fat and cholesterol, absence of fiber
Cancer of the uterus	Calories
Dental caries	Sucrose

The characteristics of these diseases are as follows:

1. The clinical manifestations usually appear in mid-adult life.
2. The precursor markers for subsequent disease may be seen in children and young adults.
3. Affluence and technology make possible a diet for everyone which is high in calories, saturated fat, sucrose, cholesterol and protein.
4. Overconsumption is a cultural and economic problem and a core part of the life-style.

There are certain advantages and disadvantages of the application of preventive nutrition which need to be evaluated. The advantages include: less strain upon the crisis-care intervention component of our disease-care delivery system, which is already overburdened; the cost of prevention has been identified to be less than that for crisis treatment; prevention allows patient choice and patient responsibility, so that they are controlling part of their own life destiny; the evidence for harm is minimal to nonexistent in using prevention and nutritional approaches; and lastly, the control of all the important degenerative diseases is possible through the implementation of an effective preventive nutrition program. The problems in this approach include: people have difficulty in changing their food habits; there is no control over the contents of manufactured, preprepared and fabricated food products (of which more and more are being consumed); and because almost 40 percent of the meals in this country are eaten in institutional settings away from the home, there is again a loss of control of the food supply by individuals.

To implement an effective preventive nutrition program sensitive to these advantages and disadvantages education of the public and the health-care practitioners in the area of nutrition and diet aimed at the prevention of disease is essential. Progress needs to be made in providing ample alternative foods to those that are highly processed and nutrient-imbalanced. Education needs to go hand-in-hand with an improved food supply. Screening for individual early-warning precursor markers to subsequent disease and the relationship of these characteristics to specific diets should be emphasized in this education. A variety of government studies have demonstrated the prevalence of these problems of overconsumption/undernutrition. These include the Ten State Nutritional Study, The Health and Nutrition Examination Survey (HANES), and The Dietary Goals of the United States Senate.[8]

The question is, "What type of training should be provided to health-care practitioners so they may be better able to recognize these early warning signs of nutritional inadequacy or excess and to implement an effective behavior modification program before symptomatic disease results?" It is clear that new types of evaluation tools need to be integrated into the health-care practitioner's general screening protocol and that these should stress early-warning recognition of nutritional inadequacies and excesses. Gallagher and Vivian have indicated what type of concepts they view as essential in the education of health-care practitioners to allow them to understand the current information in clinical nutrition as it applies to health care and prevention. These can be broken down into the three broad categories of biochemistry, food-oriented and patient-management-oriented concepts, as indicated in Table 1.3.[9]

TABLE 1.3
Classification of Twenty-Six Designated Nutrition Concepts by Subject Content Orientation

BIOCHEMICALLY- AND PHYSIOLOGICALLY-ORIENTED CONCEPTS
 Nutrient digestion, absorption, utilization
 Energy metabolism
 Alcohol metabolism
 Nutrient requirements and allowances
 Acid-base balance
 Fluid and electrolyte balance
 Nutrition and acquired immunity
 Nutrition and mental retardation
 Hormonal control of nutrient metabolism
 Nutritional research techniques

FOOD-ORIENTED CONCEPTS
 Nutritive content of foods
 Fad diets and other food and health claims
 Additives to foods

PATIENT-MANAGEMENT-ORIENTED CONCEPTS
 Psychological regulation of food intake
 Nutrient deficiencies and excesses
 Nutrient and drug interaction
 Nutritional supplements
 Tube and parenteral feedings
 Nutrition during stages of the life style
 Nutrition and fetal development
 Nutrition and pregnancy and lactation
 Nutritional management for disease states
 Nutritional management in surgery
 Dietary history elicitation and evaluation
 Nutritional status assessment
 Patient instruction for nutritional management

In development of this training, it is important that expertise be developed in the area of both prophylactic and therapeutic nutrition. Prophylactic nutrition focuses more on prevention of specific diet-related health dysfunctions by dietary revision, whereas therapeutic nutrition deals with specific nutritionally related problems in people with diagnosed physiological problem areas, such as ulcerative colitis, diabetes, coronary heart disease, cancer, anemias, sprue or any number of other nutritionally related specific disease entities.

As this formalism is developed, it is clear that a better understanding of the role that both macronutrients (protein, carbohydrate and fat) and micronutrients (the vitamins, minerals and accessory food factors) play in promoting optimal health needs to be explored. There is ever-emerging data to suggest that there are a number of nutrients within food, which are synthesized by human metabolism and therefore do not fulfill the criterion as essential nutrients, but may be used therapeutically in some individuals as accessory food factors to promote optimal health where need for that specific agent exceeds the level they can synthesize *de novo*. Examples of such types of accessory food factors are seen in Table 1.4.

TABLE 1.4
Representative Examples of Accessory Food Factors

inositol
carnitine
choline (lecithin)
dihomogamma linolenic acid
omega-3-eicosapentaenoic acid
taurine
vegetable gums
saponins

Nutrition in Everyday Practice

The question that remains from this discussion is, "What responsibility does the general practitioner in health care have as a nutrition evaluator?" Obviously, questions related to implementation of the ideal basic diet need to be addressed, as well as more specific questions such as what diets are specific for weight reduction, questions related to the positive and negative aspects of the use of therapeutic vitamin/mineral supplements, problems of potential toxicity of specific nutrients, and what, if any, justification there is to support the contention that the diversity of the human population is greater than accounted for by the Recommended Dietary Allowances, so that certain individuals may need levels of nutrients far in excess of the RDAs for optimal function based upon their genetic uniqueness. These questions will all be addressed in subsequent chapters and will provide an awareness of the vitality of the rate of growth of the information available within the science of human nutrition. This field of clinical and laboratory research in nutrition is advancing at a staggering rate, partly due to the incorporation of the tools of the immunologist, the clinical biochemist, the exercise physiologist, the cellular physiologist and the human anatomist in designing and implementing controlled studies to look at the relationship of human nutrition to human disease.

As this multifactorial, interdisciplinary approach has been employed, there has been a virtual plethora of new associations made between the aspects of nutrition and physiological function. Association does not necessarily demonstrate causality, but from this research have come new therapeutic entries into such things as the management of diabetes through nutritional alteration, prevention of coronary heart disease and the amelioration of risk to many degenerative diseases. Supporting this particular vitality are the words of the United States Dietary Goals Committee: "In the view of doctors and nutritionists consulted by the Select Subcommittee on Nutrition for the National Need, it was concluded that changes in the U.S. diet over the past thirty years have led to a wave of malnutrition of both over- and underconsumption, and this may be as profoundly damaging to the nation's health as the wide-spread contagious diseases of the early part of the century." The Dietary Goals, promulgated as the basis of recommendation of the Senate Select Committee on Nutrition and Human Needs, came to the following sweeping conclusions as to improvement of the average American diet:

1. Carbohydrate consumption (predominately as complex carbohydrate) should be increased to account for 55 to 60 percent of the energy (calorie) intake.
2. Fat consumption should be reduced overall from 40 to no more than 30 percent of the energy intake.
3. Saturated fat consumption should account for about 10 percent of the total energy intake and should be balanced with polyunsaturated and monounsaturated fats.
4. Cholesterol consumption should be reduced to about 300 milligrams a day.

5. Sugar consumption should be reduced by 40 percent to account for no more than 15 percent of the total energy intake.
6. Salt consumption should be reduced by 50 to 85 percent to approximately 3 to 5 grams per day.

These recommendations translate into the following alterations for the average American:

1. Increased consumption of fruits, vegetables, whole grains and legume products.
2. Decreased consumption of red meat and increased consumption of fish and poultry without skin.
3. Decreased consumption of foods high in fat and partial substitution of polyunsaturated oils for saturated animal fat products.
4. Substitution of low-fat milk for whole milk.
5. Decreased consumption of butter fat, eggs and other high dietary cholesterol sources.
6. Decreased consumption of sugar and hidden-sugar-rich foods.
7. Decreased consumption of salt and hidden-salt-rich foods.[10]

These Dietary Goals imply fairly sweeping changes in the American food supply, which would be difficult to implement today, due to the momentum that is already built into the providing of highly processed, fabricated foods. Governmental agencies such as the National Institutes of Health have dealt gingerly with the diet/disease link, but pressure for the NIH to take a stand is building. A battle over what we should eat to prevent disease has split the federal establishment down the middle. Congress, appalled by the rising cost of health care, sees prevention as an alternate approach to health care. Both the U.S. Department of Agriculture and Congress want to alert the public to links between diet and chronic diseases, such as diabetes, hypertension, heart disease and cancer, but officials at the National Institutes of Health are skeptical, saying that in most cases hard evidence of such a diet/disease link has not yet come to light.[11] The present position on this debate seems to be stated by the recent comment on the subject by Fredrickson of the National Institutes of Health when he said, "We have more or less become adjusted to the fact that we probably will never be able to get the ideal proof that we want as it relates to the diet-disease link. The weight of the evidence seems to be strong enough so that we can now direct people toward a kind of set of guidelines."

It is with this in mind that the chapters in this book are offered, not as ultimate solutions to the problems, but as progress reports on how to implement improved nutrition in the areas of both prophylactic and therapeutic need, where the diet/disease link has been indicated to be quite strong.

Therapeutic nutritional improvement might start with the major problem of hospital malnutrition, and the prophylactic nutrition might start with the improvement of the average American diet to help prevent in those individuals with genetic sensitivity certain nutritionally related dysfunctions.

There is recognition that an alarming number of people in hospitals are malnourished and that this condition is preventable if proper therapeutic nutrition is employed. It has become well established that good nutrition plays a major role in wound healing and in lessening the risk to infection. There might be no more important role of therapeutic nutrition than the prevention of hospital malnutrition. [12]

Implementation of an Effective Preventive Nutrition Program

It is now respected that malnutrition has for too long been identified only with classical vitamin deficiency syndromes by health practitioners and other health professionals. Although these far advanced syndromes are occasionally encountered and should not be missed, overt vitamin and mineral deficiencies are best regarded as rare medical curiosities. By contrast general undernutrition has been found to affect from one-fourth to one-half of medical and surgical patients who required hospitalization for two weeks or more and possibly from one-sixth to one-fifth of the general population in the United States. Given the lack of recognition, then, of these problems, the improvement in the implementation of preventive nutrition will only be achieved when practitioners recognize what variables should be used in screening for these nutritional inadequacies.

As pointed out by Guthrie and Guthrie, three types of data should be developed on patients as they relate to their nutritional status: those coming from biochemical, anthropometric and dietary data. [13]

As seen in Table 1.5, the assessment of nutritional status can be accomplished by utilizing a variety of basic data. Dietary recall data in conjunction with biochemical information on nutritional status and anthropometric information all need to be integrated to give rise to a profile of patients as it relates to their relative risks to specific types of nutritional inadequacies or excesses. Davis has suggested that expanded criteria for establishing nutritional adequacy ought to be considered. These criteria should utilize more information as it relates to functional measurements of the individuals' ability to thrive as contrasted to focusing on the signs of nutritional deficiency.[14]

TABLE 1.5
Variables Used in Nutritional Assessment[13]

Dietary	*Biochemical*	*Anthropometric*
Calories	Hemoglobin	Height
Protein	Hematocrit	Weight
Iron	Transferrin	Lean body mass
Calcium	Serum folate	Exercise tolerance
Thiamin	Albumin	Arm circumference
Ascorbic acid	Ascorbic acid	
Vitamin A	Carotene	
	Urinary thiamin	
	& riboflavin	
	Iodine	

These screening tools will be the subject of the discussion in Chapter 4. The basic thrust of these screening tools is to identify the biochemical individuality of patients and what their unique nutritional needs may be for optimization of function.[15] The past five years have witnessed considerable improvement in the ability to recognize unique biochemical needs, based upon specific genetically determined metabolic patterns. These concepts will frame much of the discussion of subsequent chapters and will lead the clinician into new therapeutic avenues that may have previously been unexplored.

What then does the future for nutrition and medicine hold? The following areas represent a platform upon which future directions of research and development in the relationship of nutrition to health can be built:

1. The study of scientific nutrition begins with understanding the role of the macro- and micronutrients in human physiology.
2. The recognition that people can and do live, even when their nutrition is suboptimal, but that this may be associated with increased risk to certain diseases.
3. Nutrition is for real people. Statistical humans are of little or no value in discussing specific relationships of nutrition to individual disease patterns.

4. Nutrients work together synergistically, and therefore the study of food and its impact upon health is the foundation of nutrition understanding.
5. The extent to which nutritional manipulation can prevent disease is still an unknown quantity which demands intensive exploration, but at this point in time there is adequate evidence in many directions for effective clinical and nutrition programs to prevent disease.
6. Cellular nutrition is the basic underlying concept of human nutrition. The study of biochemically and physiologically oriented concepts related to cellular nutrition is essential.
7. Hormone-nutrition interrelationships need more exploration.
8. The impact of medications upon nutritional status deserves better recognition.
9. The occurrence of specific toxicants in natural foods needs to be better recognized.
10. Contaminants and possibly toxicological constituents of our food supply system must be evaluated as they relate to the impact upon the nutrition and health status of the individual.
11. The exploration of genetics, carcinogenesis, molecular biology and tissue culture cannot develop adequately without focusing on nutritional considerations.

The future of preventive nutrition will rest not only on the recognition of better early warning precursor markers to subsequent nutritionally related dysfunctions, but also on new methods for patient behavior modification as it relates to diet. This would involve better delivery of community nutritional support through a change in our food distribution system, the foods available at institutional settings and the types of prefabricated foods.

As Connor pointed out in his outgoing presidential address before the annual meeting of the American Society of Clinical Nutrition in 1979, "I know full well that these dietary modalities are not going to be taken up by the cardiologist, or indeed by any other subspecialist of medicine. Here is a vast arena for the talents of a clinical nutritionist to be expressed if he (or she) would so incline himself (herself). . . . I strongly suggest that the issue is no longer in doubt if the clinical nutritionists will accept the challenges of the disease of overconsumption/undernutrition. The public is now demanding action by us—both to treat and prevent these diseases in individuals, families and communities."[7]

Such is the challenge to the future of preventive nutrition and the focus of this book.

REFERENCES

1. Robson, J.R.K. 1977. Food faddism. *Pediat. Clinics N. Amer.* 24: 189.
2. McCollum, E.J. 1957. *History of Nutrition.* Boston: Houghton Mifflin Co.
3. Hodges, R.E. 1977. Nutrition education in the clinical years. *Am. J. Clin. Nutr.* 30: 803.
4. Podell, R., Gary, L.R. and Keller, K. 1975. A profile of clinical nutrition knowledge among physicians and medical students. *J. Medical Educ.* 50: 888.
5. Dugdale, A.E., Chandler, D. and Baghurst, K. 1979. Knowledge and belief of knowledge in nutrition. *Am. J. Clin. Nutr.* 32: 441.
6. Olson, R.E. 1978. Clinical nutrition, an interface between human ecology and internal medicine. *Nutrition Reviews* 36: 161.
7. Connor, W.E. 1979. Too little or too much: the case for preventive nutrition. *Am. J. Clin. Nutr.* 32: 1975.
8. *Diet Related to the Killer Diseases.* 1977. Washington: U.S. Government Printing Office.
9. Gallagher, C.R. and Vivian, V.M. 1979. Nutrition concepts essential in the education of the medical student. *Am. J. Clin. Nutr.* 32: 1330.
10. Alfin-Slater, R., Anderson, J., Bozian, R.C., Brechtelshauer, D.A., Collins, M.E. and Peske, E.D. February 28, 1978. Nutrition in everyday practice. *Patient Care*, pp. 76-135.
11. Broad, W.J. 1979. NIH deals gingerly with diet-disease link. *Science* 204: 1175.
12. Butterworth, C.E. and Blackburn. G.L. March/April 1975. Hospital malnutrition. *Nutrition Today*, pp. 8-18.
13. Guthrie, H.A. and Guthrie, G.M. 1976. Factor analysis of nutritional status data from the ten state nutrition surveys. *Am. J. Clin. Nutr.* 29: 1238.
14. Davis, D. and Williams, R. 1976. Potentially useful criteria for judging nutritional adequacy. *Am. J. Clin. Nutr.* 29: 710.
15. Williams, R. 1956. *Biochemical Individuality: The Basis of the Genetotrophic Concept.* New York: John Wiley and Sons.

2

RISK FACTOR INTERVENTION
AND PREVENTIVE NUTRITION

————— ◆●► —————

JEFFREY BLAND, PH.D.

RECENTLY, the World Health Organization promulgated a goal for improved worldwide health as "an attainment by all citizens of the world by the year 2000 of a level of health that will permit them to lead socially and economically productive lives."[1]

The question that remains is how do we meet this articulated goal and by what measure can we quantify health improvement (a process which depends upon the definition of health).

Health can be defined as improvements in mortality patterns, in morbidity patterns, or in psychosocial indices of a society. Epidemiological data relating to the frequency of certain types of illnesses, mean average life span, probability of death at any decade of life, and indications of psychosocial dysfunction can all be used to argue for states of the health of a given population.

Some individuals have suggested that the health of a society is most accurately assessed by measuring such indicators as:

(1) the number of children with behavior problems,
(2) the frequency of mental retardation,
(3) the frequency of delinquency,
(4) alcohol consumption and related problems,
(5) prevalence of drug addiction,
(6) frequency of sexually-transmitted diseases,
(7) problems related to child abuse,
(8) the number of extranuptial births,
(9) suicide,
(10) teenage pregnancies.

Other indications for the health of the population may be related to changes in the incidence of certain chronic degenerative diseases and the age at which these diseases appear in the society. One could also look at days of absenteeism in certain occupations, as well as statistics related to perinatal mortality, mean average life span and the probability of survival after the age of forty, fifty or sixty years.

Alternative Health Care Philosophies

From these various perspectives, conclusions about the health of a population may be derived. Changes in morbidity and mortality patterns are generally focused on recognition of disease states. Such changes, however, are not necessarily related to levels of wellness of a population. Wellness may be more subtle as it relates to manifestations of potential productivity of individuals who make up that group.

The philosophy that encompasses levels of optimal health and productivity and focuses on wellness has been termed preventive medicine, as contrasted with those philosophies that have dealt more exclusively with disease patterns and mortality statistics, which is the crisis-care model, characterized as the predominant philosophy of Western medicine.

The process of disease control has become more highly specialized in the past thirty years through the use of high-technology intervention whose cost/benefit relationships have been questioned by a number of evaluators. Recently, the director of UNICEF, in concert with the World Health Organization, has stated, "Most conventional health-care systems are becoming increasingly complex and costly, with doubtful social relevance. They distort by dictates of medical technology in conjunction with the misguided efforts of the medical industry to provide many unnecessary medical consumer goods to society. Even affluent countries have come to realize the high costs and low health benefits of these systems."[2]

A number of critics of the present emphasis on disease care have commented that the system now focuses on specialization, centralization and high technology delivery to specific disease states and neglects some of the major areas of health care improvement which have historically been proven to have the most significant benefit in terms of health improvement to the society at large—including improved sanitation, hygiene, nutrition and life-style modification.[3]

The Prevention Model

The alternative model to that of high-technology crisis intervention is based on the old maxim of "An ounce of prevention is equal to a pound of cure," and was originally proposed in the United States in 1861 by Dobell, who advocated regular prognostic health screening of individuals to recognize early signs of potential illness. In 1925 the American Medical Association committed itself to the concept of regular check-ups, following statistics generated by the Metropolitan Life Insurance Company which declared that routine health examinations increased life expectancy 28 percent above expected mortality without an increase in cost to their clients within five years of the initiation of the program.[4]

However, in 1945 Kuh found that there was no conclusive evidence of improved health in individuals who had routine health examinations.[5] There has been criticism levied at this report because its conclusion was drawn upon data derived from screening for pathology rather than utilizing early-warning screening tools or markers of potential subsequent disease. As William Connor points out, the success of the implementation of preventive medicine is dependent upon the application of early-warning risk assessment tools which will better demonstrate the potential risk of subsequent disease before actual pathology occurs.[6] The development of better early-warning precursor markers for subsequent disease is at the forefront of effective delivery of preventive medicine and has historically been related to two schools of thought.

Multiphasic Screening Versus
Health Hazard Appraisal

The first of these is called multiphasic screening, in which, utilizing blood chemical screens, certain parameters are regularly evaluated, such as serum glucose, BUN, cholesterol, triglycerides and serum enzymes, to indicate potential organ system dysfunction. Bell found in a comprehensive evaluation of multiphasic screening that of all individuals tested 12.8 percent were found to have ailments significant enough for referral.[7] Within this particular system the benefit in relation to the cost for screening has been questioned. A number of both false positives and false negatives are seen. No test has complete predictability, sensitivity or specificity. And because of the frequency of these ambiguities, the prognostic efficiency of the procedure must be called into question. In support of multiphasic screening, Holland, when screening 1,157 people in Baltimore, found abnormals in 98 percent of the population, although 36 percent were found to be false positives by follow-up evaluation.[8]

Criticism has been levied against multiphasic screening because it is not broad-based enough. It is focused on the evaluation of existing pathology, and it uses basically passive types of testing which may not indicate the potential lack of organ reserve which can only be demonstrated through the challenge testing type of protocol. Fries has indicated that the lack of organ reserve may be one of the causes for illness when a person is subjected to a specific stressor in the environment. In this model, the particular system that has been exposed to stress with insufficient reserve is unable to mobilize enough reserve to meet the challenge and therefore suffers organ failure.[9]

The use of a challenge, or provocative, testing procedure such as the cardiac stress test allows for the exposure of weakness in the physiological fabric and measurement of the degree of reserve. A passive test, however, such as the resting EKG, will not allow measurement of that reserve.[10]

The second method that has been employed to implement early warning risk analysis is called the health hazard appraisal. This concept is built upon the actual biological age of the individual, relative to that person's chronological age. It is rooted in the concept of risk factor analysis which looks at an individual's relative risk factors to subsequent disease and takes into account the genetic background and symptoms in ascribing specific types of risk, which when accumulated give rise of a relative biological age, or probability of developing certain disease-related conditions relative to the population at large. The data for this risk

TABLE 2.1
Relative Risk of Ischemic Heart Disease
From the Framingham Study

Age at entry	MALES			FEMALES		
	BP^a	Serum cholesterol[b]	Smoking[c]	BP^a	Serum cholesterol[b]	Smoking[c]
35–44	3.6	3.5	4.8	4.7	—[d]	4.3
45–54	1.2	3.9	1.7	1.7	10.1	0.5
55–64	1.0	1.4	1.5	1.4	0.6	0.9

[a]150 - 159 Hg systolic compared to 120 - 129 mm Hg
[b]250 - 264 mg/100 ml compared to 096 - 189 mg/100 ml
[c]> 20 cigarettes per day compared to nonsmokers
[d]Insufficient data

assessment have been derived from the Geller-Gesner tables, which were tabulated from information procured from the Framingham, Tecumseh studies and the American Cancer Society screen.[11]

The Framingham statistics have been utilized to establish certain risk factors to cardiovascular mortality, as seen in Table 2.1. This is but a single example of the way that these particular data can be put together to establish a relative biological age for an individual, such that a risk factor reflects the relative incidence of that disease in a group that has that specific risk factor versus the incidence of that specific disease in the population at large.

Behavior Modification and Risk Intervention

This particular approach is heavily tied to behavior modification, which means that certain aspects of a person's life-style, once indicated as potentiating an increased risk, must be modified to decrease that relative risk. It is not a diagnostic approach focused on treating a specific disease, but rather a prognostic approach focused on reducing the probability of specific dysfunctions related to cumulative risk factors. Some risk factors cannot be changed such as maleness or age after forty, but many of the most significant are modifiable. There is great debate as to what risk factors should be included in such a health hazard appraisal format.

Smoking, weight/height ratio, stress adaptive levels, serum cholesterol, high density lipoprotein cholesterol, consumption of certain drugs, alcohol, occupation and lack of exercise are all known to correlate with relative risk of future ill health.

Hall has published a cost/benefit analysis of health hazard appraisal versus multiphasic screening (or standard health check-ups) and found that with health hazard appraisal 6.41 problems were found per patient at a cost of $2.34 per problem, whereas a history and physical with standard health evaluation identified only 2.47 problems per patient at a cost of $20.26 per problem, indicating the much higher cost/efficiency of the health hazard appraisal approach.[12]

Two recent articles have eloquently addressed the concept of health risk assessment and health hazard appraisal. Both articles indicate that the development of this approach is intimately tied to the acceptance of preventive medicine as an important cost/efficient, efficacious, health improvement modality.[13,14]

The Success of Risk Factor Intervention

A number of studies have been accomplished to examine how successful the implementation of health hazard appraisal with lifestyle modification can be in changing morbidity and mortality statistics. Three basic approaches have been employed, the first of which is built upon a medical model, the second of which is built upon a public model, and the third of which is built upon an ecological model.

The medical model is basically interventive in scope, when a person indicates particular immediate signs of disease such as elevated blood pressure and is treated with antihypertensive medication.

The public health model focuses more on education and behavior modification, designing a particular approach to that specific patient's high risks to minimize those risks.

The ecological model deals with larger social questions such as how to reduce risk by changing occupational hazards, by improving the quality of air and water, and by improving lighting and urban design to minimize specific risks to community health.

All of these approaches involve some form of prognostic screening followed by intervention. Therefore evaluation of their success involves evaluation for an intervention trial.

The work of Marmot and Winklestein indicates that within ten years, if risk factor intervention and life-style modification could be effectively delivered to 10-million males between the ages of thirty-five and sixty-four years, 45 percent of the present incidence of ischemic heart disease cases could be prevented at 100 percent participation, and a 34 percent reduction in incidence would result if only 75 percent of the population participated.[15]

The Oakland-Alameda Health Study accomplished in Oakland, California, revealed eight characteristics associated with a longer, more healthy life that could be identified as areas of emphasis in public health education and reduction of risk. These included:

(1) the consumption of a regular breakfast,
(2) six to eight hours of sleep per day,
(3) prudent weight-to-height ratio,
(4) no smoking,
(5) regular exercise,
(6) consumption of fresh foods from the four food groups,
(7) moderate alcohol consumption (less than 2 ounces per day),
(8) effective management of stress.

A person with more than five of these characteristics was found statistically to have a life span 6.7 years longer than a person with less than five of these characteristics.[16]

The Chicago Coronary Prevention Evaluation program was another prognostic program designed to explore the impact of risk factor intervention on cardiovascular mortality, utilizing nonpharmacological approaches. In this study a 25 percent reduction in risk of mortality was found after effective life-style modification and dietary revision.[17]

The largest prognostic study ever designed to evaluate the impact of risk factor intervention is the Multiple Risk Factor Intervention Trial (MRFIT), which is involving 370,000 men between the ages of thirty-five and fifty-seven years, 50 percent randomized in a treatment group, and 50 percent randomized in a control group. The treatment group receives education and counseling in the areas of risk factor minimization (reduction of blood pressure, ways of reducing blood cholesterol and cessation of smoking). It is multifactorial in approach, suggesting that chronic degenerative diseases have many contributing factors, not a single cause, and that controlling all of these factors, or delivering education and modification involving all of these factors, improves in a synergistic way the potential effectiveness of outcome.[18] The preliminary results of this study indicated a much smaller difference between the control group and intervention group in cardiovascular disease incidence than was anticipated. This was suggested to be a result of two complicating factors: many of the control group changed their lifestyles voluntarily and the treatment group received drugs to lower their serum cholesterol which was suggested to possibly increase the risk to disease in that group.[19]

In the region of North Karelia, Finland, there exists one of the highest rates of ischemic heart disease in the world. In 1972 a risk factor intervention program was implemented, with a control population that was socioeconomically matched, serving as an internal control without treatment. A 16 percent reduction in myocardial infarction was seen in men between the ages of thirty and sixty-four, with the highest decline (24 percent) occurring in men thirty to fifty-four years of age, indicating that the greatest probability of improved health occurs in the younger group of men. These facts argue strongly for the model of Fries, which says that effective risk factor intervention should be able to compress mortality.[20]

The Stanford Heart Disease Prevention Program compared three cities, similar in their socioeconomic make-up, receiving three different types of trials relating to the incidence of cardiovascular disease. Watsonville received media education and personal education in the area of risk factor intervention. Gilroy received media education only, whereas in Tracy there was no effort for media or for personal education in health improvement. After examining the data, a 20 percent reduction in relative frequency of cardiovascular disease was seen in Watsonville relative to Tracy and 16 percent reduction was found in Gilroy relative to the incidence in Tracy, providing more data to support the efficacy of risk factor intervention.[21]

The Reduction in Heart Disease: Its Cause

Looking at society at large and asking whether there is any support for the assertion that large scale risk factor intervention is effective in reducing the incidence of disease, one needs only to examine the nationwide 35 percent reduction in ischemic heart disease from 1950 to 1976. There are several potential reasons for this decline, other than life-style modification, including:

(1) advances in the treatment and management of congenital and rheumatic heart conditions,
(2) coronary care improvement and improved emergency medical facilities,
(3) new drugs and surgery, such as the coronary bypass operation,
(4) better preventive medical implementation, using risk factor, intervention, through improved diet, exercise and stress management.

Coronary bypass surgery, which now accounts for more than 80,000 procedures per year at a cost of more than one billion dollars, has only been proven to be effective in reducing angina. There is still no unequivocal data that the operation prolongs life or treats the underlying disease.[21] Equal lack of evidence surrounds management of congenital heart disease, better coronary intensive care units or drug therapy as proven causes for the observed reduction in heart disease.

According to Robert Levy, if we evaluate all of these potential reasons for the decline in ischemic heart disease, the only statistically significant factor is the reduction that can be ascribed to delivery of better preventive medicine through life-style intervention. In fact, Levy goes on to say, "In the past thirty years, the major improvement in health is in the identification of risk factors and their community acceptance."[22]

The Kaiser-Permanente Study in California, which evaluated two million people for risk factors and which included intervention by education and preventive medicine, found fewer heart attacks in that population but with little improvement in survival after an attack, indicating that the effectiveness of this system stems from preventing the end-stage crisis condition.[23]

Many individuals ask what risk prevention can actually do for them. Does it guarantee them a long healthy life? Obviously, this approach is built upon probability theory and there is no guarantee of personal health by reducing risk factors, but what can be assured is a much higher probability of preventing disease with improved probability for higher levels of health. If one waits for symptoms of disease to develop, it may be too late to manage the patient effectively or to return him back to high levels of health. In occlusive artery disease, angina (heart pain) is seen only when greater than two-thirds of the major coronary vessels are occluded with plaque. At this point heroic high technology intervention is required for the relief of symptoms, without any guarantee of effectively treating the underlying disease. In fact, if one waits for such symptoms to develop, it is known that in approximately one-fourth of new heart attack victims the very first symptom is death itself.

When comparing this against early-warning risk factor intervention, one can see a very important cost/benefit improvement. For instance, after ceasing smoking for one year, the risk of cardiovascular disease associated with smoking is reduced by 90 percent, and after five years of no smoking the risk associated with prior smoking is almost identical to that of a person who has never smoked at all.[24]

There are numbers of studies showing that diet directly influences the total cholesterol, LDL cholesterol, and HDL cholesterol, all of which are intimately involved with cardiovascular risk.[25] There is now evidence from the work of Benditt that elevated levels of LDL cholesterol may actually be related to the cause of atherosclerotic disease through the monoclonal theory of atherosclerosis.[26] It is interesting to note that the cardiovascular disease rate is declining only in those affluent countries where risk factor intervention is being successfully applied, such as the United States, Finland, Australia and Canada, and not in countries of similar medical technology that have not effectively employed risk factor intervention, such as Ireland, Scotland, West Germany and Denmark, where the rates of cardiovascular disease are actually on the increase. As Ivan Illich points out in *Medical Nemesis*, the major advances in health care over the past seventy years have come through improvements in nutrition, sanitation, hygiene and life-style modification.[3]

Implementing the Intervention Program

The conclusion is that health is not a mystery, but is related to the design of a person's own environment in a way that maximizes the biochemical strengths and minimizes weaknesses, so that the probabilities of subsequent disease are minimized. This model is built upon the concept of Roger Williams, entitled "The Genetotrophic Theory of Disease," which suggests that disease is a result of the complex interaction of genetic characteristics with environment, postulated upon a wide range of human biochemical diversity, much greater than is now generally accepted.[27] This theory explains the variable needs that different people may have for levels of specific micronutrients, such as the vitamins and minerals, far in excess of the mean average requirement for the average population, caused by their own biochemical uniqueness and individual requirements to promote proper enzymatic or physiological function. The absence of adequate amounts of a specific agent in the diet or in the environment can cause an inappropriate expression of certain genetic characteristics, resulting in suboptimal function which is eventually diagnosed as disease after going through a long period of latency prior to symptomatic dysfunction.[28]

In establishing biochemical individuality in the spirit of early-warning risk assessment, several types of data must be accumulated to describe the patient adequately. These include:

(1) anthropometric data dealing with height, weight, blood pressure, lean body mass, aerobic competency and psychosocial stress adaptability,
(2) dietary data (such as may be derived from a computerized dietary evaluation),
(3) family and personal health history,
(4) patient symptom evaluation with organ-system emphasis,
(5) biochemical assessment, including blood serum, urine and hair tissue analysis.

Advanced screening tools have only recently become available for better assessment, under a provocative testing protocol, of certain aspects of nutrition and physiological status. These include noninvasive vascular studies, urinary or red blood cell mineral status, *in vitro* erythrocyte vitamin assay systems and special serological chemistries, including such biochemical measurements as high density lipoprotein, glycohemoglobin and the zinc challenge-alkaline phosphatase test. Utilizing these tools and integrating them in a prognostic fashion allow for earlier recognition of the risk of chronic degenerative diseases. A major risk factor may be related in part to a malnutrition, seen with reasonable prevalency in the United States, the malnutrition of overconsumption/undernutrition—too much of too little.[29]

   Early-warning symptoms of nutritional inadequacy include those signs listed in Table 2.2 and Table 2.3.[30] As individuals are screened using these prognostic tools and as they become more knowledgeable concerning their own personal risk factors, it has been found that the people who are educated are the first to see improvement of health. This is predicted by the concepts of learning theory which indicate that in social improvement programs the first group to receive benefit from the improvement are those who are better educated.[31]

TABLE 2.2
Warning Signs of Nutritional Inadequacy

Organ System	Physical Signs	Nutrient Deficiency
HAIR	Becomes fine, dull, dry, brittle, stiff, straight; becomes red in Blacks, then lighter in color; may be "bleached" in Whites ("flag sign"); is easily and painlessly pluckable; outer one-third of eyebrow may be sparse in hypothyroidism (cretinism, iodine deficiency or other causes)	Protein-Calorie, Zinc
NAILS	Ridging, brittle, easily broken, flattened, spoon shaped, thin, lusterless	Iron
FACE	Brown, patchy, pigmentation of cheeks, Parotid enlargement. "Moon Face"	Protein-Calorie
EYES	Photophobia; poor twilight vision; loss of shiny, bright, moist appearance of eyes; xerosis of bulbar conjunctivae; loss of light reflex; decreased lacrimation; keratomalacia (corneal softening), corneal ulceration which may lead to extrusion of lens; Bitot's spot (frothy white or yellow spots under bulbar conjunctivae)	Vitamin A
	Palpebral conjunctivae are pale	Iron or Folate
	Circumcorneal capillary injection with penetration of corneal limbus	Riboflavin
	Tissue at external angles of both eyes which is red and moist	Riboflavin
	Angular blepharitis (or palpebritis)	Pyridoxine
	Optic neuritis	B-12

TABLE 2.2 (Continued)
Warning Signs of Nutritional Inadequacy

Organ System	Physical Signs	Nutrient Deficiency
NOSE	Nasolabial dyssebacea (exfoliation, in flammation, excessive oil production and fissuring of sebaceous glands, which are moist and red) May be found at angles of eyes, ears or other sites	Riboflavin
	Nasolabial seborrhea	Pyridoxine
LIPS	Cheilosis, inflammation of the mucus membranes of the lips and the loss of the clear differentiation between the mucocutaneous border of the lips	Riboflavin
GUMS	Interdental gingival hypertrophy	Vitamin C
	Gingivitis	Vitamin A, Niacin, Riboflavin
MOUTH	Angular stomatitis; cheilosis; angular scars	Riboflavin
	Apthous stomatitis	Folic Acid
TONGUE	Atrophic lingual papillae, sore, erythe matous	Iron
	Glossitis, painful, sore	Folic Acid
	Magenta in color, atrophic lingual papillae; filiform and fungiform papillae hypertrophy	Riboflavin
	Scarlet; raw; atrophic lingual papillae; fissures	Niacin
	Glossitis	Pyridoxine
TEETH	Caries	Fluoride, phosphorus
	Mottled enamel, fluorosis	Fluoride (excessive)
	Malposition; hypoplastic line across up- per primary incisors; becomes filled with yellow-brown pigment; caries then oc- curs and tooth may break off	Protein-Caloria
NECK	Neck mass (goiter)	Iodine

TABLE 2.2 (Continued)
Warning Signs of Nutritional Inadequacy

Organ System	Physical Signs	Nutrient Deficiency
SKIN	Xerosis (dryness of skin) Follicular hyperkeratosis ("gooseflesh," "sharkskin," "sand-paper skin"); keratotic plugs arising from hypertrophied hair follicles. Acneiform lesions	Vitamin A
	Perifollicular petechiae which produce a "pink-halo" effect around coiled hair follicles. Intradermal petechiae, purpura, ecchymoses due to capillary fragility. Hemarthroses; cortical hemorrhages of bone visualizable on X ray	Vitamin C
	Intracutaneous hemorrhages; GI hemorrhage	Vitamin K
	Pallor	Iron, folic acid
	Pallor; icterus	B-12
	Erythema early, vascularization, crusting, desquamation. Increased pigmentation (even in Blacks), thickened, inelastic, fissured, especially in skin exposed to sun; becoming scaly, dry, atrophic in intertrigenous areas, maceration and abrasion may occur. "Necklace of Casals" in neckline exposed to sun; Malar and supraorbital pigmentation	Niacin
	Edema (pitting), "Flaky paint" dermatosis, Hyperkeratosis or "Crazy pavement" dermatosis Hyperpigmentation	Protein-Calorie
	Scrotum Dermatitis, erythema, hyperpigmentation	Niacin
VULVA	Vulvovaginitis and chronic mucocutaneous candidiasis	Iron
SKELETAL	Osteoporosis (in association with low protein intake and fluoride deficiency)	Calcium
	Epiphyseal enlargement, painless. Beading of ribs ("Rachitic Rosary"). Delayed fusion of fontaneles, craniotabes.	Vitamin D

TABLE 2.2 (Continued)
Warning Signs of Nutritional Inadequacy

Organ System	*Physical Signs*	*Nutrient Deficiency*
	Bowed legs, frontal or parietal bossing of skull. Deformities of thorax (Harrison's Sulcus, pigeon breast). Osteomalacia (adults)	
	Subperiosteal hematoma. Epiphyseal enlargement, painful	Vitamin C
MUSCULAR	Hypotonia	Vitamin D
	Muscle wasting; weakness, fatigue, inactivity; loss of subcutaneous fat	Protein-Calorie
	Intramuscular hematoma	Vitamin C
	Calf muscle tenderness; weakness	Thiamin
CENTRAL NERVOUS SYSTEM	Apathy (kwashiorkor); irritability (marasmus); Psychomotor changes.	Protein
	Hyporeflexia; foot and wrist drop. Hypesthesia; parasthesia	Thiamin
	Psychotic behavior (dementia)	Niacin
	Peripheral neuropathy, symmetrical sensory and motor deficits, especially in lower extremities. Drug resistant convulsions (infants). Dementia, forgetfulness.	Pyridoxine
	Areflexia. Extensor plantar responses. Loss of position and vibratory sense. Ataxia, paresthesias	B-12
	Tremor, convulsions, behavioral disturbances	Magnesium
LIVER	Hepatomegaly (fatty infiltration)	Protein-Calorie
GASTRO-INTESTINAL	Anorexia, flatulence, diarrhea	B-12
	Diarrhea	Niacin, Protein-Calorie
CARDIO-VASCULAR	Tachycardia, congestive heart failure (high output type), Cardiac enlargement, electrocardiographic changes	Thiamin

TABLE 2.3
Guidelines for Criteria of Nutritional Status by Laboratory Evaluation

Nutrient and Units	Age of Subject (years)	Deficient	Criteria of Status Marginal	Acceptable
*Hemoglobin	6-23 mos	Up to 9.0	9.0-9.9	10.0+
(gm/dl)	2–5	Up to 10.0	10.0–10.9	11.0+
	6–12	Up to 10.0	10.0–11.4	11.5+
	13–16M	Up to 12.0	12.0–12.9	13.0+
	13–16F	Up to 10.0	10.0–11.4	11.5+
	16 + M	Up to 12.0	12.0–13.9	14.0+
	16 + F	Up to 10.0	10.0–11.9	12.0+
	Pregnant (after 6 + mos.)	Up to 9.5	9.5–10.9	11.0+
*Hematocrit	Up to 2	Up to 28	28–30	31 +
(Packed cell	2–5	Up to 30	30–33	34 +
volume in	6–12	Up to 30	30–35	36 +
percent)	13–16 M	Up to 37	37–39	40 +
	13–16 F	Up to 31	31–35	36 +
	16 + M	Up to 37	37–43	44 +
	16 + F	Up to 31	31–37	33 +
	Pregnant	Up to 30	30–32	33 +
*Serum	Up to 1	—	Up to 2.5	2.5+
Albumin	1–5	—	Up to 3.0	3.0+
(gm/dl)	6–16	—	Up to 3.5	3.5+
	16+	Up to 2.8	2.8–3.4	3.5+
	Pregnant	Up to 3.0	3.0–3.4	3.5+
*Serum	Up to 1	—	Up to 5.0	5.0+
Protein	1–5	—	Up to 5.5	5.5+
(gm/dl)	6–16	—	Up to 6.0	6.0+
	16 +	Up to 6.0	6.0–6.4	6.5+
	Pregnant	Up to 5.5	5.5–5.9	6.0+
*Serum Ascorbic Acid (mg/dl)	All ages	up to 0.1	011–0119	0.2+
*Plasma vitamin A (mcg/dl)	All ages	Up to 10	10–19	20 +
*Plasma Carotene (mcg/dl)	All ages Pregnant	Up to 20 —	20–39 40–79	40 + 80 +
*Serum	Up to 2	Up to 30	—	30 +
Iron (mcg/dl)	2.5	Up to 40	—	40 +
	6–12	Up to 50	—	50 +
	12 + M	Up to 60	—	60 +
	12 + F	Up to 40	—	40 +

TABLE 2.3 (Continued)
Guidelines for Criteria of Nutritional Status by Laboratory Evaluation

Nutrient and Units	Age of Subject (years)	Deficient	Criteria of Status Marginal	Acceptable
*Transferrin	Up to 2	Up to 15.0	—	15.0+
Saturation	2–12	Up to 20.0	—	20.0+
(percent)	12 + M	Up to 20.0	—	20.0+
	12 + F	Up to 15.0	—	15.0+
**Serum Folacin (ng/ml)	All ages	Up to 2.0	2.1–5.9	6.0+
**Serum vitamin B-12 (pg/ml)	All ages	Up to 100	—	100+
*Thiamin in	1–3	Up to 120	120–175	175+
Urine (mcg/g	4–5	Up to 85	85–120	120+
creatinine)	6–9	Up to 70	70–180	180+
	10–15	Up to 55	55–150	150+
	16 +	Up to 27	27–65	65+
	Pregnant	Up to 21	21–49	50+
*Riboflavin	1–3	Up to 150	150–499	500+
in Urine (mcg/g	4–5	Up to 100	100–299	300+
creatinine)	6–9	Up to 85	85–269	270+
	10–16	Up to 80	70–199	200+
	16+	Up to 27	27–79	80+
	Pregnant	Up to 30	30–89	90+
**RBC Trans-ketolase-TPP-effect (ratio)	All ages	25+	15–25	Up to 15
**RBC Gluta-thione Reductase-FAD-effect (ratio)	All ages	1.2+	—	Up to 1.2
**Tryptophan Load (mg Xan-thurenic acid	Adults (Dose: 100 mg/kg body weight)	25+ (6 hrs) 75+ (24 hrs)	— —	Up to 25 Up to 75
**Urinary	1–3	Up to 90	—	90+
Pyridoxine	4–6	Up to 80	—	80+
(mcg/g	7–9	Up to 60	—	60+
creatinine)	10–12	Up to 40	—	40+
	13–15	Up to 30	—	30+
	16 +	Up to 20	—	20+

TABLE 2.3 (Continued)
Guidelines for Criteria of Nutritional Status by Laboratory Evaluation

Nutrient and Units	Age of Subject (years)	Deficient	Criteria of Status Marginal	Acceptable
*Urinary N'methyl nicotinamide (mg/g creatinine)	All ages Pregnant	Up to 0.2 Up to 0.8	0.2–5.59 0.8–2.49	0.6+ 2.5+
**Urinary Pantothenic Acid (mcg)	All ages	Up to 200	—	200+
**Plasma vitamin E (mg/dl)	All ages	Up to 0.2	0.2–0.6	0.6+
**Transaminase Index (ratio) +EGOT †EGPT	Adult Adult	2.0+ 1.25+	— —	Up to 2.0 Up to 1.25

*Adapted from the Ten State Nutrition Survey
**Criteria may vary with different methodology
+ Erythrocyte Glutamic Oxalacetic Transaminase
†Erythrocyte Glutamic Pyruvic Transaminase

Reprinted from the American Journal of Public Health, November, 1973, part two, v. 63

Potential Implications on Degenerative Disease Risk

This model of early-warning risk assessment and behavior modification through intervention in specific risk factors is applicable to reducing the risk to all major, chronic degenerative diseases. It is not clear from the data available today what the exact extent is of the cost savings achievable by applying preventive medicine through risk factor intervention. All of the answers and proof of its efficacy are not in. But the data at this point are strong enough to argue effectively that to withhold the implementation of risk factor intervention because of incomplete data is comparable to not employing better sanitation back in the early 1900s because we did not yet know what organisms transmitted infectious disease or how they related to improved sanitation.

The future of multifactorial risk intervention and better prognostic screening is rich, and frames an improved philosophy of medicine with the emphasis more on keeping people well than on treating disease. Provocative testing which looks at specific organ reserves of an individual under physiological stress, rather than at the presence of end stage pathology, will allow an evolution in the successful implementation of this model. These techniques are just now becoming available. As the clinician and the laboratory researcher are better able to work together in the promotion and development of better tools for screening and for applying them in behavior modification and life-style risk factor intervention, the possible improvement in health for all segments of the population will be remarkable. This will greatly hasten achievement of the goals as established by the World Health Organization that ". . . the citizens of the world will attain by the year 2000 a level of health that permits them to lead socially and economically productive lives." The application of this model will help reduce the rate of inflation of the health-care dollar by replacing less complex technology for more costly high technology crisis intervention, as well as returning responsibility for health in large part back into the hands of the informed health-care consumer.[32]

REFERENCES

1. *Formulating Strategies for Health for All by the Year 2000: Guiding Principles and Essential Issues*. 1979. Geneva: World Health Organization Document No. EB/63/47.
2. WHO/UNICEF. *Primary Health Care: Report of the International Conference on Primary Health Care*, September, 1978.
3. Illich, I. 1975. *Medical Nemesis*, New York: Bantam Books and Toffler, A. 1981. *The Third Wave*, New York: Dell Books.
4. Dobell, H. 1921. *Lectures on the Germs and Vestiges of Disease and the Prevention of the Invasion of Disease by Periodic Examination*. London: Churchill. The value of periodic medical examinations. *Stat. Bull. Metro. Life. Insur. Co.* 2:1.
5. Kuh, C. 1945. Periodic health examination versus early sickness consultation. *Perm. Found. Med. Bull.* 3:12.
6. Connor, W. 1979. Preventive nutrition: too little or too much? *Am. J. Clin. Nutr.* 31:1131.
7. Bell, B. D. 1972. The yield of multiphasic screening. *JAMA* 222:74.
8. Holland, B. 1975. Automated multiphasic screening. *Public. Health Rep.* 90:133.
9. Fries, J. 1980. Aging, natural death and the compression of morbidity. *N. Engl. J. Med.* 303:130.
10. Bland, J. The use of the clinical laboratory in preventive medicine. *J. Int. Acad. Prev. Med.* (in press).
11. Hall, J. H. and Zwemer, J. 1979. *Prospective Medicine*. Indianapolis: Methodist Hospital.
12. Hall, J. H. 1980. The case for health hazard appraisals. Which health screening techniques are cost-effective? *Diagnosis* 2:60.

13. Saward, E. and Sorenson, A. 1978. The current emphasis on preventive medicine. *Science* 200:889.
14. Okrent, D. 1980. Comment on societal risk. *Science* 208:372.
15. Marmot, M. and Winkelstein, W. 1975. Epidemiologic observations on intervention trials for prevention of coronary heart disease. *Am. J. Epidemiol.* 101:177.
16. Beilge, A. 1973. Oakland-Alameda health survey. *Prev. Medicine* 2:67.
17. Stamler, J., Mojonnier, L., Hall, Y., et al. May 1975. Long-term findings of the Chicago coronary prevention evaluation program, 1958-1971. In: *Proc. 2nd Int. Cong. Biol. Value of Olive Oil.* Stamler, J., Hall, M., Moss, D. and Farinara, E. 1980. Prevention and control of hypertension by nutritional means. *JAMA* 243:1819.
18. The multiple risk factor intervention trial group. 1978. *Ann. N. Y. Acad. Sci.* 304:293.
19. *Public Annual Report.* MRFIT June 30, 1975 to July 1, 1976. DHEW (NIH) 77-1211.
20. Farquhar, J. W., Maccoby, N., Wood, P. D., el al. 1977. Community education for cardiovascular health. *Lancet* 1192.
21. McIntosh, H. D. and Garcia, J. A. The first decade of aorta-coronary bypass grafting, 1967-1977. *Circulation* 198; 57:405; Seides, S. and Borer, J. S. 1978. Long-term anatomic fate of coronary-artery bypass grafts. *N. Engl. J. Med.* 298:1214.
22. Levy, R. I. and Feinleib, M. 1980. Coronary artery disease: risk factors and their management. In: *Heart Disease.* Braunwals, E., ed. Philadelphia: Saunders, 1246-1278.
23. Friedman, G. D. *Decline in Hospitalizations for Coronary Heart Disease and Stroke: The Kaiser-Permanente Experience in Northern California.* U.S. Department of Health, Education, and Welfare. DHEW publication no. (NIH) 79-1610.
24. Reid, D. D. and McCartney, P. 1976. Smoking and other risk factors for coronary heart disease in British civil servants. *Lancet* 2:979.
25. Clarkson, T. B. and Lehner, D. M. 1979. A study of atherosclerosis regression. I. Design of experiment and lesion induction. *Exp. Molec. Pathol.* 30:360.
26. Benditt, E. March 1979. The origin of atherosclerosis. *Scientific American*, pp. 47-61.
27. Williams, R. 1976. *Nutrition Against Disease.* New York: Bantam Books.
28. Bland, J. 1981. *Your Health Under Siege: Using Nutrition to Fight Back.* Brattleboro, Vermont: Stephen Greene Press.
29. Kallen, D. J. 1971. Nutrition and society. *JAMA* 215:94. Page, L. and Friend, B. 1971. The changing United States diet. *Bioscience* 28:192.
30. Christakis G. 1981. How to make a nutritional diagnosis. In: *Nutrition and Medical Practice.* Barness L. A., ed. Westport, Ct.: AVI Publishing Co., pp. 9-12.
31. Levy R. 1981. The decline in cardiovascular disease mortality. In: *Annual Review of Public Health*, vol. 2. Palo Alto: Annual Reviews, Inc., p. 66.
32. Kristein M. and Wynder, E. 1977. Health economics and preventive care. *Science* 195:457.

PART II

NUTRITION FOR THE INDIVIDUAL

3

NUTRITIONAL NEEDS AND
BIOCHEMICAL DIVERSITY

DONALD R. DAVIS, PH.D.

Every individual organism that has a distinctive genetic background has distinctive nutritional needs which must be met for optimal well-being.

ROGER J. WILLIAMS, 1956

Introduction

THE CONCEPT that individual differences in nutrient requirements may have unsuspected implications for the broad fields of health and medicine was first proposed in 1950 by Roger J. Williams and his co-workers.[1] Subsequently Williams broadened and supported this concept in his classic 1956 monograph, *Biochemical Individuality.*[2] A large body of experimental data presented in this book and accumulated since its publication leads to the unavoidable conclusion that striking individual variations of 2-, 5- or 10-fold or more, commonly exist in normal human populations. Such variations are observable throughout biology, for example in anatomy, chemical composition, enzyme and endocrine activities, excretion patterns, drug responses and, of special interest here, in nutritional requirements. Although these variations cannot be denied, they have been inadequately studied and recognized, and this fact probably has delayed the understanding and solution of many human problems.

This chapter is an attempt to summarize present knowledge about variations in nutrient requirements, their consequences, causes and management. Particularly from the viewpoint of medical applications of clinical nutrition, present knowledge unfortunately is preliminary and fragmentary. However, simple awareness

41

of the pervasive existence of biological and nutritional diversity may be of great benefit to many practitioners and researchers. Such awareness will lead eventually to a more sophisticated handling of the complexities and opportunities which arise from biochemical diversity. Concepts and examples of greatest relevance to clinical applications will be emphasized. Imperfect though they may be, the gropings and successes of today's forward-looking physicians and nutritionists will lead to tomorrow's more mature science of evaluating and coping with individuality of nutrient requirements.

Diversity of Nutrient Requirements

It is universally recognized that quantitative nutrient requirements vary unpredictably among "normal, healthy" individuals, at least to some degree, and that illness, drugs and other unusual factors often increase this variation. Also recognized are rare abnormal individuals who require some 100 to 1000 times greater than average amounts of a particular nutrient due to serious inborn errors of metabolism (sometimes imprecisely termed nutrient "dependencies"). What is not generally recognized is the amount and significance of variation among "normal" individuals.

RDAs and the Food and Nutrition Board's approach

The Food and Nutrition Board of the National Academy of Sciences in its publication on Recommended Dietary Allowances (RDAs) estimates that requirements for a given nutrient generally range from about 70 percent to 130 percent of the mean requirement—a range of less than 2-fold—in 95 percent of a "normal, healthy" population.[3] This estimate is dependent on two assumptions: first, that nutrient requirements in normal, healthy people are distributed according to the mathematical Gaussian (so-called "normal") distribution, and second, that the standard deviations for nutrient requirements are generally about 15 percent of the mean (95 percent of the area of this particular curve lies between plus and minus two standard deviations of the mean).

The Board does not mention the first assumption (Gaussian distributions) or its great importance. The second assumption of 15 percent standard deviations is based primarily on a finding of a 15 percent standard deviation for *nitrogen losses* in male college students deprived of protein. (The applicability of this figure to *"protein" requirements* is far from established; still more dubious is its applicability to vitamin and mineral requirements.)

The Board's idealized approach is fundamentally questionable, because there is inadequate data to substantiate either of its two assumptions for even one of the forty-five or more known nutrients. (Strictly speaking there is no "protein" requirement, but rather amino acid requirements.)

In order to know the meaning (or lack of meaning) of any RDA, it is essential to know the actual shape of the statistical distribution of requirements for that nutrient in the population of interest, especially including that portion of the distribution near the high end. This knowledge requires reliable measurements of the requirements for that nutrient among at least a hundred selected people, preferably many hundreds. Such experiments have never been done, partly because of their difficulty. For this reason no one can know to what fraction of a "normal, healthy" population any of the RDAs apply. The Board uses the terms "nearly all" and "most."

The Food and Nutrition Board, of course, cannot benefit from non-existent data. But it could foster scientists' interest in performing crucial experiments by discouraging the prevailing uncritical acceptance of its convenient assumptions. The Board could point out that some informed observers and existing direct experimental data do not support the small range of requirements implied by its assumptions. And it could note the profound consequences when one considers the statistical risk of deficiency among any one of forty-five or more nutrients, rather than considering just one nutrient at a time. It may *seem* acceptable to run a supposed 2 to 3 percent risk of deficiency of *one* nutrient (the Board's stated goal for each RDA), but is it acceptable to run a 2 to 3 percent risk of deficiency for *each* of ten or twenty or thirty nutrients?

Evidence for diversity of requirements

Existing limited data on ranges of requirements in humans and animals were discussed by Williams in 1956[2] and were summarized by Williams and co-workers in 1973.[4] Table 3.1 is taken from the latter paper. Note that the reported ranges of human requirements for amino acids and other nutrients are from 2- to 7-fold, with an average range of 4-fold in these groups of only fifteen to fifty-five subjects. This is twice the general 2-fold range indirectly assumed by the Food and Nutrition Board.

Other observers[5,6] have also concluded that amino acid requirements apparently often vary by more than a 2-fold range; in fact, one careful analysis[6] can be interpreted as indicating ranges of 3- to 9-fold (average in excess of 5-fold) in small groups of normal college women. While some contribution from experimental or procedural errors cannot be ruled out, several researchers

TABLE 3.1
Ranges of Human Needs for Certain Nutrients[4]

Nutrient	Range of Requirements		No. of Subjects
Tryptophan	82-250 mg	(3.0-fold)	50
Valine	375-800 mg	(2.1-fold)	48
Phenylalanine	420-1,100 mg	(2.6-fold)	38
Leucine	170-1,100 mg	(6.4-fold)	31
Lysine	400-2,800 mg	(7.0-fold)	55
Isoleucine	250-700 mg	(2.8-fold)	24
Methionine	800-3,000 mg	(3.7-fold)	29
Threonine	103-500 mg	(4.8-fold)	50
Calcium	222-1,018 mg	(4.6-fold)	19
Thiamin	0.4-1.59 mg	(3.9-fold)	15

and methods have consistently yielded similar results in both sexes, and the results are in line with extensive findings of other kinds of human variability.[2]

Yew has surveyed numerous indications of several-fold human variations in ascorbic acid requirements, storage and metabolism.[7] For example, in order for 50 percent of their intake to be excreted in their urine, nine normal adult females required from 0.6 to 2.2 mg/kg of body weight daily (42 to 154 mg/70 kg). In studies of depletion on diets low in vitamin C, humans vary considerably in their ability to maintain tissue levels of the vitamin. With intakes of 10 to 12 mg/day, four of fifteen normal subjects showed drastic declines in leukocyte ascorbic acid concentration within ten days, while at the other extreme, two subjects showed no significant drop for over seventy days.

Because of the difficulty and lack of interest in experiments which focus on the variability of human nutrient requirements, little is known about the range of requirements for other vitamins or minerals in normal, healthy humans.

However, some information is available from animal studies, which are easier to control than human experiments, and they reinforce the findings in humans. Williams and Deason found evidence for a 20-fold range of needs for vitamin C in 102 male guinea pigs.[8] Earlier, Williams[2] cited experiments which showed evidence for 3- to 10-fold variations in requirements among small groups of rats (vitamin A, folic acid, choline) or monkeys (tryptophan). That these differences can be due to genetic factors is proven by numerous findings[2,9] of different requirements in different strains of rats and chickens (thiamin, riboflavin, manganese and choline). An even more striking genetic effect was discovered through an investigation of poor hatchability: bare backs and short down feathers found in some black, female chicks from a cross between two breeds of chickens. Most of the black females were found to require several times more riboflavin for normal development than their *siblings* of other colors from the same hen.[9]

Causes of diversity of requirements

Inborn genetic differences are the only known factors adequate to explain the large variations in requirements found in normal, healthy humans and animals. Genetically based variability might affect any stage of the nutritional process, including digestion, absorption, conversion to active forms, transport, storage, excretion or utilization. For example, an enzyme which requires a vitamin or mineral cofactor may have an unusually low ability to bind the cofactor or to carry out its function even when bound to the cofactor. In either case increased amounts of cofactor may enhance enzyme function. Because there are many thousands of different enzymes, each associated with a particular biochemical step, genetically based variations in nutrient requirements may be expressed (with variable intensity) in any of thousands of ways.

If a genetic impairment is sufficiently crucial and severe, it will be fatal before birth. If its nature and severity are somewhat less profound, an individual may possess a clearly "abnormal" inborn "error of metabolism" which in some cases may be more or less mitigated by nutritional adjustments. If the genetic impairment is still less severe, the afflicted individual may be "normal" but require for his or her optimum health atypical amounts of a specific nutrient (or other environmental accommodations to his or her genetic nature). There is no reason to expect a sharp or even a definable division between "abnormal defect" and "normal variation." Whether or not 5- or 10-fold variations in nutrient requirements are designated as "normal," what is important is that they be recognized and accommodated when they occur. Several examples of genetically linked increased nutrient requirements are discussed below (see Genetotrophic Disease, p. 53).

Relatively small variations in human needs may be due to numerous environmental factors such as dietary factors (many nutrients interact with each other, unsaturated fats increase vitamin E needs, heme iron reduces iron requirements), exercise level (exercise promotes retention of calcium), pollution, and environmental temperature. Many of these sources of variation are discussed by the Food and Nutrition Board.[3]

TABLE 3.2
Adult Recommended Dietary Allowances and Contents of Selected Supplements
(mg/day except as noted)

Nutrient	Recommended Dietary Allowances[a]			Nutritional Insurance Formulation[b]	Fortified Insurance Formulation[b]	Genetotrophic Research Supplement
	Men	Women	Pregnant			
VITAMINS						
Ascorbic acid	60	60	80	250	2500	1500
Biotin	(0.1-0.2)			0.3	3	
Folic acid	0.4	0.4	0.8	0.4	0.4	0.4
Niacin	18	13	15	20	200	750
Pantothenate	(4-7)			15	150	450
Riboflavin	1.6	1.2	1.5	2	20	200
Thiamin	1.4	1.0	1.4	2	20	300
Vitamin A, I.U.	3330	2670	3330	7500	15,000	15,000
Vitamin B$_6$	2.2	2.0	2.6	3	30	350
Vitamin B$_{12}$	0.003	0.003	0.004	0.009	0.09	1
Vitamin D, I.U.	200	200	400	400	400	300
Vitamin E	10	8	10	40	400	600
Vitamin K	(0.07-0.14)					
MINERALS						
Calcium	800	800	1200	250	250	450
Chloride	(1700-5100)					
Chromium	(0.05-0.2)			1	2	

	a	b	1	2	c
Copper	(-3)		1	2	1.75
Fluoride	(1.5-4)				
Iodide	0.15	0.175	0.15	0.3	0.15
Iron	10	50-80	15	30	7.5
Magnesium	350	450	200	200	300
Manganese	(2.5-5.0)		5	10	3
Molybdenum	(0.15-0.5)		0.1	0.2	
Phosphorus	800	1200	250	250	9
Potassium	(1875-5625)				
Selenium	(0.05-0.2)		0.05	0.1	
Sodium	(1100-3300)				
Zinc	15	20	15	30	30
"PROTEIN"	56 g	74 g			
OTHER					
Choline	dietary need "unproven"	250	250	500	
Linoleic Acid	3 to 10 % of total calories				

[a]Ages twenty-three to fifty, revised 1980.[3] Intended to meet or exceed the established needs of "practically all healthy people in the U.S.A." Values in parentheses are rough estimates of "safe and adequate" intakes. Vitamin A figures shown assume no vegetable carotenoid sources, for comparison with retinol-containing supplements. For this and other explanations and qualifications, see [3].

[b]Similar to formulations suggested by R. J. Williams.[4] Also contain inositol, para-aminobenzoic acid and rutin (a bioflavonoid). Some suggested ingredients, including additional amounts of folic acid, are not permitted by Food and Drug Administration regulations. These or very similar supplements are marketed by Bronson Pharmaceuticals, La Canada, Calif., and Strong, and Cobb & Arner, Covina, Calif.

[c]Used to investigate the possibility that nutritional supplements can help mentally retarded children, based on formulations of Mary B. Allen.[42]

The Board also adjusts its RDAs for various groups subdivided according to age, sex (especially iron requirements), pregnancy or lactation (see Table 3.2). These adjustments seem to be generally useful, although they are often merely interpolations or estimates which cannot be expected to apply to all individuals. Especially the estimated adjustments for elderly people are uncertain and may be quite inappropriate for the large proportion of elderly individuals who suffer from various chronic disorders or who regularly consume drugs. Such individuals are excluded from studies designed to estimate requirements and RDAs for "normal, healthy" people.

This latter point brings us to causes of diversity which were excluded in the "normal" ranges of requirements cited earlier, but which are also of great importance. Disease, stress, trauma, infection and the drugs or surgery used to treat them may all greatly affect nutritional requirements. Unfortunately, physicians, surgeons, dietitians, pharmacists, psychologists, psychiatrists and other specialists may be taught about RDAs (if at all) without emphasis on the fact that the RDAs—whatever their merits for "normal, healthy" people—specifically are not intended for most of their clients. A great need and opportunity await the efforts of scientists who will systematically explore the optimal nutrient intakes of those with cardiovascular disease, cancer, hypertension, diabetes, serious infections, kidney disorders, muscular dystrophy, cystic fibrosis or arthritis, and those who show signs of senility or who suffer mental disturbances. Similarly we need to study the most favorable intakes of those with injuries, fractures or burns, and those undergoing surgery. We already have much evidence and numerous hints that nutrient intakes considerably larger than the RDAs can aid recovery and reduce mortality in a very wide variety of circumstances such as these (see, for example, studies reviewed in References 10-13).

Whether the increased needs are primarily *caused by* the disease or disability or are a *cause of* it will determine the duration of the appropriate adjustments. Temporarily enhanced nutrient needs may serve primarily to compensate for increased utilization or losses, or to stimulate and enhance various natural mechanisms of resistance and healing. Temporarily high apparent requirements also may be caused by long-standing marginal or inadequate intakes and a slow process of restoring tissue concentrations to normal. (These are among the points which need consideration by those who evaluate reports of benefits from nutritional supplementation in excess of RDA levels.)

Drugs are another major cause of unusual nutrient requirements which should especially concern physicians. Like genetic and pathologic factors, drugs may interfere with digestion, absorption, transport, excretion or utilization of nutrients. In addition, drugs may affect appetite and customary eating patterns, and antibiotics may block intestinal synthesis of certain nutrients such as vitamin K and biotin. A few drugs, such as the folic acid antagonist methotrexate, function by inducing a nutrient deficiency, in which case the deficiency is intentional rather than accidental. Recently drug-nutrient interrelations have begun to receive attention in monographs[14-16] and in *Drug-Nutrient Interactions*, a journal founded in 1980.

Vitamin B_6, folic acid and vitamin B_{12} received the earliest recognition as nutrients commonly affected by a wide variety of drugs.[14] Table 3.3 from Roe shows a number of drugs which affect these three nutrients. Drugs which are taken for extended periods must be regarded with the greatest concern, but in most cases it is not firmly established exactly what nutritional adjustments are indicated, and official bodies have been reluctant to make recommendations. One commentator (from Hoffmann-La Roche, Inc.) has suggested that an RDA "type of daily multivitamin supplement may be necessary to avoid nutritional complications of drug therapy" where inadequate nutritional status is suspected, and that "Where drug administration has increased the vitamin need beyond that which could be obtained through diet such as in the case of vitamin B_6 and oral contraceptive steroids, it is essential for the physician to be conscious of the need for supplementation of specific nutrients."[17]

Oral contraceptive steroids represent an important example because of their long-term and widespread use. There is evidence that they affect the metabolism of calcium, phosphorus, magnesium and other minerals as well as vitamin A, thiamin, riboflavin, folic acid, vitamin B_6, vitamin B_{12}, vitamin C and vitamin E. Requirements for several nutrients seem to be increased in some users of the drugs, especially for vitamin B_6.[18] Disturbed tryptophan metabolism, depression and abnormal carbohydrate metabolism ("chemical diabetes" in severe cases) have all been repeatedly found to respond favorably to daily supplements of 20 to 50 mg of vitamin B_6 (10 to 25 times the RDA). Unfortunately, many observers and institutions generally remain unwilling to recommend vitamin B_6 or other supplements for women using contraceptive steroids until there is even more abundant proof of benefit and safety.[18]

TABLE 3.3
Drugs Which Most Commonly Produce Nutritional Deficiencies
of Vitamin B$_6$, Folate, and Vitamin B$_{12}$. Source: Roe.[14]

Deficiency	Some Interfering Drugs	Drug Use
Vitamin B$_6$	Isonicotinic acid hydrazide	Tuberculosis
	Cycloserine	Tuberculosis
	Hydralazine	Hypertension
	Penicillamine	Metal chelator
	L-dopa	Parkinson's disease
	Oral contraceptives	
	Alcohol	
Folate	Methotrexate	Cytotoxin
	Pyrimethamine	Malaria
	Diphenylhydantoin	Anticonvulsant
	Phenobarbital	Anticonvulsant
	Primidone	Anticonvulsant
	Triamterene	Diuretic
	Oral contraceptives	
	Cycloserine	Tuberculosis
	Salicylazosulfapyridine	Inflammation
	Aspirin	Inflammation
	Pentamidine	Anti-infective
	Alcohol	
Vitamin B$_{12}$	Biguanides	Hypoglycemia
	Metformin	
	Phenformin	
	Para-aminosalicylic acid	Tuberculosis
	Cholestyramine	Bile acid sequestrant
	Alcohol	

Even when a consensus may emerge regarding supplements for contraceptive and other drug users, the variability of individual responses to drugs (and nutrients) will require some experimentation for each individual to find what supplements may be worthwhile and what amounts are adequate.

"Contingent" nutrients—another variability?

Among the many thousands of chemical substances entering into the functioning of human cells, all but about forty-five are ordinarily produced internally in adequate amounts. These approximately forty-five substances are the "essential nutrients" which humans must obtain from their environment, including amino acids, minerals, vitamins and a few miscellaneous items. The thousands of other biochemicals—many contained in foods—are equally essential for *life*, but they are not dietary essentials if adequate amounts are available endogenously.

The question arises whether internal synthesis of dietary "non-essentials" is always adequate in all individuals under all circumstances. A related question is whether there may be dietary "non-essentials" which are *not* produced internally but which may be needed or beneficial under some circumstances or in particular individuals. If so, we would recognize another important source of variability in nutrient needs—substances which are nutrients only for certain individuals or under certain circumstances, substances I will call "contingent" nutrients.

There are many reasons to suspect the existence of contingent nutrients, and to keep alert for them, *particularly in the young or elderly or those with various health problems.* We know, for example, that arginine is synthesized by mammals, but not in adequate amounts during early growth in most species, making this amino acid an essential nutrient for a limited time during life. The status of another amino acid, histidine, is uncertain in humans, because we can synthesize amounts almost or roughly equal to our needs, or at least some healthy college students can.[3] Even if histidine were a "nonessential" nutrient for most humans, it would seem quite unreasonable to suppose that all individuals, whether young, elderly, injured, ill, suffering from degenerative diseases or taking drugs are fully able to meet their needs by internal synthesis. In any case these two amino acids illustrate the well-established fact that endogenous synthesis may be inadequate or marginal, even in "normal, healthy" people.

A "nonessential" amino acid, glutamine, is a possible contingent nutrient. Synthesized in certain tissues for use by others, glutamine is the dominant amino acid in serum and cerebrospinal fluid, and is the only amino acid which readily passes the blood-brain barrier. Numerous reports suggest that internal plus dietary sources may be suboptimal in certain conditions. These reports include enhanced healing of peptic ulcers,[19] reduced appetite for alcohol in rats and in human alcoholics,[20,21] IQ improvements in mentally deficient children[22] and benefits to epileptic children.[23] There is also a suggestion that glutamine deficiency may play a part in the mental retardation associated with phenylketonuria.[24]

Any of the other approximately dozen "nonessential" amino acids are also candidates as contingent nutrients which may be needed by certain individuals in amounts larger than are provided by synthesis and diet.

Another type of possible contingent nutrient is exemplified by the group of bioflavonoids. Although many efforts over four decades have failed to prove "essential" roles for any of the bioflavonoids in normal, healthy people, numerous reports, most notably in very recent years, indicate that bioflavonoids provide a wide variety of health benefits. Bioflavonoids are not known to be synthesized by humans, and their possible biochemical functions are obscure, but the amounts available from daily use of peeled oranges or tangerines (not the juice) seem to confer many benefits.[25] These include prevention of abnormal blood platelet adhesion accompanying some disorders (reducing the risk of heart attacks and strokes), stimulation of enzymes which inactivate carcinogens and other toxicants including aflatoxin, protection against "diabetic" and galactose cataracts, reduction of excessive inflammation (including thrombophlebitis), and protection against a variety of bacteria, fungi and viruses (including flu and rhinovirus).

Other candidates[26] as contingent nutrients include the food ingredients inositol, lipoic acid, para-aminobenzoic acid and coenzyme Q (the latter has been the subject of three international symposia and of over 250 reports by Karl Folkers and coworkers alone[27,28]). These candidates do not appear to be dietary essentials for "normal, healthy" humans, but they may be essential or at least useful for some others, especially for those with various health difficulties.

The Food and Nutrition Board describes possible benefits from bioflavonoids as "pharmacological,"[3] and the Food and Drug Administration has attempted to regulate bioflavonoids and other contingent nutrients as "drugs." These descriptions seem inappropriate and arbitrary. The same Board says that fluorine "can be considered an *essential* [nutrient] element . . . on the basis of its proven *beneficial* effects on dental health"[3] (emphasis added).

Whether they are in fact essential or merely beneficial, and whatever they may be called, "contingent" nutrients which are needed only under limited conditions may prove to be an increasingly important part of nutritional research and clinical practice.

Summary

Genetically based variations in nutrient requirements are the most important and troublesome ones for those who wish to promulgate RDAs or other standards for "normal, healthy" populations. But for physicians and others who regularly deal with abnormal, unhealthy *individuals*, RDAs are virtually useless and are potentially very misleading. Not only are such individuals excluded from deliberations about RDAs, they also comprise a selected population which is especially likely to possess nutrient needs substantially beyond RDA levels, for reasons of heredity, illness, trauma or medical treatments including drugs and surgery.

Genetotrophic Disease

Drawing from the then-new finding of "partial genetic blocks," Williams and coworkers postulated in 1950 that some individuals may have genetically-based, increased nutrient requirements which are not met by diets that are adequate for most individuals. If unmet, these unusual needs would lead to what they called "genetotrophic" disease (genetic disease of nourishment).

Subsequently, we have learned that genetotrophic diseases do exist, and that the efficiency of enzymatic transformations and the enzymes themselves commonly show significant variations among individuals. The genetotrophic diseases recognized so far in humans and animals generally involve profound anatomical or biochemical abnormalities found at birth or during early growth. The augmented nutrient requirements which prevent, cure or ameliorate these diseases range from only about 2-fold to many hundred-fold times the needs of most individuals.

Human examples

The best known human examples include a variety of severe metabolic diseases which respond to increased intakes of vitamin B_6,[29] and "vitamin D-resistant rickets," a group of disorders which often responds to increased intakes of vitamin D_3 or its normal metabolites.[30] In many afflicted individuals the specific hereditary biochemical impairment has been identified.

Williams cited and discussed a less severe human "familial periodic paralysis" which is accompanied by hypopotassemia.[2] During a seizure or prior to it, plasma potassium levels are abnormally low, and relief from the condition comes promptly with administration of 1 to 2.5 grams of potassium in the form of potassium chloride. Williams noted that this disorder may be considered a hereditary need for modestly augmented amounts of potassium.

Other genetotrophic diseases in humans include a variation of "maple syrup urine disease" which responds to thiamin (only 10-30 mg/day; 7-20 times the RDA), a form of methylmalonic acidemia which responds to vitamin B_{12} injections (1 mg/day; 300 times the RDA), a variation of propionic acidemia which responds to biotin (10 mg/day; about 70 times the estimated RDA), and

Hartnup's disease which involves increased requirements for niacin.[31,32]

These examples illustrate the important point that despite definite-sounding names and "diagnostic" biochemical indicators, inborn errors of metabolism "differ in their severity, the age of onset and in the involvement of [various organs]. . . . it is perhaps true to say that the rule most clearly applicable to the clinical pattern of inborn metabolic errors is the inapplicability of any general rule."[33] This diversity probably reflects variations in the exact nature and intensity of the hereditary impairment, genetic variations in the metabolic context of the impairment, as well as environmental factors including diet.

Animal Examples

Hutt has reviewed several nutritional disorders in animals which have clear genetic links.[9] The frequencies of these disorders could be greatly increased or decreased by simple selective breeding, or they could be prevented entirely by dietary improvements. Compared to the presently recognized human genetotrophic diseases, these animal examples were relatively common, and they usually responded to relatively small increases of nutrients (2- to 5-fold). The examples include rats with nose bent to one side (prevented by adjustments in the calcium:phosphorus ratio or in vitamin D intake), brain hernia in swine, slipped tendon in chickens (preventable by manganese supplementation), and riboflavin-linked bare backs and short down feathers in black chicks as mentioned earlier. Large individual variations in requirements were always in evidence, indicated by a few normal individuals even at low nutrient intakes and by a few afflicted individuals even at higher intakes.

A striking genetotrophic disease has been found in the mutant "pallid" mouse.[34] The offspring of homozygous mothers show, in addition to a pallid color, an irreversible congenital ataxia caused by defects of the inner ear. That is, about two-thirds of the offspring are afflicted when their mothers receive a customary diet. But if the mothers are given a 20-fold increase in dietary manganese, the ataxia (but not the pallid color) is prevented in all of their offspring. (This shows that the offspring of these mice vary by more than a 20-fold range in their mothers' requirements for manganese.)

Discussion

The genetotrophic nature of these diseases in animals would probably have remained undiscovered if they had occurred in humans. Elucidation of the pallid-mouse requirement for extra manganese, for example, depended on unusual conditions. The ataxic symptoms mimicked those found in earlier experiments feeding "manganese-free" diets to ordinary mice. And the symptoms happened to occur in a strain of mice marked by a distinctive coat. Feeding deficient diets to human mothers is unthinkable, and furthermore, genetotrophic diseases often do not show symptoms similar to "ordinary deficiencies" (see below) and are not accompanied by distinctive physical traits.

Note also that the presently recognized genetotrophic diseases usually involve profound abnormalities obvious at birth or shortly thereafter, and that they are often irreversible if they are not prevented during gestation. Genetotrophic diseases involving more subtle impairments, slight mental or psychological defects, or increased susceptibilities to common diseases during adulthood would be *very difficult* to recognize as such, especially if they are irreversible.

Even "ordinary deficiencies" of nutrients involving major or multiple metabolic functions may be difficult to recognize, because the symptoms are often non-specific and quite variable from person to person. But, as discussed recently by Shive and Lansford,[35] defects in nutrient *utilization* by a single enzyme, for example, may result in a syndrome unique to the functions of that enzyme. Since most nutrients have a multitude of functions, the recognition and treatment or prevention of genetotrophic conditions "represents one of the greatest challenges for nutritional research, and promises to have a significant impact on health and productivity of man. . . . Although the frequency of such . . . states is very small, the potential number of different [genetotrophic] diseases is very large and probably affects the level of performance and the health status of many individuals to some degree."[35]

Presumably the presently recognized human genetotrophic diseases represent only the most extreme (rare), easily recognized "abnormalities" from a continuous distribution of genetic variabilities which in milder, more common forms merge into what we consider "normal variations." If so, the greatest challenge before us is to learn to recognize, cope with, or prevent, the more subtle, numerically more significant forms of genetotrophic impairments.

Coping With Diverse Nutrient Requirements

Ideally, one could assess an individual's nutritional status for each nutrient, including the functional efficiency of every metabolic activity of each nutrient. This would require thousands of tests. In actual practice, we are able to measure only a few tissue levels (mainly in blood, hair or urine) and to make a very few tests of biochemical function. Although tissue concentration measurements are sometimes helpful in detecting deficiencies caused by poor diet or defective assimilation, they cannot detect impaired enzymatic activities or localized transport or utilization problems.

Skilled clinical observations

As a result, skilled clinical observation is an important, yet highly imperfect, means of detecting nutritional deficiencies. The widest possible knowledge of often neglected literature[10-16] is needed, because there are many possible manifestations and causes of nutritional lacks, and new findings frequently appear. Judgment and an investigative attitude are also important, because many manifestations are non-specific and variable among individuals.

Many physicians and nutritionists understandably have shied away from enthusiastic reports and unsophisticated observations which do not fit into the mainstream of traditional nutritional thinking, because the reports are so often unreliable. But to completely ignore these reports and other "folklore" is to lose many potentially valuable leads.

Fortunately, increasing numbers of forward looking physicians and researchers are pursuing innovative nutritional explorations. An important example comes from the 1966 and 1973 books of John Ellis, a practicing physician in a small Texas town.[36,37] Chance observations and informal explorations led him to believe that vitamin B_6 deficiency caused painfully swollen or tingling hands in many of his patients, and that ten to twenty times RDA levels of vitamin B_6 cured them. Subsequently he concluded that many other conditions responded to similar vitamin B_6 supplementation, including some forms of arthritis and rheumatism, muscle cramps, some cases of diabetes and hypoglycemia and the edemas associated with pregnancy, menstruation and contraceptive steroids. At the time all of these novel conclusions easily could be dismissed as "anecdotal" and very unlikely.

However, in recent years much research (mentioned earlier) has supported links between inadequate vitamin B_6 and side effects of the contraceptive steroids, including "chemical diabetes." And over a dozen careful investigations in cooperation with Karl Folkers and coworkers recently have demonstrated an intimate relationship of vitamin B_6 deficiency to carpal tunnel syndrome.[38,39] This "widespread" syndrome includes painful or tingling hands and is known to be associated with rheumatoid arthritis, pregnancy, oral contraceptives and diabetes.[40]

In 100 percent of twenty-two cases reported so far, vitamin B_6

deficiency was biochemically demonstrated, and 100 percent responded to pyridoxine supplementation, including one patient under double-blind conditions. Response is rather slow (twelve weeks), apparently partly due to a remarkable two-phase effect of pyridoxine. First, it promptly supplies a cofactor needed for enzyme activity (glutamic oxaloacetic transaminase). Second, as a delayed effect it stimulates synthesis of additional amounts of apoenzyme. RDA levels of supplementation help, but higher levels have been found necessary for the most rapid and complete recovery.

If these findings withstand the further test of time, Ellis's chance observations and persistent claims will have led to discovery of the remarkably simple cause, prevention and treatment for a syndrome hitherto of unknown etiology and treatable only symptomatically by surgery or cortisone. Unfortunately such simple, uniformly successful nutritional approaches cannot be expected as a rule.

Dietary improvements

Nature copes with nutritional diversity by providing a wide variety of wholesome foods which (if whole and well balanced) presumably provide sufficient amounts of nutrients to accommodate the needs of most individuals. Theoretically, individuals with needs much higher than available from raw, whole, natural foods would have tended to be removed from the population. (In modern times these theoretical considerations tend to be disrupted by sedentary lifestyles and low calorie needs, environmental changes, modern agricultural practices or drugs, and they may never have applied to elderly individuals well beyond the age of reproduction.)

As a guide to possible higher nutrient requirements and to possible dietary improvements, we may ask, what amounts of nutrients would be provided by a diet of exclusively whole, raw foods, and how do these levels compare with diets commonly consumed in modern U.S.?

The rough answer regarding most vitamins and minerals is that modern "average" diets in the U.S.A. supply approximately RDA levels, a fact which is not entirely coincidental.[3] And since these "average diets" derive over 60 percent of their calories from purified sugars, separated fats, alcohol and milled grains which supply little or no vitamins and minerals, generally speaking two to four times RDA levels of these micronutrients would be obtained from a mixed diet of whole, raw foods as available in the U.S. A notable exception is vitamin C for which intakes could be even higher. (These facts seem to be surprisingly little noticed.)

Considering that some nutritional losses of storage, cooking and processing are difficult to avoid and that purified sugars and fats are very seldom reduced to less than 10-20 percent of calories, careful dietary improvements might roughly double the broad range of vitamin and mineral intakes of "average" diets in the U.S., with greater increases possible for specific nutrients and for individuals with below average diets. Such improvements would probably be adequate, if maintained from gestation through adulthood, to meet many of the higher ranges of needs of "normal, healthy" people. And they would have the important advantage of supplying possible unknown nutrients or "contingent" nutrients about which we are presently ignorant, as well as known nutrients which are ordinarily omitted from supplements.

It would be an extremely interesting experiment to test a diet of nearly exclusively whole, minimally cooked foods for a lifetime in a selected population, and to study its reproductive record, vigor, educational and intellectual accomplishments, social adjustments, susceptibilities to diseases and longevity. Unfortunately this method of detecting subtle nutritional disorders in humans is far more difficult to carry out than it is in animals.

Nutritional supplements

Another possible way to explore and cope with nutritional diversity is by the use of nutritional supplements. In the absence of individualized information about requirements, judgments must be made about which nutrients to include and in what amounts. Many considerations may enter in. These include the contents of typical diets, the need for balance and teamwork among nutrients, ease of administration, safety and cost.[26]

Three different kinds of supplement formulations are illustrated in Table 3.2. Two are based on (recently updated) formulations for nutritional insurance which R. J. Williams has suggested and given to the public.[41] The third is a specialized formula used in recent research designed to test the hypothesis that mental retardation in children may have genetotrophic links.[42]

The "nutritional insurance" formulation contains most of what is practical and presently known to include in a convenient, low cost supplement, generally at about RDA levels. It necessarily excludes many nutrients such as amino acids and potassium which are needed in inconveniently large amounts. The amounts of calcium and other major minerals are limited for the same reason.

The "fortified insurance" formulation "contains much higher amounts of some of the vitamins and double the amount of some of the minerals and other nutrients. If one tolerates this fortified supplement well, he or she can take it indefinitely but in many cases it may be desirable to continue it at a lower level.[41] Williams suggests it for insurance purposes to those who may have higher requirements which the first supplement does not adequately supply, including those vulnerable to alcoholism.

The "genetotrophic research" supplement was used (with apparent success) in a research context with a small group of children with mental retardation and other clear abnormalities, including Down's syndrome.[42] Based on formulations of the late Mary B. Allen, it contains still higher levels of most vitamins and omits a few ingredients contained in the other formulas.

Possible toxicity, imbalances and intolerances must be kept in mind with supplements containing amounts well in excess of those present in foods. All nutrients (unlike drugs) are of course native to human metabolism, and most vitamins can be taken in very large amounts without apparent harm. However, serious toxicity has been observed in sensitive individuals taking as little as ten to twenty times RDA levels of vitamin A[43] and even less of vitamin D. These vitamins and all of the minerals are used relatively cautiously in the three supplements illustrated here.

Summary

Until convenient, detailed assessments of individual nutritional status become available, including tests for the biochemical efficiency of multitudinous metabolic activities, coping with diverse nutrient requirements in individuals seems destined to remain a less-than-satisfactory mixture of many methods. These include inadequate clinical tests, skilled clinical observations backed by extensive (but far from complete) knowledge, chance observations, using clues from questionable lore and from the nutrient contents of whole, natural diets, and individual experimentation with dietary improvements and nutritional supplements.

Conclusion

Scientists, including nutritional researchers, understandably look for order, uniformities and generalizations that may apply to "the human" or "the average rat." In this context, ever-present biological diversities may be viewed as unwelcome distractions which must be "averaged out" or otherwise excluded, sometimes at great effort. When the diversities and exceptions are small or relatively unimportant compared to major uniformities, this focus on generalizations can be extremely useful. When the diversities are large or otherwise important, however, we are left with a distorted, oversimplified concept of "the normal human" which permeates our biology, medicine, psychology, education and even our language. Progress in nutritional science for real men, women and children demands that scientists and clinicians focus on the diversities themselves in order to understand and solve problems which have their roots in diversity.

Even for "normal, healthy" people, nutritional standards such as RDAs based on average requirements are of dubious conceptual or practical utility. If we assume, as presently indicated, that 4- to 10-fold variations exist for many nutrients in small groups of normal, healthy individuals, then an analysis based on averages, Gaussian ("normal") distributions and standard deviations is simply stretched beyond its capabilities, and this fact must be recognized.

For physicians and others who deal primarily with "abnormal, unhealthy" individuals who may be ill, stressed, diseased, aged, injured or taking drugs or other medical therapy, it is still more important to recognize human nutritional diversity.

Methods to cope with nutritional diversity are far from satisfactory, to be sure, but increasing numbers of physicians and other professionals are making an effort. In spite of the foibles of error-prone enthusiasts, commercial excesses and widespread nutritional illiteracy, sound progress is being accumulated by observant clinicians and competent researchers. Outdated, simplistic assumptions that nutrients function merely to prevent "scurvy," "beriberi" and the like are being gradually overcome. High public interest helps compensate for the lack of commercial incentive for ethical pharmaceutical companies to research and promote unpatentable nutrients.

The fundamental premises of Roger J. Williams's 1950 genetotrophic hypothesis have been amply demonstrated, and we may hope that the current generation of biomedical researchers will begin to investigate the many presently obscure human health problems which may be prevented or ameliorated by nutritional improvements.

POSTSCRIPT

A new and promising approach to the assessment of individual nutritional requirements is under development by William Shive of the University of Texas. He presented his preliminary findings at the International Conference on Human Nutrition at Tianjin, China in June 1981. This method is applicable to virtually all nutrients and is based on studying the unique nutritional requirements of cultured lymphocytes of individuals. It graphically demonstrates the great biological diversity of individuals and promises to provide a new level of functional assessment of their nutritional status.

REFERENCES

1. Williams, R. J., Beerstecher, E. Jr. and Berry, L. J. 1950. The concept of genetotrophic disease. *Lancet* 1:287.
2. Williams, R. J. 1956. *Biochemical Individuality: The Basis for the Genetotrophic Concept.* New York: John Wiley & Sons. Austin, Texas: University of Texas Press. 1979.
3. *Recommended Dietary Allowances,* 9th Ed. 1980. Washington, D. C.: National Academy of Sciences.
4. Williams, R. J., Heffley, J. D., Yew, M. and Bode, C. W. 1973. A renaissance of nutritional science is imminent. *Persp. Biol. Med.* 17:1.
5. Scrimshaw, N. S. and Young, V. R. 1978. Biological variability and nutrient needs. In: *Progress in Human Nutrition,* vol. 2, *Biological and Cultural Variability.* S. Margen and R. A. Ogar, eds. Westport, CT.: AVI Publishing Co.
6. Hegsted, D. M. 1963. Variation in requirements of nutrients—amino acids. *Federation Proceedings* 22:1424.
7. Yew, M. S. 1975. Biological variation in ascorbic acid needs. *Annals N. Y. Acad. Sci.* 258:451
8. Williams, R. J. and Deason, G. 1967. Individuality in vitamin C needs. *Proc. Nat. Acad. Sci. U.S.A.* 57:1638.
9. Hutt, F. B. 1953. *Genetic Resistance to Disease in Domestic Animals.* Ithaca, N. Y.: Cornell University Press.
10. Williams, R. J. 1973. *Nutrition Against Disease: Environmental Prevention.* New York: Bantam Books.
11. Stone, I. 1972. *The Healing Factor: Vitamin C Against Disease.* New York: Grosset & Dunlap.
12. Wright, J. V. 1979. *Dr. Wright's Book of Nutritional Therapy.* Emmaus, Pa.: Rodale Press.
13. Hall, K. 1975. Orthomolecular therapy: review of the literature. *Orthomolecular Psychiatry* 4:297.
14. Roe, D. A. 1976. *Drug-Induced Nutritional Deficiencies.* Westport, CT.: AVI Publ. Co.
15. *Nutrition and Drug Interrelations.* 1978. J. N. Hathcock and J. Coon, eds. New York: Academic Press.
16. March, D. C. 1976. *Handbook: Interactions of Selected Drugs with Nutritional Status in Man.* Chicago: Amer. Dietetic Assoc.
17. Brin, M. 1978. Drugs and environmental chemicals in relation to vitamin needs. In: *Nutrition and Drug Interrelations.* J. N. Hathcock and J. Coon, eds. New York: Academic Press.
18. Rose, D. P. 1978. Effects of oral contraceptives on nutrient utilization. In: *Nutrition and Drug Interrelations.* J. N. Hathcock and J. Coon, eds. New York: Academic Press.
19. Shive, W., Snider, R. N., DuBilier, B., Rude, J. C., Clark, G. E. and Ravel, J. O. 1957. Glutamine in treatment of peptic ulcer. *Texas State J. of Med.* 53:840.
20. Shive, W. 1964. Glutamine as a general metabolic agent protecting against alcohol poisoning. In: *Biochemical and Nutritional Aspects of Alcoholism.* New York: The Christopher D. Smithers Foundation.

21. Fincle, L. P. 1964. Experiments in treating alcoholics with glutamic acid and glutamine. In: *Biochemical and Nutritional Aspects of Alcoholism*. New York: The Christopher D. Smithers Foundation.
22. Rogers, L. L. and Pelton, R. B. 1957. Effect of glutamine on IQ scores of mentally deficient children. *Texas Rep. Biol. Med.* 15:84.
23. Tower, D. B. 1955. Nature and extent of the biochemical lesion in human epileptogenic cerebral cortex. *Neurology* 5:113.
24. Perry, T. L., Hansen, S., Tischler, B., Bunting, R. and Diamond, S. 1970. Glutamine depletion in phenylketonuria: a possible cause of the mental defect. *N. Engl. J. Med.* 282:761.
25. Robbins, R. C. 1980. Medical and nutritional aspects of citrus bioflavonoids. In: *Citrus Nutrition and Quality*. S. Nagy and J. A. Attaway, eds. ACS Symposium series 143. Washington, D.C.: Am. Chem. Soc.
26. Williams, R. J. 1975. *Physicians' Handbook of Nutritional Science*. Springfield, IL.: Charles C. Thomas.
27. Folkers, K., Watanabe, T. and Kaji, M. 1977. Critique of coenzyme Q in biochemical and biomedical research and in ten years of clinical research on cardiovascular disease. *J. Molec. Med.* 2:431.
28. *Biomedical and Clinical Aspects of Coenzyme Q*. 1977. Folkers, K. and Yamamura, Y., eds. New York: Elsevier.
29. Mudd, S. H. 1971. Pyridoxine—responsive genetic disease. *Federation Proc.* 30:970.
30. DeLuca, H. F. 1979. *Vitamin D—Metabolism and Function*. New York: Springer-Verlag.
31. Wong, P. W. and Hsia, D. Y. 1973. Inborn errors of metabolism. In: *Modern Nutrition in Health and Disease*. 5th ed. R. S. Goodheart and M. E. Shils., eds. Philadelphia: Lea & Febiger.
32. Hommes, F. A. and Van Den Berg, C. J., eds. 1973. *Inborn Errors of Metabolism*. New York: Academic Press.
33. Bickel, H. The clinical pattern of inborn metabolic errors with brain damage. In *Inborn Errors of Metabolism*.
34. Erway, L., Hurley, L. S. and Fraser, A. 1966. Neurological defect: manganese in phenocopy and prevention of a genetic abnormality of the inner ear. *Science* 152:1766.
35. Shive, W. and Lansford, E. M., Jr. 1980. Roles of vitamins as coenzymes. In: *Human Nutrition—A Comprehensive Treatise*. vol. 3B. R. Alfin-Slater and D. Kritchevsky, eds. New York: Plenum Publishing Co.
36. Ellis, J. M. 1966. *The Doctor Who Looked at Hands*. New York: Vantage Press.
37. Ellis, J. M. and Presley, J. 1973. *Vitamin B₆: The Doctor's Report*. New York: Harper & Row.
38. Folkers, K., Ellis, J., Watanabe, T., Saji, S. and Kaji, M. 1978. Biochemical evidence for a deficiency of vitamin B_6 in the carpal tunnel syndrome based on a crossover clinical study. *Proc. Nat. Acad. Sci. U.S.A.* 75:3410.
39. Ellis, J., Folkers, K., Watanabe, T., Kaji, M., Saji, S., Caldwell, J. W., Temple, C. A. and Wood, F. S. 1979. Clinical results of a crossover treatment with pyridoxine and placebo of the carpal tunnel syndrome. *Am. J. Clin. Nutr.* 32:2040.
40. Taylor, N. 1971. Carpal tunnel syndrome. *Am. J. Phys. Med.* 50:192.
41. Williams, R. J. 1981. *The Prevention of Alcoholism through Nutrition*. New York: Bantam Books.

42. Harrell, R. F., Capp, R. H., Davis, D. R., Peerless, J. and Ravitz, L. 1981. Can nutritional supplements help mentally retarded children? An exploratory study. *Proc. Nat. Acad. Sci. U.S.A.* 78:574.
43. Davis, D. R. 1978. Using vitamin A safely. *Osteopathic Medicine* 3:31. Reprinted in *J. Int. Acad. Preventive Med.* 5:38.

4

ASSESSMENT OF THE MALNUTRITION
OF
OVERCONSUMPTION/UNDERNUTRITION

———————◀●▶———————

JEFFREY BLAND, PH.D.

NUTRITIONAL assessment has traditionally been recognized as a function of the dietitian in clinical practice; however, recent documentation of the substantial incidence of malnutrition of the overconsumption/undernutrition type has established the need for increasingly sophisticated and comprehensive assessment programs utilized by standard health practitioners. Historically, clinicians have tended to recognize and acknowledge only the more extreme nutritional aberrations. Subtle forms of nutritional depletion have evaded significant attention, primarily because of the limited knowledge and availability of clinical nutritional assessment techniques.[1]

The current state of nutrition knowledge affords the clinician better opportunities to recognize the early warning signs to subsequent nutritionally related diseases, leading them into implementation of support programs. The notion that it is wise to identify and act upon problems at an early stage is hardly novel, but it has only been recently that we have had the tools available for better recognition at an early stage of the signs of undernutrition. Guthrie and Guthrie have pointed out that in reviewing the Ten State Nutrition Surveys three broad categories of data are needed to assess the nutritional status of an individual patient, these being dietary, anthropometric and biochemical information.[2]

As Jensen and Dudrick point out, "No single test or measurement can identify or classify malnutrition, but the comprehensive profile of anthropometric, biochemical and immunological indica-

64

tors can identify patients with nutritional aberrations. Although the clinical relevance of each index remains to be established, the use of a battery of tests permits the early recognition of nutritionally depleted states, which have formerly gone undetected."[3]

This assessment program should allow the inspection of adequacy both of the macronutrients (protein, carbohydrate and fat) and of the micronutrients (vitamins, minerals, potential accessory food factors). The integration of a prognostic screening profile, which allows early recognition of signs, symptoms and laboratory data indicating nutritional inadequacy, is at the core of delivering improved, individualized, therapeutic nutritional programs. Table 4.1 lists the types of information which can be accumulated on a patient in the formation of this prognostic nutritional screening profile in the areas of anthropometric, dietary and biochemical data.

TABLE 4.1
Variables Used in Nutritional Evaluation

Dietary	*Biochemical*	*Anthropometric*
food frequency	erythrocyte	height/weight
diet diary	transketolase	lean body mass
	EGOT	biographical
	glutathione reductase	symptoms & signs
	serum	family history
	protein	stress evaluation
	albumin/globulin	exercise tolerance
	uric acid	hair pluckability
	blood urea nitrogen	blood pressure
	creatinine	axillary body
	cholesterol/HDL	temperature
	triglycerides	
	glucose	
	hemoglobin A1c	
	fibrinogen	
	alkaline phosphatase	
	free thyroxine	
	ultrafilterable calcium	
	gamma glutamyl transpeptidase	
	complete blood count with	
	differential whole blood or	
	serum trace elements	
	urinalysis	
	ketones	
	indican	
	trace minerals	
	sodium	
	hair trace elements	
	fecal analysis (malabsorption)	
	salivary sediment	

Many new diagnostic screening tests are introduced into the health-care system each year. Evaluating them can be difficult and there has been a tendency in the past few years to reject these screening tools because they lead to rapid cost escalation in the health-care community.[4]

As any new assessment tool is added to the profile, the question of its sensitivity, specificity and predictive value needs to be addressed. The sensitivity of a test is defined as the percentage of all people with the specific problem who have a positive test, whereas the specificity is the percentage of all people without a specific condition who have a negative test. The predictive value of a test is defined as the fraction of all positive tests that truly represent a case of the dysfunction. A valuable new contributor to a nutrition screening program should have reasonably high sensitivity, specificity, and be of high predictive value in picking up nutritionally related dysfunction early enough that modification of diet can make a significant difference in the improvement of the health of the individual. Several authors have developed criteria for inclusion of such new screening tests with the following being representative of such criteria:[5,6]

1. The condition sought should be an important health problem.
2. There should be an accepted nutritional approach for treatment of patients with a recognized problem.
3. Facilities for recognition and treatment should be available.
4. The screening test should be acceptable to the population.
5. There should be an agreed policy on whom to treat as patients.
6. The cost of case finding, including recognition and treatment, should be economically balanced in relation to possible expenditure on medical care as a whole.
7. The test should be able to recognize a latent or early symptomatic stage.

There are historically a number of tests, signs and symptoms which adequately fulfill all of these criteria; however, new tests which have only recently become available to the health-care community at large may fail in one or more of these criteria. The objective is to develop a screening protocol which would include the minimum number of variables that would give the greatest prognostic screening sensitivity, specificity and predictive value as it relates to the malnutrition of overconsumption/undernutrition. Although many leaders in the field have developed methods of indexing and quantifying degree and type of malnutrition, it is found that many of these assessment techniques have proved to be too arduous or not well understood by most clinicians and not in widespread use for this reason.[7,8]

As pointed out by Wright[9] and Kovach,[10] education appears to be the major tool in improvement of health-care practitioners' appropriate use of available nutritional screening tools. As Habicht points out, nutritional monitoring and surveillance require the ability to measure changes in the prevalence or the risk of a specific disease.[11] The concept of risk is just now being recognized as an important determinant in the implementation of an effective preventive nutritional program. Due to the uncertainties that are encountered in the establishment of a relative risk to a nutritionally related disease entity, it is important that considerable redundancy be developed in the screening program to identify patterns of suggested risk. This data base should be built upon epidemiological evidence which shows prevalence in certain populations of a specific nutritionally related disease with the nutritional inadequacy or excess.[14]

Selection of the appropriate reference population and use of evaluative criteria that are more suggestive of functional adequacy, rather than the absence of disease, should be the determinants in such a screening program. Once collected, these data can then be used in the implementation of a behavior modification program to lower the relative risk to a specific disease entity. Such is the focus of the *M*ultiple *R*isk *F*actor *I*ntervention *T*rial (Mr. Fit), which represents a randomized clinical trial, sponsored by the National Heart, Lung and Blood Institute in an attempt to determine the efficacy of modification of multiple risk factors in reducing coronary heart disease mortality, with specific emphasis on reducing elevated blood cholesterol, elevated blood pressure and cigarette smoking.[15] It was found in this study that the identification of specific dietary habits and the relationship of these dietary habits to biochemical and anthropometric variables were at the crux of implementing an effective behavior modification program in the attempt to reduce the risk to coronary heart disease.[16]

Accurate Retrieval of Dietary Data

There are several ways that a health practitioner can assess a patient's daily nutritional intake, or relative dietary habits. These include a diet diary, which keeps a record of a patient's actual dietary intake for a specified period of time, generally three to seven days in length, a food frequency questionnaire, which indicates the relative frequency in portions per week that certain foods are eaten, or a nutrition scan, which outlines the number of meals per week that contain certain foods. The nutrition scan, advocated by Christakis, asked four questions of the patient:[17]

1. How many times per week do you have the following for breakfast in usual portions?
   a. citrus fruit
   b. whole grain cereals
   c. eggs
   d. pancakes, waffles
   e. coffee, milk (whole, 2 percent fat, or skim)
2. Of the 14 lunches and dinners you eat a week, how many are:
   a. beef, lamb, pork or organ meats (liver, heart, kidneys)
   b. poultry (chicken, turkey or duck)
   c. fish, shellfish
3. How many times a week do you eat or drink:
   a. bread, rolls
   b. vegetables of all types
   c. cheese
   d. legumes
   e. pasta
   f. fruit
   g. butter
   h. margarine
   i. vegetable oil/salad dressings
   j. ice cream
   k. alcoholic beverages
   l. snacks
   m. cookies
   n. nuts
   o. raisins
   p. soft drinks
4. How much water do you drink daily?

   This nutrition scan is incomplete and permits only a broad view of the eating pattern of the patient; however, it only takes five minutes and can provide a rough estimate of the following:

1. Adequacy of intake of the six major food groups, which include:
   dairy products
   meat, poultry and fish
   grain products
   starchy vegetables
   nonstarchy vegetables
   citrus fruits
   noncitrus fruits

2. The relative proportions of saturated and polyunsaturated fats in the diet;
3. Adequacy of dietary protein with regard to amount and sources;
4. Estimate of whether dietary cholesterol is excessive because of overintake of eggs, organ meats, red meats, shellfish, butter, ice cream and cheese;
5. Estimate of whether fiber is adequate through intake of whole grain cereals, vegetables and fruit;
6. Whether snacks, alcohol or salt intake is excessive.

A more quantifiable reflection of dietary intake can be achieved by looking at either the dietary history from a food frequency questionnaire or a diet diary. A comparison of the accuracy of these two dietary study methods indicates advantages and disadvantages of each.[18] The data of Young and colleagues would indicate that a longer record than three days of the dietary intake is necessary to achieve reasonably good average data concerning the patient's nutrient intake.[19] A food frequency questionnaire asks patients to indicate on a prescribed list of foods from the various food families how they consume them in the portion sizes indicated per week. It is a convenient method of accumulating dietary data, and generally has less "ownership" of certain foods by the patient filling out the questionnaire than by the diet diary, where each food must be indicated as it is consumed. The advantage to the food frequency questionnaire is that certain foods that may otherwise be subconsciously omitted in a diet diary—that is, foods the patients feel that they don't want known with regard to the frequency of consumption may more likely be included in the frequency questionnaire than in the diet diary.

The disadvantage, however, is that patients often forget what foods they actually have been consuming, and that there are seasonal and temporal differences in the food consumption patterns, which may lead to considerable errors in the responses to the food frequency questionnaire. These would not be seen in the diet diary where the patient is actually tabulating each food that's consumed, including snacks, during the prescribed period.

Both of these methods of data accumulation are amenable to computer processing, which is the only practical way to generate quantifiable information concerning average daily nutrient intake. As pointed out by Witschi and colleagues, the computer interactive method of dietary evaluation is convenient, because of its quick input, the relative ease of retrieval, the number of calculations that can be done, and computations concerning specific macronutrient/micronutrient intakes.[20]

One thing that should be pointed out is that the validity of this evaluation is only as good as the data base that is stored within the computer file as it relates to the nutrient values of foods. Although Widdowson and McCance,[21] Bransby et al[22] and Grover et al[23] cite large differences between calculated and chemically analyzed nutrient values, Tekkarinen[24] noted close agreement if the tabulated data contained values obtained from analysis of local foods. Recently, Hertzler and Hooper suggested that with the advent of computers and better analytical methods, nutrient data bases are becoming more comprehensive, reliable, and suitable for various uses.[25]

The most recent revision of the data base from which quantified diet survey information can be derived is that of the United States Department of Agriculture's *Nutrient Value of Foods, Revision, 1977* and *The Composition of Foods, Revised Handbook* from the United States Department of Agriculture, 1979.[26,27]

The use of a computer-based food information retrieval system allows immediate feedback and interpretation which has been proven instrumental in eliciting dialogue between the health practitioner and the patient regarding food and motivating behavioral change in the patient. Immediate access to the data base encourages further discussion about suitable substitute foods and about nutritional modification. Because of these advantages, there may be an increasing use of computer-based dietary evaluation in the offices of health practitioners, both as an aid to quantify a patient's dietary habits and as a tool in implementing effective behavior modification.

Huncher[28] regarded incomplete knowledge of food composition as one of the greatest handicaps in coping with dietary and nutritional problems, and the use of the in-office computer may help improve this level of knowledge.

There are still some significant holes in the nutritional data offered in the currently available handbooks on the nutrient value of foods. Included in this list of nutritional information on foods which is difficult to find are amounts and types of dietary fiber in individual foods, types and quantities of various sugars in foods, and the level of specific microtrace elements in foods, such as chromium and selenium.

If computerized data evaluation of a food frequency questionnaire or diet diary is not practical, then at least the evaluation of a patient's nutrition status by a nutrition scan or dietary score should be determined for every patient. A modification of the dietary score concept has been developed by Guthrie and Scheer and can serve also as a simple scoring system for rapid evaluation of dietary adequacy as the basis for education or counseling.[29] In this system, points are assigned whenever a serving of a food item appears in the diet, with two points being given for each of two items in both the milk and protein food groups and one point for each of four items in both the fruit or vegetable groups and the cereal or bread group. With this scoring system, equal weights are attributed to each of four food groups. This system may have limitations due to its lack of consideration of the way the food may have been stored or prepared and the difficulty of putting some fabricated foods into the diet which may not appear within the traditional four food families (fabricated foods, such as orange drink, which only remotely resemble the nutrient content of the food they mimic).

Variations in the various methods discussed for quantifying nutrient data have been analyzed, and it has been demonstrated that even under the best of conditions no more than plus or minus 20 percent correspondence of nutrient intake with the patient's actual dietary intake can be achieved.[30] In most cases this is acceptable in order to establish dietary trends and to focus on the major areas of need for dietary revision, particularly as they relate to comparing the patient's diet with the Dietary Goals established by the United States Senate.

Anthropometric Assessment Tools

The relationship of the average daily diet to the status of the individual is at the fore of providing competent nutritional evaluation. Evaluation of lean body mass by caliper skin fold methods, arm circumference, hydrostatic weighing, potassium-40 determination or deuterium oxide partitioning are important in establishing the relative ratio of muscle and bone to body fat. Lange and McGaw calipers have been suggested as one convenient method for establishing lean body mass.[31,32] Values of lean body mass for healthy individuals have been established by Keys[33] and are in a range of 85 to 90 percent lean body mass for men and 80 to 85 percent lean body mass for women. The body mass index is a crude indicator of lean body mass and is given as the weight in pounds divided by the height in feet squared.[34] Values of the body mass index less than 4.5 or greater than 5.1 may be associated with either reduced or excessive fat stores, respectively, with increased risk to certain health-related problems.

A second component of the anthropometric assessment is functional fitness testing, which explores the aerobic competency and exercise tolerance of the individual. Several methods are available, including maximal exercise tolerance testing, submaximal exercise tolerance testing on a treadmill, stationary bicycle or other instruments used for ergometry, or more simplistic methods such as the Canadian Step Test.[35] The Canadian Step Test involves the patient dressed in loose fitting clothes in a room at approximately 70° Fahrenheit, 21° Centigrade, stepping up and down onto a standard riser at the rate of 90 steps per minute for five minutes, then following the recovery pulse after three minutes and using standard tables establishing a fitness score for that individual, based upon his or her age. This, along with blood pressure and resting pulse, can serve as a useful screening tool for vascular sufficiency and general fitness level.

These data can be correlated, then, with the physical signs and symptoms of the patient, as they relate to the chronic signs of nutritional inadequacy, as discussed in Chapter 2, Table 2.2.

Expanded Criteria for Judging Nutritional Adequacy

Davis and Williams suggest that expanded biochemical and physiological criteria for judging nutritional adequacy may need to be implemented to fully indicate early warning signs of nutritional inadequacy.[36] Standard biochemical testing of an individual generally proceeds by way of measuring the concentration of a specific analyte in a biological fluid or tissue and from this determination establishing whether the patient falls within or outside a normal reference range. One of the limitations of this standard testing protocol, as it relates to screening for chronic states of inadequacy, is that this procedure focuses on the existence of constituents which are present in the biological fluid as it relates to end-organ failure, or pathology, and not as a result of indication of the relative reserve of the specific organ to accommodate functional stress.

Fries has pointed out that increased risk to illness occurs as the result of the loss of organ reserve.[37] Homeostasis and health are obtained by an organism's adjustment within limits of the compensating mechanisms against stress in organ systems such as heart, lungs, kidney and liver. In young adult life the functional capacity of human organs is four to ten times that required to sustain life. The existence of this organ reserve enables the stressed organism to restore homeostasis when it is deranged by an external threat. It has been found that organ reserve declines in almost a linear rate, beginning at the age of thirty, with different slopes of rate of loss for different individuals.[38]

Nutritional status has been found to be one of the parameters which influences the rate of loss of organ reserve. Suboptimal nutrition contributes to an increased rate of loss of organ reserve, thereby resulting in increased risk to degenerative disease at a specific age.[39] Screening programs which would then be able to evaluate functional organ reserve would better be able to prognosticate relative risk to degenerative diseases than testing or screening protocols which focused exclusively on the existence or absence of pathology.

A method that has been employed to assess the reserve in a specific organ system is that of the provocative (or stress) test, which challenges the patient to mobilize reserve in response to the challenge. Examples of this type of testing protocol, as opposed to traditional end-point analyses that have been used, are the cardiac stress test and the oral glucose tolerance test. In the cardiac stress test certain cardiac abnormalities, which were not seen in the resting EKG, are only obviated when putting the cardiovascular system under an imposed stress, allowing examination of its ability to manifest reserve.[40]

In preventive nutrition, one is screening for inherent metabolic insufficiencies or individual biochemical uniquenesses, which may be present before a symptomatic observed pathology has arisen, and the need to consider reserves under stress may be much more important than in the diagnosis of frank disease states. This relates closely to Williams's concept of the genetotrophic theory of disease[41] in which the genetic pattern of the afflicted individual requires an augmented supply of one or more nutrients such that when these nutrients are adequately supplied, the disease is ameliorated. Table 4.2 lists a number of the well-recognized vitamin-dependent disorders which may be classified under the concept of the genetotrophic theory of disease.[42]

TABLE 4.2
Vitamin Dependent Genetotrophic Diseases

Thiamin	*Cobalamine*
Leigh's disease	Methylmalonic aciduria
Maple syrup urine	Homocystinuria
Pyruvic decarboxylase deficiency	
Pyridoxine	*Niacin*
Homocystinuria	Hartnup's disease
Xanthurenic aciduria	
Cystathioninuria	

Please see Table 2.3 on pp. 34–36 for Guidelines for Criteria of Nutritional Status by Laboratory Evaluation.

Recently, Harrell, Capp and Davis have reported a controlled study done with mentally retarded children which supports the hypothesis that certain types of mental retardation are in part genetotrophic in origin and respond to specific nutrient supplementation, based upon the biochemical need of the individual.[43]

The Erythrocyte as a Tool For Nutritional Assessment

Given, then, the need to screen for subclinical nutrient deficiencies, which may not be evident by the appearance of standard symptoms of vitamin deficiency diseases, new methods have been developed to allow better exploration of the state of nutritional reserves at the biochemical level in a specific individual. This approach is much more in concert with the concept of individualized nutritional screening and the ultimate recognition of a specific patient's unique nutritional needs for improved status.

Studies of healthy school children in New York showed low circulating thiamin levels attributed to dietary habits, present in 6 percent of Chinese, 52 percent of Caucasians and 68 percent of blacks.[44]

Lonsdale and Shamberger have found that patients whose symptoms were apparently neurotically functional were suffering from vitamin undernutriture, even though they were consuming diets which may have been adequate according to the RDA levels of the B-complex vitamins. Symptoms included such things as abdominal and chest pain, sleep disturbances, personality change, insomnia, intermittent diarrhea alternating with constipation, chronic debilitating fatigue, headache and aggressive personality change—all of unknown organic origin. They were able to recognize this particular syndrome by use of the erythrocyte transketolase test as an indicator of a chronic nutritional deficiency state.[45] This test, developed by Brin and colleagues, measures the activity of the erythrocyte enzyme transketolase, which is dependent upon a specific coenzyme derived from dietary thiamin (vitamin B_1).[46] The protocol involves the examination of activity of the erythrocyte transketolase in the presence and absence of thiamin pyrophosphate. If, in this *in vitro* test, there is a considerable activation of enzyme turnover when thiamin pyrophosphate is added, it demonstrates that the enzyme is working far from saturation with its respective vitamin-derived coenzyme and that the patient may be suffering from undernutriture with regard to that specific nutrient. The greater the degree of activation, the more the suggested vitamin insufficiency, even in the face of what would be considered adequate dietary intake, or even circulating serum levels.[47]

Lonsdale and Shamberger conclude from their study with regard to the nature of chronic vitamin undernutriture that "the reversal of the metabolic disturbance that resulted from [this deficiency state] appeared to be much slower than is generally associated with vitamin-deficiency states, and our experience suggested that such states may well be seen in an affluent, modern society, and possibly may be more dangerous [than frank vitamin deficiency syndrome] since personality changes were frequently aggressive in nature and correction of the metabolic abnormalities slow."

Similar type of testing protocol can also be used for the determination of the status of riboflavin, using the enzyme glutathione reductase, and pyridoxine, using the enzyme glutamate-oxalate transaminase.[48]

Individuals may require enhanced levels of intake of a specific micronutrient in order to promote proper enzyme function, based upon their unique genetic control of enzyme structure, coenzyme binding and absorptive capacity. An example of this is seen in patients with the Wernicke-Korsakoff syndrome who have been shown to have a genetically determined diminution of the binding of the coenzyme thiamin pyrophosphate to the respective apoenzyme which predisposes them to thiamin deficiency syndrome at a much earlier stage than other individuals who do not carry this genetic need for enhanced thiamin intake.[49]

Recent studies of Anderson and colleagues suggest that apparently healthy, normal individuals may differ significantly in the rates at which their red cells convert pyridoxine, and perhaps riboflavin, to their coenzymes, and that vitamin metabolism may be under genetic control.[50,51] While studying pyridoxine metabolism in red cells, they observed that 7 percent of normal subjects were slow converters of pyridoxine, having significantly lower rates for the conversion to pyridoxal pyrophosphate. These *in vitro* enzyme vitamin challenge tests can be very useful for picking up undernutriture problems that may have been missed by other standard screening procedures. These procedures may also be useful in determining the dose of specific nutrients necessary to compensate for metabolic uniqueness. In a recent study on rural school boys, it was observed that after administering riboflavin at levels close to four times the Recommended Dietary Allowance for one month, 50 percent of the children had enzymatic evidence of riboflavin deficiency before supplementations judged by the degree of the unsaturation of the enzyme glutathione reductase that had previously been noted.[52]

These erythrocyte enzyme tests have found great use in defining certain clinical responsiveness to vitamin therapy, including carpal tunnel syndrome with vitamin B_6,[53] lassitude and fatigue related to undernutrition in geriatric patients,[54] oral contraceptive-induced depression related to B_6 inadequacy,[55] and increased risk to atherosclerosis in pyridoxine-responsive homocystinuria.[56,57]

Loading Tests for the Assessment of Nutritional Status

There are a number of oral challenge tests that have been utilized effectively for the establishment of nutritional status. These include the tryptophan loading test for determination of vitamin B_6 adequacy, the ascorbic acid loading test for determining vitamin C adequacy, the vitamin A loading test and the oral zinc tolerance test.

The tryptophan loading test for B_6 adequacy is based upon the concept that for the proper metabolism of dietary tryptophan it necessitates adequate vitamin B_6. Insufficiencies of vitamin B_6 upon an oral tryptophan load are accompanied by an increased urinary spill of the tryptophan metabolite xanthurenic acid. An oral test load of 2 to 5 grams of L-tryptophan results in little or no increase in the xanthurenic acid excretion in individuals who have been receiving adequate levels of vitamin B_6.[53,54] The dose of L-tryptophan that has been used in clinical studies is between 50 to 100 milligrams per kilogram of body weight. The larger load dose of tryptophan may be important for detecting and evaluating very early stages of vitamin B_6 insufficiency.[55]

The collection of twenty-four-hour urine samples is in many cases not feasible; therefore, as an alternative, although a less satisfactory procedure, subjects are given the test load of tryptophan and urine collected for the following six-hour period.[56] Xanthurenic acid values in excess of 25 mg for the six-hour collections are an indication of B_6 insufficiency. The abnormal excretions of xanthurenic acid are reduced to normal with the administration of relatively large doses of pyridoxine. Inspection of Table 4.3 will give the values for abnormal tryptophan loading tests to measure B_6 adequacy.

Vitamin C status has been evaluated by the lingual vitamin C test, based upon the procedure of Giza *et al*, and it was found that the vitamin C reserves of the body could be estimated by observing the time of decolorization of an aqueous solution of 2,6-dichloroindophenol by the tongue.[57] This procedure has been utilized extensively by Cheraskin and associates, who have published over twenty-five reports on the subject.[58] Studies of King and Little, however, concluded that the procedure was not specific for ascorbic acid and had little value when used to evaluate vitamin C

TABLE 4.3
Current Guidelines for Criteria of
Nutritional Status for Laboratory Evaluation

Nutrient and Units	Age of Subject (years)	Deficient	Criteria of Status Marginal	Acceptable
*Hemoglobin	6–23 mos.	Up to 9.0	9.0–9.9	10.0+
(gm/dl)	2–5	Up to 10.0	10.0–10.9	11.0+
	6–12	Up to 10.0	10.0–11.4	11.5+
	13–16M	Up to 12.0	12.0–12.9	13.0+
	13–16F	Up to 10.0	10.0–11.4	11.5+
	16+M	Up to 12.0	12.0–13.9	14.0+
	16+F	Up to 10.0	10.0–11.9	12.0+
	Pregnant (after 6+ mos.)	Up to 9.5	9.5–10.9	11.0+
*Hematocrit	Up to 2	Up to 28	28–30	31+
(Packed cell	2–5	Up to 30	30–33	34+
volume in	6–12	Up to 30	30–35	36+
percent)	13–16M	Up to 37	37–39	40+
	13–16F	Up to 31	31–35	36+
	16+M	Up to 37	37–43	44+
	16+F	Up to 31	31–37	33+
	Pregnant	Up to 30	30–32	33+
*Serum	Up to 1	—	Up to 2.5	2.5+
Albumin	1–5	—	Up to 3.0	3.0+
(gm/dl)	6–16	—	Up to 3.5	3.5+
	16+	Up to 2.8	2.8–3.4	3.5+
	Pregnant	Up to 3.0	3.0–3.4	3.5+
*Serum	Up to 1	—	Up to 5.0	5.0+
Protein	1–5	—	Up to 5.5	5.5+
(gm/dl)	6–16	—	Up to 6.0	6.0+
	16+	Up to 6.0	6.0–6.4	6.5+
	Pregnant	Up to 5.5	5.5–5.9	6.0+
*Serum Ascorbic Acid (mg/dl)	All ages	Up to 0.1	0.1–0.19	0.2+
*Plasma vitamin A (mcg/dl)	All ages	Up to 10	10–19	20+
*Plasma Carotene (mcg/dl)	All ages	Up to 20	20–39	40+
	Pregnant	—	40–79	80+

TABLE 4.3 (Continued)
Current Guidelines for Criteria of
Nutritional Status for Laboratory Evaluation

Nutrient and Units	Age of Subject (years)	Criteria of Status Deficient	Marginal	Acceptable
*Serum Iron (mcg/dl)	Up to 2	Up to 30	—	30+
	2.5	Up to 40	—	40+
	6–12	Up to 50	—	50+
	12+M	Up to 60	—	60+
	12+F	Up to 40	—	40+
*Transferrin Saturation (percent)	Up to 2	Up to 15.0	—	15.0+
	2–12	Up to 20.0	—	20.0+
	12+M	Up to 20.0	—	20.0+
	12+F	Up to 15.0	—	15.0+
**Serum Folacin (ng/ml)	All ages	Up to 2.0	2.1–5.9	6.0+
**Serum vitamin B_{12} (pg/ml)	All ages	Up to 100	—	100+
*Thiamin in Urine (mcg/g creatinine)	1–3	Up to 120	120–175	175+
	4–5	Up to 85	85–120	120+
	6–9	Up to 70	70–180	180+
	10–15	Up to 55	55–150	150+
	16+	Up to 27	27–65	65+
	Pregnant	Up to 21	21–49	50+
*Riboflavin in Urine (mcg/g creatinine)	1–3	Up to 150	150–499	500+
	4–5	Up to 100	100–299	300+
	6–9	Up to 85	85–269	270+
	10–16	Up to 80	70–199	200+
	16+	Up to 27	27–79	80+
	Pregnant	Up to 30	30–89	90+
**RBC Trans-ketolase-TPP effect (ratio)	All ages	25+	15–25	Up to 15
**RBC Gluta-thione Reductase-FAD-effect (ratio)	All ages	1.2+	—	Up to 1.2
**Tryptophan Load (mg Xanthurenic acid excreted)	Adults (Dose: 100 mg/kg body weight)	25+ (6 hrs) 75+ (24 hrs)	— —	Up to 25 Up to 75

TABLE 4.3 (Continued)
Current Guidelines for Criteria of
Nutritional Status for Laboratory Evaluation

Nutrient and Units	Age of Subject (years)	Deficient	Criteria of Status Marginal	Acceptable
***Urinary1–3	Up to 90	—	90 +	
Pyridoxine	4–6	Up to 80	—	80 +
(mcg/g	7–9	Up to 60	—	60 +
creatinine)	10–12	Up to 40	—	40 +
	13–15	Up to 30	—	30 +
	16 +	Up to 20	—	20 +
*Urinary	All ages	Up to 0.2	0.2–5.59	0.6 +
N'methyl	Pregnant	Up to 0.8	0.8–2.49	2.5 +
nicotinamide				
(mg/g				
creatinine)				
**Urinary	All ages	Up to 200	—	200 +
Pantothenic				
Acid (mcg)				
**Plasma	All ages	Up to 0.2	0.2–0.6	0.6 +
vitamin E				
(mg/dl)				
**Transaminase				
Index (ratio)				
+ EGOT	Adult	2.0 +	—	Up to 2.0
†EGPT	Adult	1.25	—	Up to 1.25

*Adapted from the Ten State Nutrition Survey
**Criteria may vary with different methodology
+ Erythrocyte Glutamic Oxalacetic Transaminase
†Erythrocyte Glutamic Pyruvic Transaminase

nutritional status.[59] Because of this controversy, the procedure requires further evaluation by additional investigators before any final recommendations can be made regarding the usefulness and validity of the test.

An oral vitamin C loading test has been used as a clinically more acceptable way of determining vitamin C sufficiency. In the vitamin C tolerance test, ascorbic acid is administered orally at 15 mg of ascorbic acid per kilogram of body weight, and the ascorbic acid level in the serum is determined three hours later, or urinary spill of ascorbic acid in the collected six-hour sample is determined.[60] A total urinary spill in the collected urine sample of less than 50 percent of the original oral load indicates vitamin C insufficiency.

One other test which has been used recently to correlate with clinical aspects of vitamin C chronic insufficiency is the leucocyte ascorbic acid test. This test is slightly more sophisticated and involves the determination of leucocyte ascorbic acid concentration.[61] Miller and colleagues have recently found that reduced leucocyte ascorbate is correlated with increased risk to coronary artery disease and may represent an important screening tool for vitamin status in this area.[62]

Absorption of the fat-soluble vitamins can be determined in part by the vitamin A loading test, which is accomplished by administering 1,000 IU of vitamin A per kilogram of body weight and then taking blood samples at one, two, and three hours and determining serum vitamin A levels. An enhancement of serum vitamin A over three hours less than 30 percent indicates a potential fat-soluble vitamin malabsorption syndrome.[63]

Lastly, the oral zinc tolerance test is a method that is used for assessing zinc adequacy. This test makes use of the fact that zinc is the central metal atom in the serum enzyme alkaline phosphatase, and as zinc status is compromised the activity of alkaline phosphatase is considerably reduced. In a patient suffering from the symptoms of zinc insufficiency, which may include impaired wound healing, retarded growth and development in youngsters, altered sense of taste or smell, dermatitis of various types, vitamin A nonresponsive night blindness, increased dental caries or reduced immune function, the fasting serum alkaline phosphatase level is determined. If in the adult it is 30 units per liter or less, an oral zinc challenge is given (30 mg of elemental zinc as the sulfate heptahydrate daily for three days). At the end of the third day the activity of alkaline phosphatase in the serum is once again determined. If the activity has more than doubled from the first baseline alkaline phosphatase activity prior to zinc supplementation, this confirms the zinc insufficiency.[64] It should be recalled that this test is only applicable to adults, due to the elevation of alkaline phosphatase in the serum samples of children, because of incomplete formation of the epiphyses of the bones.

The use of serum levels of various vitamins in assessing nutritional adequacy may prove of some use in the frank cases of nutritional deficiency, but it is of less than optimal value in monitoring chronic nutritional insufficiency which may be better assessed under the challenge or provocative testing protocol, or by utilizing erythrocyte enzyme levels, as previously discussed. These problems in nutritional assessment are nicely discussed by Sauberlich.[65]

The work of Pearson also discusses various uses of biochemical appraisal techniques in determining nutritional status and points to the importance of provocative or challenge tests in picking up chronic inadequacy.[66,67]

Determination of Serum Vitamin Levels

The serum vitamins and other essential nutrients have recently been more conveniently measured by using an assay technique developed by Baker *et al.*[68] This assay technique makes use of the fact that certain species of protozoa have distinctive nutritional requirements and thereby can be used as a tool for nutritional assessment. Protozoa such as *Ochromonas danica* have been shown to be thiamin and biotin dependent, whereas *Tetrahymena thermophilia* have been shown to be vitamin B-complex and amino acid dependent. These protozoa can then be grown on the serum of individuals whose vitamin status is to be assayed and by the growth characteristics and the use of control curves the level of vitamin or essential nutrient within the serum can be determined.[69] Again, it should be recalled that there may be cases in which the level of vitamin or nutrient within the serum assessed by this method may not directly relate to this biochemical use, because of changes in coenzyme binding efficiency, cellular transport or the presence of antagonists, and the provocative testing methods may prove more useful in picking up these chronic malutilization problems.

Assessment of Nutritional Trace Elements

The bulk of living matter consists of hydrogen, carbon, oxygen, nitrogen and sulfur, with other elements such as sodium, magnesium, phosphorus, chlorine, potassium and calcium being needed in reasonably high levels. An additional class of essential nutrients is made up of the essential trace elements, which are required by humans in amounts ranging from 50 mcg to 18 mg per day. These elements act as catalytic or structural components of larger molecules, such as proteins, and have specific functions that are indispensable for life. The search during the past twenty-five years has identified six essential trace elements whose functions were previously unknown as necessary for human function.[70]

In addition to the long-known deficiencies of iron and iodide, more recently, the deficiencies of chromium, copper, zinc and selenium have been identified in western populations. As Mertz points out, "Marginal or severe trace element imbalances can be considered risk factors for several diseases of public health importance."[71] Deficiency symptoms and biochemical functions of these trace elements are as shown in Table 4.4. Determining the

TABLE 4.4
Biochemical Functions and Manifestations of
Deficiency of Essential Trace Elements

Element	Site of Action	Key Biochemical Function	Signs of Deficiency
Chromium	Glucose toler-ance factor	Glucose metabo-lism mediates insulin effects on membrane	Impaired glucose tolerance
Cobalt	Coenzyme B_{12}	Biologic methylation	Pernicious anemia Methylmalonic aciduria
Copper	Metalloenzymes (ferroxidase, cytochrome oxidase, lysyl oxidase, tyro-sinase, etc.)	Mitochondria function Collagen metabolism Melanin formation	Menke's syn-drome, Anemia, leukopenia, neutropenia
Iodine	Tyroglobulin thyroxine	Cellular oxidation	Thyroid diseases
Manganese	Pyruvate carbox-ylase and many other enzymes	Oxidative phos-phorylation, Fatty acid me-tabolism, Muco-polysaccharide synthesis	Defective growth Reproductive dysfunction Collagen problems Central nervous system disorders
Molybdenum	Flavoenzymes (e.g., xanthine oxidase)	Xanthine hypoxanthine metabolism	Growth retardation Impaired urease clearance (chicks)
Selenium	Glutathione Peroxidase	Degration of intracellular peroxides	Liver necrosis (rats) "White muscle" disease (lambs)
Vanadium	Hemovanadin	Oxygen transport	Impaired bone and lipid metabolism
Zinc	Metalloenzymes (e.g., alcohol dehydro-genase, DNA polymerase)	Metabolism of lipids, carbo-hydrates and nucleic acids	Hypogonadism, poor wound healing Uremic impotence

sufficiency of these elements is a difficult job clinically. Symptoms, along with biochemical information, may be very helpful. Serum, urine, salivary and hair mineral levels have all been utilized in recognition of essential trace element insufficiencies. Erythrocyte and hair element levels have been used for suggested intracellular information concerning element status, whereas serum, urine and salivary levels have a stronger relationship to extracellular levels of the respective element.

Hair trace element levels were first used to assess potential excess body burden of the toxic minerals, such as lead, cadmium and arsenic. Kopito showed that hair lead levels in children were useful for screening for chronic lead exposure before the symptoms of acute lead toxicity developed.[72] More recently, hair has been suggested as a useful screening tool for picking up essential mineral status, and may be a useful adjunct screening tool for trace mineral nutriture or metabolic imbalances.

Hair trace elements which are now recognized to have potential clinical importance in screening for trace mineral metabolic disturbances in humans include: zinc, chromium, copper, selenium and to a lesser degree calcium and magnesium.[74] Strain was one of the first investigators to point out that low hair zinc levels, less than 110 parts per million, are suggestive of zinc deficiency in humans.[75] Klevay has confirmed that hair zinc may be a useful indicator of metabolic problems encountered with either dietary zinc insufficiency or the unavailability of physiologically active zinc in pivotal tissues.[76]

Recently, a case was reported of a seventeen-year-old man who had suffered a traumatized head injury and after hospitalization had developed a decubitus ulcer, eczema and low immune status.[77] Hair samples indicated levels of zinc in excess of 360 parts per million (normal range 160 to 260 ppm) and upon oral zinc supplementation his hair zinc over the course of the next eight weeks returned to normal range and his immune challenge index returned to normal with clearance of his eczema and healing of his decubitus ulcer. The explanation for an elevated hair zinc being associated with tissue zinc insufficiency is that zinc is a pivotal trace element in controlling protein synthesis and hair is a rapidly growing protein; therefore, in low zinc status situations hair protein is being synthesized more slowly and the hair stays in the follicle for a longer period of time saturating with the low serum zinc and producing an elevated hair zinc concentration. After administration of oral zinc, protein synthesis is increased, leading to less time in residence in the follicle and less saturation with zinc, producing a normal hair zinc level. The conclusion of this work is that both elevated hair zinc and reduced hair zinc may be associated with zinc insufficiency and need should be confirmed by additional laboratory testing.

The usefulness of hair trace element analysis is as a screening, not a diagnostic tool. The technique is not significantly refined at this point to justify its use in diagnosis of any essential trace element or toxic element imbalance, but is a very convenient, reasonably inexpensive screening tool for looking at mineral imbalances and then confirming the presence of such imbalances by additional accepted diagnostic tests.

Bergmann has recently found that mothers who give birth to infants with spina bifida cystica have statistically higher hair zinc levels than women who give rise to normal-birth children. They speculate that the differences in zinc indicate an abnormality of zinc availability and metabolism in the mothers of infants with spina bifida.[78]

Hambidge *et al* have found that the concentration of chromium in the hair is lower in children with juvenile diabetes mellitus than in control children.[79] These investigators have also found that the chromium levels of multiparous women are lower than those of parous women.[80] These observations were recently confirmed by Saner, who looked at the effect of parity on maternal hair chromium concentration and the changes in chromium levels during pregnancy. He concluded that hair chromium in multiparous women is lower than that of nulliparous women, and depending upon chromium nutrition, hair chromium of pregnant women shows a decrease with advancing pregnancy; however, the women who were on a higher intake during pregnancy showed less decrease in hair chromium during the pregnancy. Lastly, from these studies he points out that if adequate amounts of chromium are not taken during pregnancy, deficiency may result with increasing parity, and this may be recognized by changes in hair chromium levels as a screening tool.[81] Chromium has importance in human metabolism as the central element in glucose tolerance factor, which is stored in the liver and secreted upon an oral glucose load of either starch or sugar and facilitates the tissue sensitivity to insulin in the cellular uptake of glucose.[82] Chromium has been shown when administered orally to improve carbohydrate metabolism in infants, presumably through the improvement of glucose tolerance factor status.[83]

Selenium deficiency was first recognized to be coincident with Keshan disease, seen in China as a cardiomyopathy in children. Recently, the first Occidental cases in the United States of selenium deficiency have been illustrated in children who have hepatosplenomegaly, cardiomyopathy and wasting disease.[84] In screening the children with Keshan disease, no child with the disease was found to have hair selenium greater than 0.12 parts per million, with a normal range in human hair from 0.2 to 15 ppm.[85]

Lastly, hair copper has been suggested to be indicative of liver copper stores.[86] This assertion has been challenged by the work of Epstein *et al*, and Bradfield and coworkers.[87,88] The work of Deming and Weber and Porter does seem to show a relationship between low hair copper and altered copper metabolism.[90,91] At this point, the significance of hair copper in assessing copper metabolism demands further investigation to clarify these discrepancies.

The advantage of hair element testing over other methods of trace element assessment is that hair is reasonably easy to procure, is biologically stable, can be analyzed relatively easily with concentrations of the elements 5- to 10-fold higher than in other tissues or fluids, and provides a running record in the first inch and a half of growth from the scalp as to what the patient's past three months' metabolic status with regard to that element is. Recently, it was found that a woman who had given birth to a child with birth defects very similar to those found in animals held on zinc-deprived diets during the first trimester after conception had hair zinc levels that were extremely low coincident with that time in her pregnancy. In detailing her history, it was found that during the first three weeks after conception she had been on a very primitive diet, which was very low in zinc, and that this zinc deprivation at a time during the first few weeks of her pregnancy, before she knew of her pregnancy, may have contributed to a fetal compromise.[92]

Newer methods of trace element assessment are becoming available, which should allow for better recognition of these nutritionally related problems. Recently, salivary sediment zinc has been found to be very useful in confirming zinc deficiency.[93]

Urinary and serum levels of several of the trace elements are also useful in assessing mineral status, although serum tends to be one of the last fluids to change concentration during a short term deficiency state and may provide marginal usefulness in picking up chronic short term deficiency states.[94]

The direction of the field in assessing trace element status is going more toward the use of provocative testing such as the oral zinc challenge test which examines the physiological activity of the specific enzymes which require a trace element for activity, and also intracellular assessment tools such as erythrocyte trace element level determination. As these tools become more widely available and better understood, it should allow for the recognition of many trace element chronic deficiency symptoms which are now not being recognized.

Additional Biochemical Tests
for Recognizing Nutritional Inadequacy

The importance of serological parameters and complete blood count with differential for screening for chronic nutritional inadequacy has received increased attention recently. A comprehensive series of articles was published in *The Lancet* in 1974, detailing various serological screening tests for subsequent disease and the benefits and liabilities of using these, the available standard chemistries, for determining relative risk to disease.[95,96,97,98,99,100]

These articles pointed out that the risk to nutritionally related diseases such as cardiovascular disease, anemia, diabetes and inherited metabolic diseases may be in part evaluated by the use of specific serum analyte testing. The use of the blood urea nitrogen-to-creatinine ratio coupled with serum total protein, albumin-to-globulin ratio allows exploration of dietary protein sufficiencies. Elevation of the BUN-to-creatinine ratio (> 20 to 1) has been found to be an indication of excessive dietary protein, whereas a reduced BUN-to-creatinine ratio (< 20 to 1) is generally related to dietary protein insufficiency in the absence of frank organicity. Reduced albumin-to-globulin ratios with lowered total protein are highly indicative of protein/calorie or protein malnutrition. In the same spirit the serum cholesterol/triglyceride/high density lipoprotein cholesterol levels can be used to monitor an individual's lipid metabolism and its relationship to the diet. Elevation of total serum cholesterol with a reduced HDL, so that the cholesterol-to-HDL ratio increases above 5 to 1, is statistically correlated with increased risk to cardiovascular disease. A lowered cholesterol-to-HDL ratio, on the order of 3 to 1, has been statistically demonstrated to be associated with half the risk of the average population to coronary heart disease. Elevated triglycerides in the absence of elevated cholesterol may be a result of sucrose sensitivity with the individual consuming excessive dietary sucrose.[101]

Elevated glycohemoglobin (glycosylated hemoglobin) with reduced high density lipoprotein cholesterol is associated with increased risk to maturity-onset diabetes and arteriosclerotic disease.[102] Elevated serum uric acid levels have been identified to be associated with a diet high in purines found commonly in rich foods such as cheese, sardines, yeast and shellfish. Elevated ionized serum calcium levels have been associated with nutritionally induced secondary hyperparathyroidism and may indicate a dietary calcium/phosphorus imbalance, due to the ingestion of a low-calcium, high-phosphorus laden diet. This condition encourages bone resorption and soft tissue calcification and can be reviewed through the use of ionized (or ultrafiltrable) serum calcium.

In the complete blood count, a rise in mean corpuscular volume may indicate an early warning of risk to vitamin B_{12} and folic acid insufficiencies and has been demonstrated as a useful screening tool for this condition.[103] Elevated eosinophils have been identified to be useful as a screening tool for potential food allergy, although it is recognized that some foods may produce hypersensitivity in biochemically disposed individuals.[104] Salivary immunoglobulins have also been identified recently as being useful as screening tools for specific nutrient insufficiencies that are related to immune B cell activation, such as vitamin C, and this may open a whole new area of nutritional assessment, as more information is gained.[105] Elevated fibrinogen concentrations have been suggested as a risk factor to cardiovascular disease,[106] and elevated leucocyte counts have been associated with increased risk to myocardial infarction.[107]

Food allergy has also recently been examined by looking at IgE specific antibodies in serum and a specific food-related antigen. The radioallergosorbent procedure has been developed to screen for various specific food families, which the patient may be allergic to, by an *in vitro* serum blood test.[108]

Lastly, malabsorption syndrome, as it relates to either hypochlorhydria or pancreatic insufficiency, can be evaluated by a pH sensitive telemetering capsule technique,[109,110] or by examining the urinary excretion of indoxyl sulfate (indican), a product of maldigestion and malabsorption of dietary tryptophan.[111]

These miscellaneous nutritionally related screening tests are as summarized in Table 4.5.

Integration for a Prognostic Profile

During the first half of this century the health and average life span of Americans have improved considerably. Epidemics of infectious diseases have ceased to be a serious threat, and acute nutritional diseases have been reduced. More recently, however, the increasing age of the population and certain life-style habits have brought about increasing rates of chronic illnesses. Evidence accumulated during the last twenty years indicates that the most important of modern diseases are caused by a variety of factors,

TABLE 4.5
Additional Biochemical Tests
for Recognizing Nutritional Inadequacy

Complete Blood Count with Differential

elevated mean corpuscular volume	deficiency of folic acid or vitamin B_{12}
elevated eosinophils	potential food allergies
elevated leucocytes	increased risk to myocardial infarction (particularly in smokers)

Serum Analysis
BUN/creatinine ratio

above 20:1	dietary protein excess
below 8:1	dietary protein deficiency

albumin/globulin ratio

elevated	immune insufficiency—zinc, vitamin C, selenium deficiency
reduced	protein-calorie malnutrition infection

cholesterol/HDL ratio

5:1	"normal" risk to heart disease
8:1 to 11:1	twice the normal risk
<3:1	one-half the normal risk

triglycerides

elevated	sucrose sensitivity
glycohemoglobin (> 8%)	carbohydrate intolerance
uric acid elevation	sensitivity to "rich" foods vascular disease essential fatty acid need
IgE antibody elevation	potential food allergy

Heidelberg gastrogram

positive test	hypochlorhydria with malabsorption

Urinary Indoxyl Sulfate (indican)

positive test	malabsorption of dietary protein

Oral Loading Tests

tryptophan	B_6 sufficiency
ascorbic acid	vitamin C saturation
vitamin A	pancreatic sufficiency (fat absorption)
zinc tolerance test	zinc status *in vivo*

most significantly by reckless personal social habits, such as improper diet, excessive drinking, smoking, drug abuse, lack of exercise, unsafe driving and working conditions, and inadvertent and deliberate environmental pollution.[112] Given this, the urgency is upon health practitioners in an ever-increasing way to develop better ways of evaluating patients' health status prognostically and implementing effective behavior modification programs to reduce the risk to subsequent disease. This urgency has led to the development of many new screening tools for the assessment of nutritional status; however, one should not jump to the conclusion that just because a test is new it is necessarily cost/efficient and gives useful information. Recently, serum ferritin and transferrin saturation have been used to screen for anemias, which were presumably not being recognized by other screening tests. Hershko *et al* have recently suggested however, that reduced serum ferritin and transferrin saturation had less predictive value than the traditional, less expensive test of mean corpuscular hemoglobin and serum hemoglobin.[113] There is a very subtle balance to be maintained between improvement in chronic nutritional screening tools and overuse of laboratory testing at the expense of the health-care system. The direction in the field of nutritional assessment is to develop better early warning precursor markers to subsequent disease by employing provocative or challenge methods of testing which will expose deficiencies in organ reserves. Intracellular measurements of nutrient utilization rather than extracellular measurements of nutrient concentration will be used more in the future with emphasis on functional capacity. There is still a considerable amount of uncertainty about what is the most efficacious screening profile to establish nutritional status, but it can be said with surety that an integrated approach which focuses on prognostic rather than diagnostic functions, utilizing anthropometric, biochemical and dietary data will best result in a comprehensive and successful evaluation program. The use of this profile not only should be helpful in recognizing individual biochemical differences from patient to patient that need specific nutritional management, but also should help as a behavior modification tool to motivate patients to life-style changes in their best health interest.

Continued questions about the cost/benefit ratio of evaluating patients for nutritional status will be aired, as this newly developing field receives more attention. It is difficult at times to evaluate, in the absence of long-term statistical data, the success that a preventive nutritional program has in improving the cost/efficiency of the health-care dollar. Questions such as, "What is the success of improved nutrition in reducing the likelihood of an expensive surgical procedure like coronary bypass surgery?" are still the focus of many of the critics of nutritional and life-style modification therapies. The most common statement, "Even if we could identify what patients are at risk to specific nutritionally related problems, we could not motivate them to change," is a self-fulfilling prophecy that prevents effective management and effective delivery of preventive nutrition programs. It is hard to know what has been prevented when the patient is or was not diseased.

The good effect that would follow a commitment to a preventive focused program to the same extent as we have committed ourselves to high technology medical intervention through improved public education, professional commitment in education, and integrated approaches towards behavior modification has yet to prove unequivocally its efficacy. The first step along this road of acceptance is to develop a successful nutritional screening profile, framed in the spirit of recognizing biochemical individuality, and that will identify those people who are at highest risk to the various forms of nutritional inadequacy associated with the malnutrition of overconsumption/undernutrition. As Kirstein, Arnold, and Wynder point out, "In view of the epidemiologic research indicating that the incidence of cardiovascular disease, many cancers, and other chronic diseases may be significantly reduced through preventive care, the potential social and economic benefits to be realized through preventive medicine seem staggering. While there is much yet to learn about preventive intervention, putting into effect what is currently known would provide substantial social benefits."[114]

REFERENCES

1. Sauberlich, H.E., Dowdy, R.P. and Skala, J.H. 1974. *Laboratory Test for Assessment of Nutritional Status*. Cleveland, OH: CRC Press.
2. Guthrie, H.A. and Guthrie, G.M., 1976. Factor analysis of nutritional status data from ten state nutritional surveys. *Am. J. Clin. Nutr.* 29: 1238.
3. Jensen, T. and Dudrick, S.J. 1981. Implementation of a multidisciplinary nutritional assessment program. *J. Am. Dietetic Assoc.* 79: 258.
4. Swets, J.A., Pickett, R.M., Whitehead, S.F., Getty, D.J., Schnur, J.A. and Freeman, B.A. 1979. Assessment of diagnostic technologies. *Science*, 205: 753.
5. North, A.F. 1977. Current status and future role of health screening. *South. Med. J.*, 70: 1232.

6. Rose, G. and Barker, D.J.P. 1978. Screening. *Br. Med. J.* 2:1417.
7. Kaminski, M.V. and Winborn, A.L. 1978. *Nutritional Assessment Guide*. Midwest Nutrition Education and Research Foundation.
8. Clark, D.G. and Sigman, R. 1979. A simple form for nutritional evaluation. *J. Proc. Clin. Nutr.* 3: 157.
9. Wright, R. 1980. Nutritional assessment. *J. Am. Med. Assoc.* 244: 559.
10. Kovach, K.M. and Huerta, E. 1981. Nutritional assessment: a commentary. *J. Am. Med. Assoc.* 245: 1911.
11. Habicht, J.P. 1980. Some characteristics of indicators of nutritional status for screening and surveillance. *Am. J. Clin. Nutr.* 33: 531.
12. *Report on Methodology of Nutritional Surveillance*. 1976. Joint FAO/UNICEF/WHO Expert Committee. WHO Tech. Report Series no. 593.
13. Habicht, J.P. and McDowell, A.J. 1978. National nutrition surveillance. *Federation Proc.* 37: 1181.
14. Rogan, W.J. and Gluden, B. 1978. Estimating prevalence from the results of a screening test. *Am. J. Epidemiol.* 107: 71.
15. Tillotson, J.S., Gordon, D. and Kassim, N. 1981. Nutrient data collection in the multiple risk factor intervention trial. *J. Am. Dietetic Assoc.* 78: 235.
16. Farrand, M.E. and Mojonnier, L. 1980. Nutrition in the multiple risk factor intervention trial: background. *J. Am. Dietetic Assoc.* 76: 347.
17. Christakis, G. 1981. Adult nutritional diagnosis. In *Nutrition and Medical Practice*. L. Barness, ed. Westport, CT: AVI Publishing.
18. Young, C.M., Chalmers, F.W., Chruch, H.N., Clayton, M.M., Tucker, R.E., and Foster, W.D. 1952. A comparison of dietary study methods. Dietary history vs. seven-day record. *J. Am. Dietetic Assoc.* 28: 124.
19. Young, C.M., Hagan, G.G. and Foster, W.D. 1952. A comparison of dietary study methods. Dietary history vs. seven-day record vs. 24-hour recall. *J. Am. Dietetic Assoc.* 28: 218.
20. Witschi, J., Kowaloff, H., Bloom, S. and Slack, W. 1981. Analysis of dietary data: An interactive computer method for storage and retrieval. *J. Am. Dietetic Assoc.* 78: 609.
21. Widdowson, E. M. and McCance, R.A. 1943. Food tables. Their scope and limitations. *Lancet* 1: 230.
22. Bransby, E.R., Daubney, C.G. and King, J. 1948. Comparison of nutrient values of individual diets found by calculation from food tables and by chemical analysis. *Br. J. Nutr.* 2: 232.
23. Groover, M.E., Boone, L. and Wolf, S. 1967. Problems in quantitation of diet surveys. *J. Am. Med. Assoc.* 201: 8.
24. Pekkarinen, M. 1967. Chemical analysis in connection with dietary surveys in Finland. *Voeding* 28: 1.
25. Hertzler, A.A. and Hoover, L.W. 1977. Development of food tables and use with computers. *J. Am. Dietetic Assoc.* 70: 20.
26. Reeves, J.B. and Weinraunch, J.L. 1979. Composition of foods: fats and oils—Raw, processed, prepared. *Rev. USDA Agric. Handbook* no. 8-4.
27. Agric. Research Service 1977. Nutrition value of foods. *Rev. USDA Home and Garden Bull.* no. 72.
28. Hunscher, H.A. and Macy, I.G. 1951. Dietary study methods. Uses and abuses of dietary study methods. *J. Am. Dietetic Assoc.* 27: 558.

29. Guthrie, H.A. and Scheer, J.G. 1981. Validity of a dietary score for assessing nutrient adequacy. *J. Am. Dietetic Assoc.* 78: 240.
30. Beaton, G.H., Milner, J., Corey, P. and Little, J.A. 1979. Sources of variance on 24-hour dietary recall data: Implications for nutrition study design and interpretation. *Am. J. Clin. Nutr.* 32: 2546.
31. Hines, J.H. and Roche, A.F. 1980. Fat areas as estimates of body fat. *Am. J. Clin. Nutr.* 33: 2093.
32. Franklin, B.A., Buskirk, E.R. and Mendez, J., 1970. Validity of skinfold predictive equations on lean and obese subjects. *Am. J. Clin. Nutr.* 23: 267.
33. Keys, A. 1980. "Overweight, obesity, coronary heart disease and mortality." *Nutr. Reviews,* 38: 297.
34. Keys, A. 1980. *Seven Countries: A Multivariate Analysis of Death and Coronary Heart Disease.* Cambridge, MA: Harvard University Press.
35. Astrand, R. and Rhyming, K. June, 1967. A simple test for determining aerobic fitness level. *J. Exercise Physiology,* pp. 1213-1216.
36. Davis, D. and Williams, R.J. 1976. Potentially useful criteria for judging nutritional adequacy. *Am. J. Clin. Nutr.* 29: 710.
37. Fries, J.F. 1980. Aging, natural death, and the compression of morbidity. *N. Engl. J. Medicine* 303: 130.
38. Strehler, B.L. and Mildvan, A.S. 1960. General theory of mortality and aging. *Science* 132: 14.
39. Farquhar, J.W. 1978. *The American Way of Life Need Not Be Hazardous to Your Health.* New York: W.W. Norton.
40. Kemp, G.L. 1972. Value of treadmill stress testing in variant angina pectoris. *Am. J. Card.* 30: 752.
41. Williams, R.J., Beerstecher, E., Jr. and Berry, L.G. 1950. The concept of genetotrophic disease. *Lancet* 287.
42. *Brain Dysfunction in Metabolic Disorders,* M. Plum, ed. 1974. vol. 53. New York: Raven Press.
43. Harrell, R.F., Capp, R.H., Davis, D.R., Peerless, J. and Ravitz, L.R. 1981. Can nutritional supplements help mentally retarded children? An exploratory study. *Proc. Natl. Acad. Sci. U.S.A.* 78: 574.
44. Baker, H.O., Frank, S., Feingold. S., Christakis, G. and Ziffer, H. 1967. Vitamins, total cholesterol and triglycerides in 642 New York City school children. *Am. J. Clin. Nutr.* 20: 850.
45. Lonsdale, D. and Shamberger, R.J. 1980. Red cell transketolase as an indicator of nutritional deficiency. *Am. J. Clin. Nutr.* 33: 205.
46. Wolfe, S.J., Brin, M. and Davidson, C.S. 1958. The effect of thiamine deficiency on human erythrocyte metabolism. *J. Clin Invest.* 37: 1476.
47. Brin, M. 1962. Erythrocyte transketolase in early thiamine deficiency. *Ann. N.Y. Acad. Sci.* 98: 528.
48. Bayoumi, R.A. and Rosalki, S.B. 1976. Evaluation of methods of coenzyme activation of erythrocyte enzymes of detection of deficiency of vitamins B_1, B_2 and B_6. *Clinical Chemistry* 22: 327.
49. Blass, J.P. and Gibson, G.E. 1977. Abnormality of a thiamin-requiring enzyme in patients with Wernicke-Korsakoff syndrome. *N. Engl. J. Medicine* 297: 1367.
50. Anderson, B.B., Perry, G.M. Modell, G.B. and Mollin, D.L. 1979. Abnormal red cell metabolism of pyridoxine with thalassemia. *Br. J. Haematol.* 41: 497.

51. Clements, J.E. and Anderson, B.B. 1980. Glutathione reductase activity and pyridoxine phosphate oxidase activity in the red cell. *Biochim. Biophys. Acta* 632: 159.
52. Bamji, M.S. and Radharah, G. 1979. Relationship between biochemical and clinical indices of B-vitamin deficiency. A study in rural school boys. *British J. Nutr.* 41: 431.
53. Miller, L.T. and Linkswiler, H. 1967. Effect of protein intake on the development of abnormal tryptophan metabolism by men during B_6 depletion. *J. Nutr.* 93: 53.
   Folkers, K., Ellis, J., Watanabe, T. and Kaji, M. 1978. Biochemical evidence for deficiency of vitamin B_6 in the carpal tunnel syndrome based on a crossover clinical study. *Proc. Natl. Acad. Sci.* 75: 3410.
54. Yess, N., Price, J.M. and Linkswiler, H. Vitamin B_6 depletion in man: urinary excretion of tryptophan metabolites. *J. Nutr.* 84: 229.
   Hoorn, R.K.J. and Westernik, D. 1975. Vitamin B_1, B_2 and B_6 deficiencies in geriatric patients measured by coenzyme stimulation of enzyme activities. *Clini. Chem. Acta* 61: 151.
55. Canham, J.E., Baker, E.M., Sauberlich, H.E. and Plough, I.C. 1969. Dietary protein—its relationship to vitamin B_6. *Ann. N.Y. Acad. Sci.* 166: 16.
   Rose, D.P., Strong R., Folkand, J. and Adams, P.W. 1973. Erythrocyte aminotransferase activities in women using oral contraceptives and the effect of vitamin B_6 supplementation. *Am. J. Clin. Nutr.* 26: 48.
56. Sauberlich, H.E., Canham, J.E., Baker, E.M. and Herman, Y.F. 1970. Human vitamin B_6 nutriture. *J. Sci. Ind. Res.* 29: 528.
   Kim, Y.J. and Rosenberg, L.E. 1974. On the mechanism of pyridoxine-responsive homocystinuria. *Proc. Natl. Acad. Sciences* 71: 4821.
57. Giza, T and Weclawowiez, J. 1910. Perlingual method for evaluating the vitamin C content of the body. *J. Vit. Res.* 30: 327.
   Pyridoxine-responsive homocytinuria. 1981. *Nutr. Reviews* 39: 16.
58. Ringsdorf, W.M. and Cheraskin, E. 1962. A rapid and simple lingual test for ascorbic acid. *General Practice* 25: 106.
59. King, D.R. and Little, J.W. 1970. Lingual ascorbic acid test. *J. Oral Med.* 25: 107.
60. Dutra de Oliverta, J.E. and Darby, W.J. 1959. Clinical usefulness of the oral ascorbic acid tolerance test in scurvy. *Am. J. Clin. Nutr.* 7: 630.
61. Loh, H.S. and Wilson C.W. 1971. An improved method for the measurement of leucocyte ascorbic acid concentrations. *Int. J. Vit. Nutr. Res.* 41: 90.
62. Ramirez, J. and Flowers, N. 1980. Leukocyte ascorbic acid and its relationship to coronary artery disease in man. *Am. J. Clin. Nutr.* 33: 2079.
63. Kahan, J. 1969. The vitamin A absorption test: Studies on humans without disorders in the alimentary tract. *Scand. J. Gastroent.* 4: 313.
64. Sullivan, J.F., Jetton, M.M. and Burch, R.E. 1979. A zinc tolerance test. *J. Lab. Clin. Med.* 93: 485.
65. Sauberlich, H.E. 1971. Problems of assessment of nutritional states: an overview of biochemical methodologies. In *Problems of Assessment and Alleviation of Malnutrition in the U.S.* Hansen, R.G. and Munro, H.N., eds. Washington, D.C.: U.S. Govt. Printing Office, Pub. no. 916.086.

66. Pearson, W.N. 1962. Biochemical appraisal of vitamin nutritional status in man. *J. Am. Med. Assoc.* 180: 49.
67. Pearson, W.N. 1966. Assessment of nutritional status: biochemical methods. In *Nutrition, A Comprehensive Treatise, vol. III*. Beaton, G.H. and McHenry, E.W., eds. New York: Academic Press.
68. Baker, H. and Frank, O. 1968. *Clinical Vitaminology: Methods and Interpretation*. New York: John Wiley.
69. Hutner, S.H., Bacchi, C.J., Shapiro, A. and Baker, H. 1980. Protozoa as tolls for nutrition research. *Nutrition Reviews* 38: 361.
70. Mertz, W. 1981. The Essential Trace Elements. *Science* 213: 1332.
71. Mertz, W. 1970. The Essential Trace Elements. *Fed. Proc.* 29: 1482.
72. Kopito, L. and Schwachman, H. 1967. Hair lead in the hair of children with chronic lead exposure. *N. Engl. J. Medicine* 276: 949.
73. Maugh, T. 1978. Hair: A diagnostic tool to complement blood, serum, and urine. *Science* 202: 1271.
74. Bland, J. 1981. Trace element nutrition in *Contemporary Developments in Nutrition*. Worthington-Roberts, B., ed. St. Louis: Mosby.
75. Strain, W.H., Steadman, L.T. and Lankau, C.A. 1967. Analysis of zinc levels in hair for the diagnosis of zinc deficiency in man. *J. Lab. Clin. Med.* 68: 244.
76. Klevay, L.M. 1978. Hair as a biopsy material. *Arch. Intern. Medicine* 138: 1127.
77. Pekarek, R.S., Sandstead, H.H., Jacob, R.A. and Barcome, D.F. 1979. Abnormal cellular immune response during acquired zinc deficiency. *Am. J. Clin. Nutr.* 32: 1466.
78. Bermann, K.E., Makosh, G. and Tews, K.H. 1980. Abnormalities of hair zinc concentration in mothers of newborn infants with *spina bifida*. *Am. J. Clin. Nutr.* 33: 2145.
79. Hambidge, K.M., Canab, B.C. and Rodgerson, D. 1969. Concentration of chromium in the hair of normal children and children with juvenile diabetes mellitus. *Diabetes* 17: 517.
80. Hambidge, K.M. and Rodgerson, D.O. 1969. Comparison of hair chromium levels of multiparous and nulliparous women. *Am. J. Obstet. Gynecol.* 103: 320
81. Saner, G. 1981. The effect of parity on maternal hair chromium concentration and the changes during pregnancy. *Am. J. Clin. Nutr.* 34: 853.
82. Mertz, W. 1969. Chromium occurrence and function in biological systems. *Physiol. Rev.* 49: 163.
83. Hopkins, L.L., Ransome-Kuti, O. and Majaj, A.A. 1968. Improvement of impaired carbohydrate metabolism by chromium (III) in malnourished infants. *Am. J. Clin. Nutr.* 21: 203.
84. Collipp, P.J. and Chen, S.Y. 1981. Cardiomyopathy and selenium deficiency in a two-year-old girl. *N. Engl. J. Medicine* 304: 1304.
85. Chan, F.I. June, 1979. Selenium deficiency and Keshan disease. *Chinese J. Medicine*, pp. 107–109.
86. McKenzie, J.M. 1978. Alteration of zinc and copper concentration of hair. *Am. J. Clin. Nutr.* 31: 470.
87. Jacob, R.A., Klevay, L.M. and Logan, G.M. 1969. Hair as an index of hepatic metal in rats: copper and zinc. *Am. J. Clin. Nutr.* 31: 477.
88. Epstein, O., Boxx, M.B., Lyon, D. and Sherlock, S. 1980. Hair copper in primary biliary cirrhosis. *Am. J. Clin. Nutr.* 33: 965.
89. Bradfield, R.B. and Soohoo, T. 1960. Effect of hypochromotricihia on hair and zinc during kwashiokor. *Am. J. Clin. Nutr.* 33: 1315.

90. Deeming, S.B. and Weber, C.W. Hair analysis of trace minerals in human subjects as influenced by age, sex and contraceptive drugs. *Am. J. Clin. Nutr.* 31: 1175.
91. Porter, K.G., Munier, D.M. and Hemes, M.L. October 8, 1977. Anemia and low serum copper during therapy. *Lancet*, p. 774.
92. Hurley, L. 1981. Privileged communication. Univ. Calif./Davis.
93. Freeland-Graves, J.H. and Hendrikson, J.H. 1980. Alterations in zinc absorption and salivary sediment zinc after a lacto-ovo-vegetarian diet. *Am. J. Clin. Nutr.* 33: 1757.
94. Dulka, J.J. and Risby, T.H. 1976. Ultratrace minerals in some environmental and biological systems. *Anal. Chem.* 48: 643.
95. Whithy, L.G. 1974. Screening for disease: Definitions and criteria. *Lancet* 2: 819.
96. Sackett, D.L. 1974. Screening for disease: Cardiovascular diseases. *Lancet* 2: 1364.
97. Elwood, P.C. 1974. Screening for disease: Anemia. *Lancet* 2: 1364.
98. Malius, J.M. 1974. Screening for disease: Diabetes. *Lancet* 2: 1367.
99. Knox, E.G. 1974. Screening for disease: Multiphasic screening. *Lancet* 2: 1434.
100. Bailey, A. 1974. Screening for disease: Biochemistry for well populations. *Lancet* 2: 1434.
101. MacDonald, I., Keyser, A. and Pacy, D. 1978. Some effects in man of varying loads of glucose, sucrose and fructose on various metabolites in the blood. *Am. J. Clin. Nutr.* 31: 1305.
102. Calvert, G.D., Graham, J.J., Mannik, T., Wise, P.H. and Yeats, R.A. July 1978. High density lipoprotein cholesterol and glycohemoglobin A_1 in the diabetic. *Lancet*, p. 68.
103. Markington, D. 1980. Early rise of mean corpuscular volume and vitamin B_{12} status. *J. Am. Medical Assoc.* 245: 1110.
104. Butterworth, A.E. and David, J.R. 1981. Eosinophil function. *N. Engl. J. Medicine* 304: 154.
105. Anderson, R. and Van Wyk, H. 1981. The effect of ascorbate ingestion on levels of salivary IgA in adult volunteers. *Am. J. Clin. Nutr.* 34: 6.
106. Meade, T.W., Chakrabarti, R. and Brozovic, M. 1980. Haemostatic function in cardiovascular beds: early results of a prospective study. *Lancet* 1: 1050.
107. Zalokar, J.B., Richard, J.L. and Claude, J.R. 1981. Leukocyte count, smoking and myocardial infarction. *N. Engl. J. Medicine* 304: 465.
108. Stiehm, E.R. and Fundenberg, H.H. 1966. Serum levels of immune globulins in health and disease: a survey. *Pediatrics* 37: 715.
109. Stavney, L.S., Hamilton, T., Sircus, W. and Smith, A.N. 1969. Evaluation of the pH-sensitive telemetering capsule in the estimation of gastric secretory capacity. *Am. J. Digest. Disease* 10: 753.
110. Yarbourgh, D.R., McAlhany, J.C. and Weidner, M.G., Jr. 1969. Evaluation of the Heidelberg pH capsule. *Am. J. Surgery* 117: 185.
111. Bryan, G.T. 1966. Urinary excretion of indoxyl sulfate (indican) by human subjects ingesting a diet containing variable quantities of L-tryptophan. *Am. J. Clin. Nutr.* 19: 113.
112. Gori, G.B. and Richter, B.J. 1978. Macroeconomics of disease prevention in the United States. *Science*, 200: 1124.
113. Hershko, C., Bar-Or, D., Gaziel, Y. and Isak, G. 1981. Diagnosis of iron deficiency anemia in a rural population of children. Relative

usefulness of serum ferritin, red cell protoporphyrin, red cell indices, and transferrin saturation. *Am. J. Clin. Nutr.* 39: 1600.

114. Kristein, M., Arnold, C.B. and Wynder, E. Health economics and preventive care. *Science* 195: 457.

PART III

PREVENTIVE AND
THERAPEUTIC NUTRITION

5

WEIGHT MANAGEMENT: DIET AND EXERCISE

————————◄●►————————

WILLIAM D. MCARDLE, PH.D.
AND JOHN R. MAGEL, PH.D.

The Problem

OBESITY is a condition characterized by an excess accumulation of body fat. While the standard for obesity is often established as a percentage of body *weight* above some ideal weight-for-height, the criterion for obesity is always in relation to excessive fatness. Among Americans, an estimated 60 to 70 million adults and at least 10 million teenagers are overfat by a total of 2.3 billion pounds.[1,2] This excess fat represents an energy equivalent of 5.7 trillion kcal, or the potential energy in 1.3 billion gallons of gasoline. This is sufficient energy to power 900,000 automobiles per year or provide the total annual electrical needs of Boston, Chicago, San Francisco and Washington, D.C.[2]

The genesis of obesity may begin in early childhood[3] or develop slowly in adulthood.[4] Middle-aged men and women invariably weigh more than their college-aged adult counterparts of the same height.[5] In the western world, the average thirty-five-year old male gains between 0.2 and 0.8 kg of fat each year until the sixth decade of life.[6] The fat content of twenty-seven adult men increased an average of 6.5 kg over a twelve-year period, from age thirty-two to forty-four. This was equal to the group's total gain in body weight over the duration of the study.[7] Only four of the twenty-seven men did not gain weight. The extent to which gains in body fat during adulthood represent a normal biological pattern is unknown. However, observations of older individuals maintaining very active lifestyles suggest that this pattern can be attenuated significantly.[8]

The overfat condition is the result of an imbalance between

caloric intake and caloric expenditure. Until recently, the major cause for weight gain was believed to be simply a problem of overeating. If this were true, the easiest way to reduce body fat would be to decrease food intake. However, it is not that simple. The treatment procedures devised so far, be they dietary, surgical, drug or behavioral, either alone or in combination, have not been particularly successful in controlling obesity on a long-term basis.

The scientific literature dealing with weight loss in obese patients reveals that initial success in weight loss bears little relation to prolonged control of body size and shape, and nearly 90 percent of dieters soon regain lost pounds. In a ten-year follow-up of participants in weight control programs using careful dietary restriction, the drop-out rate varied from 20 to 80 percent.[9] Of those who remained in the program, no more than 25 percent lost as much as twenty pounds, and only 5 percent lost forty pounds or more. Clearly, the causes for excessive energy storage in humans are numerous, complex, and often overlapping. The problem is intimately related to genetic, environmental, psychological and social factors. Recent research also suggests that individual differences in specific factors such as eating patterns, body image, resting metabolic rate, basal body temperature, hypothalamic control, levels of cellular adenosine triphosphatase and other enzymes and brown fat may predispose a person to excessive fat gain. It is also becoming increasingly clear that the lack of adequate energy expenditure in daily physical activity is an important predisposing factor of obesity. In this regard, regular vigorous exercise, either alone or in combination with dietary modification, can play an important role in the prevention or treatment of obesity.

Health risks of obesity

It is difficult to determine quantitatively the importance of excess body fat as a risk to good health. Evidence is lacking to support the contention that a moderate gain in body fat is, in itself, harmful. While excessive body fat has received great notoriety as a coronary heart disease risk factor, available research suggests either that only a modest relationship exists,[10] or that the relation is co-dependent with such factors as hypertension, diabetes or cigarette smoking.[11] Angiographic findings and autopsy studies have not revealed a strong association between body fatness *per se* and the extent of atherosclerosis.[12,13,14] However, obesity is often associated with multiple atherogenic traits, and excessive weight gain in middle age contributes significantly to the risk of heart disease.[10] This may be related to the fact that extra pounds can mean a greater risk of developing high blood pressure as well as elevated serum lipids, impaired glucose tolerance and abnormal uric acid values. In the presence of these factors, obesity assumes a much stronger role as a health risk.

Weight loss with accompanying fat reduction frequently normalizes cholesterol and triglyceride levels and has a beneficial effect on blood pressure. In fact, the normally observed relationship between age and blood pressure is partially explained by the fact that as we grow older we have a tendency to put on weight. Although being too fat may not be a primary heart disease risk factor, its role as a secondary contributing factor cannot be denied. Table 5.1 summarizes the far-reaching, health related correlates of obesity.[15,16,17] It is not clear to what degree obesity causes these problems or is simply a byproduct of a particular medical condition.

TABLE 5.1

Health Related Correlates of Obesity

1. Hypertension and increased risk of stroke
2. Impairment of cardiac function
3. Diabetes mellitus
4. Renal disease
5. Decreased glucose tolerance and insulin resistance
6. Pulmonary disease
7. Problems with anesthesia during surgery
8. Osteoarthritis and gout
9. Endometrial cancer
10. Abnormal lipid and lipoprotein concentrations

Being too fat is often accompanied by changes in personality and behavior which can be manifested as depression, withdrawal, self-pity, irritability and aggression. In addition, obesity impairs exercise and sports performance and can make one more susceptible to injury and the dangers of heat stress via an impaired heat tolerance.

Balancing energy input with energy output: the energy balance equation

For most active adults body weight remains relatively stable, despite the fact that the annual food intake averages close to one ton. This relative stability in body weight is impressive considering the fact that only a slight but regular increase in daily food intake causes a substantial weight gain if energy expenditure remains unchanged. For example, eating an extra apple each day increases the yearly caloric intake by an amount equivalent to about seven pounds of body fat, while an additional slice of apple pie daily will account for the calories in 35 pounds of excess body fat. It is only when the number of calories ingested as food exceeds the daily energy requirements that excess calories are stored as fat in adipose tissue. Conversely, for weight loss to occur, an energy deficit must be created either by decreasing the energy intake (dieting) or increasing the energy output (exercising). To prevent an increase in body fat and maintain body weight, the weight control program must establish an equilibrium between energy input and energy output.

The dynamics of weight loss, weight gain and maintaining a stable body weight are summarized by the principles embodied in the "energy balance equation." Any imbalance in either the energy output or energy input side of the equation will cause the body weight to change.

Energy Input = Energy Output — Stable Body Weight
Energy Input > Energy Output — Increase in Body Weight
Energy Input < Energy Output — Decrease in Body Weight

There are three ways to "unbalance" the energy balance equation for weight loss: (1) reduce caloric intake *below* daily energy requirements, (2) maintain regular food intake and *increase* caloric output through additional physical activity *above* daily energy requirements, and (3) combine methods (1) and (2) by *decreasing* daily food intake and *increasing* daily energy expenditure.

Consider the sensitivity of the energy balance equation in regulating overall energy balance. Suppose caloric intake exceeds output by 100 kcal per day. Then the surplus number of calories consumed in a year would be 365 days × 100 kcal or 36,500 kcal. Because one pound of fatty tissue contains about 3,500 kcal, this is equivalent to a gain of 10.4 pounds of fat in one year. (Each pound of adipose tissue is about 87 percent fat or 454 grams × 0.87 = 395 grams; 395 grams × 9 kcal per gram = 3,555 kcal per pound.) On the other hand, if daily food intake is reduced just 100 kcal and energy expenditure increased 100 kcal by jogging about 1 mile each day, then the monthly caloric deficit would amount to a weight loss of 1.7 pounds (approx. 6,000 kcal) of fat. This is the equivalent of a reduction of about 21 pounds of fat in one year!

Dieting for Weight Control

How it works

This approach to weight loss creates an imbalance in the energy balance equation by reducing energy intake, usually by about 500 to 1,000 kcal a day, below the daily energy expenditure. Suppose an obese woman who consumes 2,800 kcal daily and maintains body weight at 175 pounds wishes to lose weight. She maintains her regular level of activity but reduces daily food intake to 1,800 kcal to create a 1,000 kcal deficit each day. In seven days the total caloric deficit would equal 7,000 kcal, the energy equivalent of two pounds of body fat. Two pounds a week is the recommended maximum weight loss for individuals not under close and frequent medical supervision. (In extreme situations greater weight loss can be obtained but only when the patients are followed carefully, both metabolically and physiologically.) The "two pounds-a-week" guideline is based partially on the fact that those who have been successful in achieving and maintaining a desirable body weight lost no more than one to two pounds a week during the period of caloric deficit. In addition, caloric restriction of greater than 1,000 kcal per day for a sedentary person is poorly tolerated over prolonged periods, and this form of semistarvation greatly increases the chances for poor nourishment.

Actually, our dieting woman would lose considerably more than two pounds during the first week of caloric restriction because the body's carbohydrate reserves would be used up first. This nutrient contains fewer calories and holds significantly more water (2.7 grams of water per gram of glycogen) compared to fat. This is why short periods of caloric restriction prove encouraging to the dieter, but result in a large percentage of water and glycogen loss per unit weight reduction, with only a minimal decrease in body fat.[18] As weight loss continues, however, a larger proportion of body fat is used to make up the energy deficit created by food restriction. To lose an additional three pounds of fat, the lowered caloric intake would have to be maintained for an additional 10.5 days.

While the mathematics of weight loss through caloric restriction is straightforward, it depends upon several basic assumptions which, if not followed, reduce the effectiveness of dieting. The first assumption is that the person's energy expenditure remains relatively unchanged throughout the period of caloric restriction. This is often not the case as the body has a considerable capacity to resist unbalancing the energy balance equation. For example, dieting frequently causes lethargy and thus reduces one's daily activity level. In addition, as body weight is decreased, the energy cost of moving the body is reduced proportionately. Consequently, the energy output side of the "energy balance equation" becomes smaller. Also, physiologic and metabolic changes occur during caloric restriction which affect the rate of weight loss. One such calorie-sparing, energy-efficient change is in the resting metabolism. It is well established that severe caloric restriction depresses resting metabolism perhaps by as much as 45 percent,[19,20] and this may become more apparent with repeated bouts of dieting so that the resting metabolism falls more with each subsequent attempt to reduce calorie intake. In fact, the decrease in resting metabolism is often greater than the decrease attributable to the weight loss. This actually conserves energy and causes the diet to be less effective. As a result, weight loss reaches a plateau becoming significantly less than that predicted from energy balance expectations.[21] This "slowing up" of the theoretical weight loss curve often leaves the dieter frustrated and discouraged.

Types of Diets

Well-balanced, low-calorie diets—A calorie-counting approach to weight loss can provide a well-balanced diet containing all the essential nutrients. The general recommendation is that low-calorie diets be composed of approximately 15 percent protein, 30 percent fat (with reduced saturated fats), and the remainder consisting predominantly of unrefined, complex carbohydrates. Fruits, vegetables and whole grains are high in fiber. The fiber may add to a feeling of fullness and speeds the transit of food through the digestive tract so that fewer calories are absorbed. Calories do count; the key, however, is to keep within specified daily limits as determined both by the amount and rate of fat loss desired. If the diet is nutritionally sound, what one eats is not as important as how much is eaten (that is, how many calories are consumed). If a true caloric deficit exists, weight loss will occur quite independently of the diet's composition.

A practical guide to sound nutrition during dieting is to categorize foods that make similar nutrient contributions, and provide daily servings from each category. The key is *variety*. This can be achieved by use of the Four Food Group Plan illustrated in Table 5.2. As long as the recommended number of servings from each group is obtained, and the food is prepared and cooked properly, the proper foundation for good nutrition is assured.

Table 5.3 presents examples of three daily menus formulated from the guidelines of the basic diet plan shown in Table 5.2.[22] The menus are nutritionally sound, even though the energy value of each is considerably below the average adult requirement. Be-

TABLE 5.2
The Four-Food-Group Plan,
A Basic Plan for Good Nutrition

Food Category	Examples	Recommended Daily Servings[c]
1. Milk and milk products[a]	Milk, cheese, ice cream, sour cream, yogurt	2
2. Meat and high-protein[b]	Meat, fish, poultry, eggs—with dried beans, peas, nuts, or peanut butter as alternatives	2
3. Vegetables and fruits	Dark green or yellow vegetables; citrus fruits or tomatoes	4
4. Cereal and grain food	Enriched breads, cereals, flour, baked goods, or whole-grain products	4

[a]If large quantities of milk are normally consumed, *fortified* skimmed milk should be substituted to reduce the quantity of saturated fats.
[b]Fish, chicken and high-protein vegetables contain significantly less saturated fats than other protein sources.
[c]A basic serving of meat or fish is usually 100 g or 3.5 oz of edible food, 1 cup (8 oz.) milk; 1 oz cheese; ½ cup fruit, vegetables, juice; 1 slice bread; ½ cup cooked cereal or 1 cup ready-to-eat cereal.

cause the emptying of fat from the stomach takes about 3½ hours after ingestion, some fat in the diet usually helps delay the onset of "hunger pangs" and contributes to the feeling of satiety after a meal. Therefore, reducing diets containing some fat are often considered more successful than "fat free" diets.

Starvation (fasting) diets—A starvation diet or therapeutic fast may be recommended in cases of severe obesity in which body fat exceeds 40–50 percent of body weight. Such diets are usually prescribed for up to three months, but only as a "last resort" prior to undertaking more extreme medical approaches which include various surgical treatments. This form of dieting must be closely supervised, usually in a hospital setting.[23,24,25] The starvation approach to weight loss is predicated on the hope that abstinence from food will break established dietary habits and this, in turn, can improve the long-term prospects for successful weight loss.

TABLE 5.3
Three Daily Menus Formulated From Guidelines
Established by Four-Food-Group Plan[a,b]

3 MEALS A DAY	*5 MEALS A DAY*	*6 SMALL MEALS A DAY*
Breakfast	**Breakfast**	**Breakfast**
½ cup unsweetened grapefruit juice	½ grapefruit	½ cup orange juice
1 poached egg 1 slice toast	⅔ cup bran flakes	¾ cup ready-to-eat cereal
1 teaspoon butter or margarine	1 cup skim or low-fat milk or other	½ cup skim milk
½ cup skim milk	beverage	tea or coffee, black
tea or coffee, black		
	Snack	**Mid-Morning Snack**
Lunch	1 small package raisins	⅓ cup low fat cottage cheese
	½ bologna sandwich	
2 ounces lean roast beef		**Lunch**
½ cup cooked summer squash	**Lunch**	
1 slice rye bread		2 ounces sliced turkey on
1 teaspoon butter or margarine	1 slice pizza	1 slice white toast
1 cup skim milk	carrot sticks	1 teaspoon butter or margarine
10 grapes	1 apple	2 canned drained peach halves
	1 cup skim or low-fat milk	½ cup skim milk

Dinner

3 ounces poached haddock
½ cup cooked spinach
tomato and lettuce salad
1 teaspoon oil + vinegar or lemon
1 small biscuit
1 teaspoon butter or margarine
½ cup canned drained fruit cocktail
½ cup skim milk

Total Calories: about 1,200

Snack

1 banana

Dinner

baked fish with mushrooms (3 oz.)
baked potato
2 teaspoons margarine
½ cup broccoli
1 cup tomato juice or skim or low-fat milk

Total Calories: about 1,400

Mid-Afternoon Snack

1 cup fresh spinach and lettuce salad
2 teaspoons oil + vinegar or lemon
3 saltines

Dinner

1 cup clear broth
3 ounces broiled chicken breast
⅓ cup cooked rice with
1 teaspoon butter or margarine
¼ cup cooked mushrooms
½ cup cooked broccoli
½ cup skim milk

Evening Snack

1 medium apple
½ cup skim milk

Total Calories: about 1200

[a]Each menu provides *all* essential nutrients; the energy or caloric value of the diet can be easily increased by increasing the size of the portions, the frequency of meals, or the variety of foods consumed at each sitting.
[b]From McArdle, W. D. et al. *Exercise Physiology: Energy, Nutrition and Human Performance*. Philadelphia: Lea and Febiger, 1981.

An evaluation of fasting was provided by a study of 207 obese patients hospitalized for weight reduction.[23] The results showed that the longer the patient was able to fast, the more extensive was the weight loss. Of the total group, seventy-nine reduced to within 30 percent of their ideal weight in one uninterrupted fast. The patients were then followed to note any weight gain over time. Weight loss was generally maintained for one and a half years by the majority of the patients regardless of the extent of the weight loss. Unfortunately, within two or three years, 50 percent of the fasters reverted back to their original weight, and nine years later fewer than 10 percent weighed less than they had prior to the start of such drastic dieting. It is interesting that the patients felt that the weight loss, although temporary, was worth the effort, as it resulted in better health and quality of life. The patients found that employment was facilitated and earnings increased during this weight loss period.

The possible advantages and disadvantages of prolonged fasting can be summarized as follows:

ADVANTAGES

1. Severe feelings of hunger become depressed in about seven days and craving for food decreases.

2. There is an initial rapid decrease in body weight, with slower yet progressive decreases in weight when fasting is maintained for one or two months duration.

3. A significant weight loss may convince the patient that compulsive eating behaviors can be controlled, thus reversing the usual positive caloric imbalance.

4. Fasting may be more successful than adhering to a less severe, semi-starvation diet plan.

DISADVANTAGES

1. Some patients experience a dramatic postural hypotension when assuming an upright position. Typical symptoms are dizziness and fainting.

2. Possible development of gout. This can lead to recurrent attacks of acute arthritis which usually lasts for several hours, but may continue for days or weeks if no treatment is given. Also, there may be acute inflammation and swelling of tissues.

3. Development of anemia. Lethargy and depressed physical activity are often present.

4. Impairment of renal function due to the build-up of waste products from the breakdown of body tissues.

5. Loss of hair.

6. Muscle irritability and cramping.
7. Headaches and emotional disturbances.
8. Generalized state of malnutrition.
9. In addition to fat loss, a significant percent of the weight loss is due to the loss of lean tissue.[25,26]
10. If a person fasts for several days and then attempts to exercise, deterioration in performance occurs. Since sufficient carbohydrates are not consumed in the starvation diet, the glycogen storage depots in the liver and muscles will be rapidly reduced to such low levels as to cause impairment in most tasks requiring heavy, vigorous exercise as well as sustained muscular effort.[27]

Clearly, in view of the limited long-term success as well as potential side effects, starvation is not the "diet" of choice or proper approach to weight control for most individuals.

Protein diets—The use of high-protein diets is part of the movement for a quick and easy method of weight loss. It has served as "the last chance diet"[28] for the obese as well as those who are less overweight. Among the reasons advanced for the widespread popularity of these diets is the belief that a diet consisting predominantly of protein will cause rapid weight loss and bring about results when all other approaches have failed. Protein diets are extolled as causing suppression of appetite through fat mobilization and the formation of ketone bodies. This effect has yet to be supported with careful research. It is also argued that the elevated SDA effect of dietary protein as well as its relatively low coefficient of digestibility ultimately reduces the net calories available from this food compared to an isocaloric well-balanced meal. This calorigenic effect of protein ingestion is believed to be due largely to digestive processes as well as the extra energy required by the liver to assimilate amino acids. Although this point may have some validity, many other factors must be considered in formulating a sound program for weight loss—not to mention the potentially harmful strain on kidney and liver function, and accompanying dehydration, electrolyte imbalance and lean tissue loss resulting from excessive protein intake.

Well-balanced nutrition requires a blend of carbohydrate, fat and protein as well as appropriate quantities of vitamins and minerals. In addition, if physical activity is used in conjunction with dietary modification, it is important to maintain carbohydrate intake to provide fuel for both rapid and sustained forms of exercise.[29] Also, if a person is reasonably active, the potential SDA effect of any food represents only a small portion of the total daily energy expenditure.

Protein-sparing fast. During fasting, the body essentially exhausts its carbohydrate reserves within one to three days. This brings about an increased catabolism of protein in lean tissue to make up the caloric deficit as well as to provide an alternative source for glucose synthesis by the liver. The protein-sparing diet is advocated to counter the muscle wasting brought on by fasting. The diet allows 500–800 kcal of protein and a small amount of carbohydrate. The belief is that this dietary protein is just enough to minimize the body's catabolism of lean tissue during caloric deprivation. This approach, however, has not been shown to be more effective in preserving lean tissue than an isocaloric well-balanced diet.[30,31] A limited use of the protein-sparing fast may show promise in treating certain insulin resistant and obese diabetic patients.[32,33] However, it may not be any more effective than a well-balanced, low-calorie diet combined with regular exercise. Regular physical activity enhances insulin utilization while, at the same time, promoting fat loss and lean tissue maintenance.[34,35,36]

A number of medical complications can occur in the obese as well as the non-obese person who maintains one of the many versions of the nutritionally unbalanced high-protein, low-carbohydrate diet. As of June, 1978 fifty-eight deaths had been associated with the modified-fast, low-calorie, high-protein diets; sixteen due to cardiac arrhythmias and cardiac arrest. While a cause and effect relationship has yet to be proven between this diet and such lethal side effects,[37,38] its effectiveness for prudent weight control certainly should be viewed cautiously. Table 5.4 summarizes some of the complications resulting from high protein diets.

TABLE 5.4

Some Potential Medical Complications of High-protein Diets

Death	Neuromuscular
Cardiac	Peroneal palsy
Arrhythmias	Muscle weakness resembling
Perhaps myocarditis	polymyositis
Myocardial infarction	Gastrointestinal
Cerebral ischemia	Acute cholecystitis or pancreatitis or
Pancreatitis	both during refeeding
Cardiovascular	Diverticulitis
Cardiac	Perhaps appendicitis
Arrhythmias	Renal Stones
Perhaps myocarditis	
Myocardial infarction	Fluid and Electrolyte
Thrombophlebitis	Volume contraction
Acid-Base	Potassium loss leading to hypokalemia
Ketoacidosis	

Low-Carbohydrate, High-Fat (Ketogenic) Diets—Advocates of the low-carbohydrate, high-fat diet emphasize carbohydrate restriction while ignoring the total content of the diet. It is argued that with minimal carbohydrate for energy the body must metabolize predominantly fat. This supposedly generates sufficient ketone bodies to cause urinary loss of these unused calories to account for significant weight loss, despite an allegedly high caloric intake. It is argued that this caloric loss will be so great that the dieter can eat all he or she wishes, as long as carbohydrates are restricted. While such a diet appears attractive, the claims for a metabolic advantage for effective weight loss compared to conventional well-balanced, low-calorie diets have not been supported. In general the diet is without scientific merit. For one thing, the calories lost via urinary excretion of ketones are at most about 100 to 150 kcal a day.[39] This would account for only a small weight loss of approximately one pound every month. Also, it is difficult for individuals to make dramatic alterations in diet composition. High-fat diets are not very palatable. Thus, while being potentially high in calories, the total caloric intake from these diets may actually be low, since food intake remains low.[40]

The ketogenic, high-fat, potentially atherogenic diet may cause a relatively rapid initial weight loss due largely to dehydration as the body adjusts to utilizing its stored fat. This is brought about by temporary sodium loss and extra solute load on the kidneys which increases the excretion of urinary water. Such water loss is of no lasting significance in a program designed to reduce body fat. When compared to a standard well-balanced diet, the ketogenic diet shows no advantage in facilitating losses in body fat.[41]

Aside from being highly questionable in terms of effectiveness, the high-fat, low-carbohydrate diet can be condemned as being potentially hazardous in a number of ways.[42] The diet can raise serum uric acid levels, lower potassium levels (which facilitates undesirable cardiac arrhythmias), cause acidosis, aggravate kidney problems due to the extra solute burden placed on the renal system, elevate blood lipids (thus increasing a primary heart disease risk factor), deplete glycogen reserves and contribute to a fatigued state, and cause relative dehydration. The diet is definitely contraindicated during pregnancy as adequate carbohydrate metabolism is essential for proper fetal development.

Low-carbohydrate diets are frequently associated with a negative nitrogen balance as the body uses the protein in lean tissue as a primary fuel to maintain blood glucose. This process of gluconeogenesis provides a metabolic option for augmented carbohydrate synthesis in the face of depleted glycogen stores. However,

TABLE 5.5
Some Popular Weight Loss Methods

Type of method	Principle	Advantages	Disadvantages	Comments
Surgical procedures	Alteration of the gastrointestinal tract changes capacity or amount of absorptive surface	Caloric restriction is less necessary	Risks of surgery and post-surgical complications include death	Radical procedures include stapling of the stomach and removal of a section of the small intestine (a jejunoilieal bypass)
Fasting	No energy input assures negative energy balance	Weight loss is rapid (which may be a disadvantage) Exposure to temptation is reduced	Ketogenic A large portion of weight lost is from lean body mass Nutrients are lacking	Medical supervision is mandatory and hospitalization is recommended
Protein-sparing modified fast	Same as fasting except protein intake helps preserve lean body mass	same as above	Ketogenic Nutrients are lacking Some unconfirmed deaths have been reported, possibly from potassium depletion	Medical supervision is mandatory Popular presentation was made in Linn's *The Last Chance Diet*
One-food-centered diets	Low-caloric intake favors negative energy balance	Being easy to follow has initial psychological appeal	Being too restrictive means nutrients are probably lacking Repetitious nature may cause boredom	No food or food combination is known to "burn off" fat Examples include the grapefruit diet and the egg diet

TABLE 5.5

Some Popular Weight Loss Methods

Type of method	Principle	Advantages	Disadvantages	Comments
Low-carbohydrate/high-fat diets	Increased ketone excretion removes energy-containing substances from the body. Fat intake is often voluntarily decreased; a low-caloric diet results	Inclusion of rich foods may have psychological appeal. Initial rapid loss of water may be an incentive	Ketogenic. High-fat intake is contraindicated for heart and diabetes patients. Nutrients are often lacking	Popular versions have been offered by Taller and Atkins; some have been called the "Mayo," "Drinking Man's," and "Air Force" diets
Low-carbohydrate/high-protein diets	Low-caloric intake favors negative energy balance		Expense and repetitious nature may make it difficult to sustain	If meat is emphasized, the diet becomes one that is high in fat. The Pennington diet is an example
High-carbohydrate low-fat diets	Low-caloric intake favors negative energy balance	Wise food selections can make the diet nutritionally sound	Initial water retention may be discouraging	

From: Reed, P. B. *Nutrition: An Applied Science.* St. Paul, Minn: West, 1980.

this produces a temporary reduction in the body's protein, especially the protein in muscle tissue.[43]

The principles, and advantages and disadvantages of some popular weight loss methods are summarized in Table 5.5

Factors affecting weight loss through dieting

When caloric intake is below the daily energy requirement, the initial decrease in body weight occurs primarily from water loss and a corresponding depletion of the body's carbohydrate reserves. With further weight loss, a larger proportion of body fat is metabolized to supply the caloric deficit created by restricting food intake or increasing physical activity.

Provided the diet is nutritionally sound, what one eats matters less than how many calories are consumed. There is simply no compelling evidence to support the contention that the popular "fad" diets have any advantage over a calorically-restricted, well-balanced diet. Weight loss occurs with reduced caloric intake regardless of the diet's composition of carbohydrate, protein, and fat. When obese patients consumed either a high-fat diet or high-carbohydrate 800 kcal diet, weight loss on each diet was nearly identical, as was the percentage of fat tissue lost during a ten-day period.[44] These findings illustrate an important principle of dieting and weight control; no "magic metabolic mixture" assures a more effective weight loss than a well-balanced, low-calorie diet, even though a low-calorie diet high in fat content may seem more filling and perhaps produce less hunger. Anyone contemplating a diet that deviates from a well-balanced, low-calorie diet should do so only under close medical supervision.

Adequate hydration should be maintained at all times during caloric restriction in a weight loss program. While restricting water intake causes a relatively large initial weight loss, this is due to a loss in body water. The total quantity of fat loss is independent of the water intake.[18] The important point is that the caloric equivalent of weight loss increases as a function of the duration of caloric restriction. This is the major reason why it is crucial to maintain a caloric deficit over time, because diets of short duration cause a larger percentage of water and carbohydrate loss per unit of weight loss with only a minimal decrease in body fat. The caloric equivalent of weight loss more than doubles after two months compared to the first four or five days of dieting.

Exercise for Weight Control

Is overeating the cause of weight gain?

The relative contribution of physical inactivity and excessive caloric intake to obesity are not clear. In the past, it was generally accepted that the obese condition was the result of excessive food intake. Clearly, then, the effective approach to weight control would be some form of caloric restriction through dieting. However, this view of obesity is overly simplistic as available evidence indicates that excess weight gain throughout life often closely parallels reduced physical activity rather than an increased caloric intake.[45] For example, obese infants do not characteristically consume more calories than the recommended dietary standards or counterparts of normal weight.[46] It is also noted that the infant offspring of obese parents display less spontaneous movements than infants of normal weight parents. This suggests the possibility that such subdued movement patterns are abnormal and may reflect inherited characteristics.[47]

Time-in-motion photography to document activity patterns of elementary school children clearly showed that overweight school children were considerably less active than their normal-weight peers, and that excess weight was not related to food intake.[48] The caloric intake of obese high school girls and boys was actually below their non-obese peers.[48,49,50] This observation that fat people often eat the same or even less than thinner ones is also true for adults as they become less active and slowly begin to add weight.[51,52,53] In fact, one is hard pressed for evidence that groups of overweight individuals actually eat more on the average than people of normal weight. Consequently, to further reduce caloric intake in an effort to cause weight loss would seem neither prudent nor appropriate as the only method to combat the overfat condition.

What is becoming increasingly clear is that people who maintain a physically active lifestyle or who become involved in endurance exercise programs maintain a desirable level of body composition.[8,26,53] Within this framework, a strong case can be made for habitual, lifelong, vigorous physical activity for individuals of all ages.

Physical activity

Physical activity has by far the most profound effect on human energy expenditure. At rest, the brain and skeletal muscles consume about the same total quantity of oxygen, even though the brain weighs only three and one-half pounds while muscle mass constitutes almost 50 percent of the body weight. The situation is quite different with vigorous exercise, however, as the energy generated by muscles can increase nearly 120 times in sprint-type exercise while the oxygen consumption of the brain remains essentially unchanged. World class athletes nearly double their daily caloric outputs as a result of two to three hours of hard training. In fact, most people can generate metabolic rates that are eight to ten times above the resting value during sustained, "big muscle" exercises like running, bicycling and swimming.[29] Complementing this increased metabolic rate during exercise is the observation that vigorous exercise will raise the resting metabolic rate for up to fifteen hours after exercise.

It is only recently that exercise for weight control has come into prominence. This is because two arguments have generally been raised against the exercise approach. One is the belief that exercise inevitably causes an increase in appetite, so that any caloric deficit is rapidly made up by a proportionate or even greater increase in food intake. The second argument is that the calorie-burning effects of exercise are so small that the moderate exercise makes only small "dent" in the body's fat reserves compared to fasting or semi-starvation. The truth is that regular exercise offers an important option for unbalancing the energy balance equation to produce a significant caloric deficit.

Exercise effects on appetite

It appears that physical activity is necessary for the normal functioning of feeding control mechanisms. A fine balance between energy expenditure and food intake is not maintained in sedentary people.[52,53] For these people, the caloric intake generally exceeds the daily energy requirement. This lack of precision in regulating food intake at the low end of the physical activity spectrum may account for the "creeping obesity" commonly observed in highly mechanized and technically advanced societies. For individuals who engage regularly in physical activity, appetite control is in a reactive zone in which it is simpler to match food intake with the daily level of energy expenditure.

In considering the effects of exercise on appetite and food consumption, a distinction should be made between the type and duration of the exercise. Lumberjacks, farm laborers, and certain athletes consume about twice the daily calories as average sedentary people. Woodcutters who spend four to six hours a day in heavy labor unconsciously adjust their calorie intake to balance the energy output and consume between 4,000 and 7,000 kcal daily, the average intake being about 5,500 kcal. Because these workers are usually quite lean, high caloric intakes are necessary to balance the extremely high caloric expenditure required during lumberjacking and logging.[54] The same is true for athletes whose physical training is particularly strenuous and time-consuming.[55] Endurance athletes such as marathon runners, cross-country skiers and cyclists consume about 5,000 kcal each day. Yet some of these athletes are the leanest in the world![29,56] Clearly, this extreme caloric intake is required just to meet the energy requirements of the training and is not at all related to an accumulation of body fat.

Among individuals who train for relatively short periods of time, the appetite-stimulating effect of exercise is not readily apparent.[57,58,59] Women engaged in swim training averaged about 15 percent greater caloric intake than collegiate tennis players during the training and competitive seasons.[58] Neither group, however, consumed many more calories during the season than before or after it. In another study,[60] obese young men participated in a three phase physical conditioning program consisting of five weeks of exercise, five weeks of sedentary living and another five-week exercise period. Despite variations in energy output, daily caloric intake was essentially unchanged throughout the experiment and significant reductions in body weight and body fat were observed with exercise. These modifications in body size were attributed to the calorigenic effect of exercise, since caloric intake did not change.

Data have been reported which suggest that a light to moderate increase in physical activity above the sedentary range may actually depress the appetite and reduce food intake in both animals and humans. For example, sedentary animals show a decrease in food intake with up to one hour of daily exercise.[61] For humans, the food intake was evaluated for an industrial population in West Bengal, India.[62] The dietary composition of these people was quite uniform, but the physical activity level ranged from sedentary to very heavy. As shown in Table 5.6, for persons in occupations classified as moderately heavy and heavy for physical activity, the daily food intake increased proportionately with the intensity of work. For these active workers, however, body weight was well below the people in the sedentary range. Of considerable importance is the observation that for workers in occupations requiring relatively light physical activity the daily food intake (and body weight) was actually lower than for sedentary people. Similar observations have been made for young women and men who decreased their consumption of total calories as a result of a moderate exercise program.[63,64] For both groups, body fat was reduced significantly. These results are nearly identical to findings with animals and support the contention that light exercise in previously sedentary individuals does not necessarily stimulate the appetite, and may even depress food intake.[26]

TABLE 5.6

Effect of Exercise on Caloric Intake and Body Weight

Job Classification	Daily Caloric Intake (kcal)	Body Weight (lbs)
Sedentary	3,300	148
Light work	2,600	118
Medium work	2,800	114
Heavy work	3,400	113
Very heavy work	3,600	113

Modified from: Mayer, J. et al. Relation between caloric intake, body weight, and physical work; studies in an industrial male population in West Bengal. *Am. J. Clin. Nutr.* 4: 169, 1956.

Exercise effects on energy expenditure

An argument frequently raised against exercise as a means for weight control concerns the number of calories that can be expended through regular exercise. For example, one must chop wood for seven hours, run thirty-five miles, golf for twenty-hours, play badminton for nineteen hours or perform mild calisthenics for twenty-two hours just to expend the calories in one pound of body fat. Small wonder that such a commitment seems overwhelming and discourages the overfat individual planning to lose twenty to thirty pounds or more. While facts form the basis for this attack against exercise for weight control, the same facts support a strong counterattack in favor of exercise. For one thing, the caloric effect of exercise does not depend on one exercise bout. If golf is played only two hours (about 350 kcal/day), two days a week (700 kcal), then five weeks or ten golfing days would be needed to lose one pound of fat. Assuming one could play year round, devoting two days a week to this form of exercise would result in a ten-pound loss of fat during the year, provided the food intake remained fairly constant. The point is that the calorie-expending effects of exercise are cumulative; a caloric deficit of 3,500 kcal is equivalent to a one-pound loss of fat whether or not the deficit occurs rapidly, or systematically over a long period. When this is combined with the fact that a modest increase in regular physical activity may even depress food intake in pre-viously sedentary people, exercise takes on important dimensions as an effective tool for weight control.

Tabled values for energy expenditure are available from which one can estimate the caloric cost of a variety of occupational, recreational and sports activities.[29,65,66] These values are "averages" which are applicable under "average" conditions when applied to the "average" person of a given body weight. While they provide a good approximation for establishing the caloric cost of different physical activities, some variation is to be expected due to individual differences in style and technique of performance, environmental factors such as terrain, temperature and wind resistance, as well as the intensity of participation.

Effect of body weight—Body weight is an important factor which affects the energy expended in many forms of exercise. The energy cost of a particular exercise is generally greater for heavier people, especially in weight-bearing exercise like walking and running where the person must transport his or her body weight during the activity (Table 5.7). Here, the energy expended in moving one's weight is directly proportional to body weight.[67]

TABLE 5.7

Energy Cost of Walking (kcal. hr^{-1})
in Relation to Speed and Body Weight[a]

Speed mph	Weight in Pounds						
	80	100	120	140	160	180	200
2.0	114	132	155	174	192	210	228
2.5	138	162	186	210	228	252	270
3.0	162	186	216	240	264	288	318
3.5	186	216	252	276	300	324	366
4.0	210	246	282	312	348	384	420

[a]From DeVries, H.A. Physiology of Exercise. Iowa: Wm. C. Brown Co., 1980.

The energy cost of cross-country running, for example, ranges between 8.2 kcal per minute for a 50-kilogram (110-pound) person to almost twice as much at 16.0 kcal for a person weighing 98 kilograms (215 pounds). However, if the energy requirement is expressed in relation to body weight as kcal $kg^{-1}.min^{-1}$ this difference is essentially eliminated and the energy cost averages about 0.164 kcal.$kg^{-1}.min^{-1}$. By expressing energy cost in this manner (that is, per unit of body weight) the differences between individuals are greatly reduced regardless of age, race, sex and body weight. However, the *total* calories expended by the heavier person are still considerably larger than a lighter counterpart, simply because the body weight must be transported in the activity—and this requires proportionately more energy. With weight-supported exercise such as stationary bicycling, the influence of body weight on the energy cost is less extreme.[67] Certainly, for heavy people desiring to use exercise in a program for weight loss, weight-bearing forms of exercise can provide a considerable caloric expenditure.

Table 5.8 presents values for the net energy expended during running for one hour at various speeds. Running speeds are expressed as kilometers per hour, miles per hour, as well as the number of minutes required to complete one mile at a particular running speed. The bold face values are the net calories expended to run one mile for a given body weight. This energy requirement is fairly constant and independent of running speed. Thus, for a person who weighs 62 kg (136 pounds) running a twenty-six-mile marathon requires about 2,600 kcal whether the run is completed in just over two hours or four hours.

For a heavier person, the energy cost per mile increases proportionately. For example, if a 102-kg (225-pound) person jogs five miles each day at any comfortable pace, 163 kcal will be expended for each mile completed, or a total of 815 kcal for the five-mile run. Increasing or decreasing the running speed simply alters the physiologic overload and length of the exercise period; it has little effect on the total energy expended.

Effects of regular exercise on weight loss and body composition

Regular aerobic exercise, even without dietary restriction, brings about favorable changes in body weight and body composition. The effectiveness of an exercise program for weight loss is linked to the degree of obesity at the start. As a general rule, persons who are obese lose weight and fat more readily than normal or lean counterparts.[57,68,69,70,71] In addition, exercise provides significant positive "spin off" in that it alters body composition (reduced fat and maintenance or even small increase in lean tissue) in such a way that the resting level of energy expenditure is increased. This reduces the body's tendency to store calories. Regular exercise also stimulates improved function of various physiologic systems,[29] and may also enhance the health status of the cardiovascular system[72,73,74].

When considering exercise for weight control, factors such as frequency, intensity and duration, as well as the specific form of

TABLE 5.8
Net Energy Expenditure Per Hour for Horizontal Running[a]

BODY WEIGHT kg	lbs	km.hr⁻¹ / mph / min per mile / kcal per mile	8 / 4.97 / 12:00	9 / 5.60 / 10:43	10 / 6.20 / 9:41	11 / 6.84 / 8:46	12 / 7.46 / 8:02	13 / 8.08 / 7:26	14 / 8.70 / 6:54	15 / 9.32 / 6:26	16 / 9.94 / 6:02
50	110	80	400	450	500	550	600	650	700	750	800
54	119	86	432	486	540	594	648	702	756	810	864
58	128	93	464	522	580	638	696	754	812	870	928
62	137	99	496	558	620	682	744	806	868	930	992
66	146	106	528	594	660	726	792	858	924	990	1056
70	154	112	560	630	700	770	840	910	980	1050	1120
74	163	118	592	666	740	814	888	962	1036	1110	1184
78	172	125	624	702	780	858	936	1014	1092	1170	1248
82	181	131	656	738	820	902	984	1066	1148	1230	1312
86	190	138	688	774	860	946	1032	1118	1204	1290	1376
90	199	144	720	810	900	990	1080	1170	1260	1350	1440
94	207	150	752	846	940	1034	1128	1222	1316	1410	1504
98	216	157	784	882	980	1078	1176	1274	1372	1470	1568
102	225	163	816	918	1020	1122	1224	1326	1428	1530	1632
106	234	170	848	954	1060	1166	1272	1378	1484	1590	1696

[a]The table is interpreted as follows: For a 50 kg person, the net energy expenditure for running for 1 hour at 8 km.hr⁻¹ or 4.97 mph is 400 kcal. This speed represents a twelve-minute per mile pace. Thus, in one hour 5 miles would be run and 400 kcal would be expended. If the pace was increased to 12 km.hr⁻¹, 600 kcal would be expended during the hour of running.

[b]Running speeds are expressed as kilometers per hour (km.hr⁻¹), miles per hour (mph), and minutes required to complete each mile (min per mile). The values in boldface type are the net calories expended to run one mile for a given body weight, independent of running speed.

From McArdle, W.D. et al. *Exercise Physiology: Energy, Nutrition and Human Performance*. Philadelphia: Lea and Febiger, 1981.

exercise must be considered. Since a pound of body fat contains approximately 3,500 kcal, the exercise program must establish this negative caloric balance to bring about a one-pound fat loss. Continuous, big muscle aerobic activities that have a moderate to high caloric cost such as walking, running, rope skipping, cycling and swimming are ideal. Many recreational sports and games are also effective in reducing body weight, although precise quantification of energy expenditure during such activities is difficult. These rhythmic forms of exercise burn considerable calories, stimulate lipid metabolism, reduce body fat, establish favorable blood pressure responses and generally promote cardiovascular fitness. In addition, there is generally no selective effect of running, walking or bicycling; each is equally effective in altering body composition provided the duration, frequency and intensity of exercise are similar.[75] A 300 kcal extra daily caloric output with moderate jogging for thirty minutes will cause a one-pound fat loss in about twelve days. Over a year's time, this represents a total caloric deficit equivalent to approximately thirty pounds of body fat!

Generally, the total energy expended is the most important factor influencing the effectiveness of the exercise program for weight control.[53,76,77] In fact, a dose-response relationship has been demonstrated with weight loss being directly related to the time spent exercising.[76] Thus, an overfat person who starts out at a light exercise intensity with slow walking can accrue a considerable caloric expenditure simply by extending the duration of the exercise. This effect of duration will offset the inability (and inadvisability) of the previously sedentary, obese person to exercise at high intensities. Also, the energy cost of weight-bearing exercise such as walking is proportional to body weight so that the overweight person will burn up considerably more calories to perform the same task than will a person of normal weight.

The importance of exercise duration for weight loss is illustrated by a study of three groups of men who exercised for twenty weeks by walking and running for either fifteen, thirty, or forty-five minutes per session.[71] Compared to a sedentary control group, the three exercise groups significantly decreased their body fat, skinfolds and waist girth. When comparisons were made between the three groups, the forty-five-minute training group lost more body fat than either the thirty- or 15-minute group. This was attributed to the greater caloric expenditure of the longer exercise period.

Start slowly—The initial stage of the exercise program for a previously sedentary, overfat patient is developmental in nature and should not include a high total energy output. During this time patients should be urged to adopt longterm goals, personal discipline, and a restructuring of both eating and exercise behaviors. It is often counterproductive to include unduly rapid training progressions as many obese patients initially show psychological resistance to physical training.[78] During the first few weeks, slow walking is replaced by intervals of walking/jogging which eventually lead to continuous jogging. At least eight to ten weeks are required before real changes can be observed. Behavioral approaches should also be applied to cause meaningful lifestyle changes in physical activity.[66] For example, walking, or bicycling can replace the use of the auto, stair climbing can replace the elevator, and manual tools can replace power tools.

The effectiveness of regular exercise for weight loss is shown in Table 5.9. In this study,[64] six sedentary, obese young men exercised five days a week for sixteen weeks by ninety minutes of walking on a motor driven treadmill at each session. The men lost an average of almost six kilograms of body fat which represented a decrease in percent body fat from 23.5 to 18.6. In addition, physiological fitness and work capacity improved, as did the level of high density lipoprotein and the high/low density lipoprotein ratio which increased 15.6 percent and 25.9 percent, respectively. Similar observations for changes in body fat with exercise have been made for obese women[68,76] as well as previously sedentary middle-aged men.[79]

TABLE 5.9

Changes in Body Composition and Blood Lipids in Six Obese Young Adult Men with a Sixteen-week Walking Program[a]

Variable	*Pre-training*[b]	*Post-training*	*Difference*
Body weight, kg	99.1	93.4	− 5.7[c]
Body density, g. ml⁻¹	1.044	1.056	+ 0.012[c]
Body fat, %	23.5	18.6	− 4.9[c]
Fat weight, kg	23.3	17.4	− 5.9[c]
Lean body weight, kg	75.8	76.0	+ 0.2
Sum of skinfolds, mm	142.9	104.8	− 38.1[c]
HDL cholesterol, mg. 100 ml⁻¹	32	37	+ 5[c]
HDL/LDL cholesterol	0.27	0.34	0.07[c]

[a]From Leon, A.S. et al. Effects of a vigorous walking program on body composition, and carbohydrate and lipid metabolism of obese young men. *Amer. J. Clin. Nutr.* 33:1776, 1979.
[b]Values are means
[c]Statistically significant at the 0.05 level.

Regularity is the key—Training frequency is also important when considering exercise for weight reduction. In a summary of six studies that investigated optimal training frequency,[80] it was observed that training two days a week did not change body weight, skinfolds or percent body fat. Three and four day a week training, however, had a significant effect. Subjects who trained four days a week reduced their body weight and skinfold fat significantly more than the three day per week group. However, reductions in percent body fat were similar for both groups.

Within the framework of available research, it appears that at least three days of training per week are required to bring about changes in body composition through exercise.[81,82] There is some indication that more frequent training may even be more effective. More than likely, this effect is the direct result of the added caloric output provided by the extra training. While it is difficult to speculate precisely as to a threshold energy expenditure for weight reduction and fat loss, it is generally recommended that the calorie-burning effect of each exercise session should be at least 300 kcal.[75,82] This can be achieved with twenty to thirty minutes of moderate to vigorous running, swimming or bicycling, or walking for forty to sixty minutes. Exercise programs of lower caloric cost usually show little or no effect on body weight of body composition.

Weight training for weight loss. Standard strength training programs are generally ineffective for weight loss.[83,84] This is because the energy cost of each specific exercise as well as the total energy expended in a workout is relatively low.[85] However, by modifying the standard approach to strength training it is possible to increase the caloric cost of exercise and bring about favorable changes in body weight and body fat.[86,87,88,89] This approach, called circuit weight training, deemphasizes the heavy local muscle overload of weight lifting for strength in favor of a more general physical conditioning. The person lifts a weight that is between 30–50 percent of his or her maximum strength. The weight is lifted between fifteen and twenty-two times in a thirty-second period. After a fifteen-second rest, the person moves to the next weight lifting station and so on until the entire circuit is completed. The circuit is repeated several times to allow for twenty to thirty minutes of continuous exercise. The energy cost of such circuits is usually similar to that observed jogging at five miles per hour.[86]

Diet plus exercise: the ideal combination

Weight loss principles are based on a reduction in calories consumed, and increase in the number of calories expended in physical activity, or a combination of both. For men and women, combinations of exercise and diet offer considerably more flexibility for achieving a negative caloric balance and accompanying fat loss than either exercise alone or diet alone.[68,90] In fact, the addition of exercise to the weight control program may facilitate more permanent weight loss compared to total reliance on caloric restriction.[53,92,93]

Consider an obese person who desires to reduce body weight by twenty pounds through exercise and diet. In order to maintain a prudent weight loss of about one pound a week, twenty weeks would be required to achieve the twenty-pound fat loss. With this goal, the average weekly deficit would have to be 3,500 kcal while the daily deficit must average 500 kcal.

One-half hour of moderate exercise (about 350 "extra" kcal) performed three days a week adds 1,050 kcal to the weekly caloric deficit. Consequently, the weekly caloric intake would have to be reduced by only 2,450 kcal instead of 3,500 kcal in order to lose the desired one pound of fat each week. If the number of exercise days is increased from three to five, food intake need only be reduced by 250 kcal each day. If the duration of the five day per week workouts was prolonged from thirty minutes to one hour then no reduction in food intake would be necessary for weight loss to occur, because the required 3,500 kcal deficit would have been created entirely through exercise. With greater levels of physical activity food intake could actually be increased and weight loss would still occur as long as a caloric deficit was maintained. Clearly, physical activity can be used by itself or in combination with mild dietary restriction to bring about an effective loss of body fat. This approach is likely to produce fewer of the feelings of intense hunger and psychological stress that occur with a program of weight loss which relies exclusively on caloric restriction.

Perhaps of equal or even greater importance is the fact that exercise in a weight reduction program provides protection against the significant loss in lean tissue observed with weight loss by diet alone.[94,95,96,97] The maintenance of lean tissue with exercise may be partly due to the fact that aerobic exercise training enhances the mobilization and breakdown of fat from the body's energy depots.[98] In addition, exercise tends to increase the rate of protein synthesis in skeletal muscle while at the same time retarding its rate of breakdown.[99] This protein-sparing effect thus causes a greater portion of the caloric deficit to be made up by fat catabolism. Without exercise, caloric restriction will bring about protein breakdown as the labile amino acids in skeletal muscle are recruited to contribute to the body's energy needs.[100,101]

To evaluate the degree that exercise favorably modifies the composition of weight lost, three groups of adult women were maintained on a daily caloric deficit of 500 kcal for 16 weeks.[35] The diet group reduced daily food intake by 500 kcal, while women in the exercise group increased their energy output by 500 kcal through participation in a supervised walking and exercise program. The women using diet plus exercise created their daily 500 kcal deficit by reducing food intake by 250 kcal and increasing energy output 250 kcal through exercise. In terms of weight loss, there was no significant difference between the three groups as each group lost approximately five kilograms (11 pounds). This shows that as long as a caloric deficit is created body weight will be reduced, regardless of the method used to create the imbalance. In terms of reducing body fat, however, combining diet and exercise was the most effective approach to weight loss. Expressed as a percent of initial fatness, the diet plus exercise group reduced by 13.1 percent; the exercisers reduced by 12.6 percent, and the diet group reduced body fat by 9.3 percent. The most interesting observation concerned lean body weight. While the exercise and combination groups *increased* their lean body weight by 0.9 and 0.5 kilograms (2 pounds and 1 pound) respectively, the dieters *lost* 1.1 kilograms (2.42 pounds) of lean tissue! It might be argued that this lean tissue loss was possibly due to a reduced protein intake during food restriction. However, the women in the diet group had an average protein intake of 71.3 grams per day which would be more than adequate to prevent a protein deficiency. Although more research in this area is needed, it does appear that when weight is reduced by diet alone, more lean tissue is lost (and less fat) compared to a similar weight loss brought about by the appropriate use of exercise.

Spot reduction—does it work?

Spot reduction involves localized exercise to reduce fat stores in areas of greatest deposition. The underlying basis for this fat loss technique rests on the belief that by exercising a specific body area, more fat will be selectively reduced from that area than if exercise of the same caloric intensity was performed by a different muscle group. In a practical sense, large numbers of situps would be recommended for a person with an excessively fat abdominal area. It is believed that, in some way, disuse of a muscle group causes a disproportionate storage of local subcutaneous fat and, conversely, an increase in a muscle's activity facilitates a relatively great fat mobilization from these specific storage sites.

While the promise of spot reduction with exercise is especially attractive from an aesthetic standpoint, a critical evaluation of the research does not support this idea.[102,103,104,105] Current knowledge of energy supply indicates that exercise stimulates the mobilization of fatty acids from the fat depots throughout the body, and that areas of greatest fat concentration probably supply the greatest amount of this energy. There is simply no evidence that fatty acids are released to a greater degree from the fat pads directly over the exercising muscle.

In an attempt to examine critically the claims for spot reduction, comparisons were made of the circumferences and subcutaneous fat stores of the right and left forearms of high caliber tennis players.[102] As expected, the circumference of the dominant or playing arm was significantly larger than the non-dominant arm. This was the result of a modest muscular hypertrophy associated with the muscular overload provided by tennis. However, measurements of skinfold thickness showed that there was no difference between arms in the quantity of subcutaneous forearm fat. Clearly, prolonged exercise of the playing arm was not accompanied by reduced deposits specifically in that arm.

There is no doubt that the negative caloric balance created through regular exercise can significantly contribute to a reduction in total body fat. However, this fat is not reduced selectively from the exercised areas but, rather, from total body fat reserves and from the areas of greatest fat concentration.

REFERENCES

1. Gunby, P. 1978. Research on the riddle of obesity gains new scientific weight. *JAMA* 239: 1727.
2. Hannon, B. M. and Lohman, T. G. 1978. The energy cost of overweight in the United States. *Am. J. Pub. Health* 68: 765.
3. Charney, H. C. et al. 1976. Child antecedents of adult obesity. *New Engl. J. Med.* 295: 6.
4. Novak, L. O. 1972. Aging, total potassium, fat-free mass, and cell mass in males and females between ages 18 and 85 years. *J. Gerontology* 27: 438.
5. Pollock, M. L., et al. 1976. Prediction of body density in young and middle-aged men. *J. Appl. Physiol.* 40: 300.
6. Parizkova, J. 1974. Body composition and exercise during growth and development. In: *Physical Activity: Human Growth and Development*. G. L. Rarick, ed. New York: Academic Press.
7. Chien, S., et al. 1975. Longitudinal measurements of blood volume and essential body mass in human subjects. *J. Appl. Physiol.* 39: 818.
8. Pollock, M. L. 1974. Physiological characteristics of champion american track athletes, 40 to 75 years of age. *J. Gerontology* 29: 645.

9. Stunkard, A. J. and McLaren-Hume, M. 1959. The results of treatment of obesity: a review of the literature and report of a series. *Arch. Int. Med.* 103:79.
10. Rabkin, S. W., et al. 1977. Relation of body weight to the development of Ischemic heart disease in a cohort of young North American men after a 26 year observation period: The manitoba study. *Amer. J. Cardiol.* 39: 452.
11. Keys, A. 1975. Coronary heart disease: the global picture. *Atherosclerosis*, 22: 149.
12. Spain, D. M., et al. 1963. Weight, body type, and prevalence of atherosclerotic heart disease in males. *Am. J. Med. Sci.* 245: 63.
13. Cramer, K., et al. 1966. Coronary angiographic findings in correlation with age, body weight, blood pressure, serum lipids, and smoking habits. *Circulation* 33: 888.
14. Keys, A. 1970. Physical activity and the epidemiology of CHD. In: *Physical Activity and Aging, Medicine and Sport.* D. Brunner, ed. University Park Press.
15. Bray, G. A. and Beltune, J. E. 1974. *Treatment and Management of Obesity.* New York: Harper & Row.
16. Angel, A. 1978. Pathophysiologic changes in obesity. *Can. Med. Assoc. J.* 119: 1401.
17. Angel, A. and Roncari, D. A. K. 1978. Medical complications of obesity. *Can. Med. Assoc. J.* 119: 1408.
18. Grande, F. 1961. Nutrition and energy balance in body composition studies. In: *Techniques for Measuring Body Composition.* Washington, D. C.: National Academy of Sciences, National Research Council.
19. Miller, D. S. and Parsonage, S. 1975. Resistance to slimming: adaptation or illusion. *Lancet* 1: 773.
20. Appelbaum, N. 1975. Influences of level of energy intake on energy expenditure in man. In: *Obesity in Perspective.* G. Bray, ed. Washington, D.C.: U. S. Government Printing Office.
21. Warnold, I., et al. 1978. Energy expenditure and body composition during weight reduction in hyperplastic obese women. *Am. J. Clin. Nutr.* 31: 750.
22. Smith, N. J. 1976. *Food for Sport.* Palo Alto, Calif.: Bull Publishing Co.
23. Drenick, E. J. and Johnson, D. 1977. Therapeutic fasting in morbid obesity—long term follow-up. *Arch. Int. Med.* 13: 1381.
24. Drenick, E. J. 1975. Weight reduction by prolonged fasting. In; *Obesity in Perspective.* G. Bray, ed. Bethesda, Maryland: United States Department of Health, Education, and Welfare.
25. Keys, A., et al. 1970. *The Biology of Human Starvation.* Minneapolis, Minn.: University of Minnesota Press.
26. Oscai, L. B. 1973. The role of exercise in weight control. In: *Exercise and Sports Sciences Reviews.* J. H. Wilmore, ed. New York: Academic Press.
27. Bergstrom, J., et al. 1967. Diet, muscle glycogen, and physical performance. *Acta. Physiol. Scand.* 71: 140.
28. Linn, R. and Stuart, S. L. 1977. *The Last Chance Diet.* New York: Bantam Books.
29. McArdle, W. D., et al. 1981. *Exercise Physiology: Energy, Nutrition and Human Performance.* Philadelphia: Lea and Febiger.

30. Van Itallie, T. B. and Yang, M. V. 1977. Diet and weight loss. *New Engl. J. Med.* 297: 1158.
31. Ball, M. F., et al. 1967. Comparative effects of caloric restriction and total starvation on body composition in obesity. *Ann. Int. Med.* 67: 30.
32. Bistrian, B. R., et al. 1977. Metabolic aspects of a protein-sparing fast in the dietary management of Prader-Willi obesity. *New Engl. J. Med.* 296: 774.
33. Bistrian, B. R., et al. 1976. Nitrogen metabolism and insulin requirements in obese diabetic adults on a protein-sparing modified fast. *Diabetes* 25: 494.
34. Mann, G. V., et al. 1977. Diet and obesity. *New Engl. J. Med.* 296: 812.
35. Zuti, W. B. and Golding, L. A. 1976. Comparing diet and exercise as weight reduction tools. *Physician Sportsmed.* 4: 49.
36. Costill, D. L. 1979. Interaction of skeletal muscle metabolism and hyperlipidemia in diabetics. In: *Heart Disease and Rehabilitation.* M. L. Pollock and D. H. Schmidt, eds. Boston: Houghton Mifflin.
37. Marliss, B. 1978 . Protein diets for obesity: metabolic and clinical aspects. *Can. Med. Assoc. J.* 119: 1413.
38. Cyborski, C. K. 1978. Deaths associated with the protein-sparing diet. *JAMA* 239: 971.
39. Azar, G. J. and Bloom, W. L. 1963. Similarities of carbohydrate deficiency and fasting. II. Ketones, nonesterified fatty acids, and nitrogen excretion. *Arch. Int. Med.* 112: 338.
40. Yudkin, J. and Craig, M. 1960. The treatment of obesity by the high-fat diet. The inevitability of calories. *Lancet* 2: 939.
41. Lewis, S. B., et al. 1977. Effect of diet composition on metabolic adaptations to hypocaloric nutrition: Comparison of high carbohydrate and high fat isocaloric diets. *Amer. J. Clin. Nutr.* 30: 160.
42. American Medical Association. 1973. A critique of low-carbohydrate ketogenic weight reduction regimens (A review of Dr. Atkins' diet revolution). *JAMA* 224: 1418.
43. Felig, P. and Wahren, J. 1971. Amino acid metabolism in exercising man. *J. Clin. Invest.* 50: 2703.
44. Kinsel, L. W., et al. 1964. Calories do count. *Metabolism* 3: 195.
45. Chirico, A. M. and Stunkard, A. J. 1976. Physical activity and human obesity. *New Engl. J. Med.* 263: 935.
46. Beaton, G., et al. 1979. An examination of factors believed to be associated with infantile obesity. *Amer. J. Clin. Nutr.* 32: 1997.
47. Hollenberg, C. H. 1978. Human obesity—a survey and suggestion. *Can. Med. Assoc. J.* 199: 1383.
48. Bullen, B. A., et al. 1964. Physical activity of obese and non-obese adolescent girls appraised by motion picture sampling. *Amer. J. Clin. Nutr.* 14: 211.
49. Huenemann, R. 1972. Food habits of obese and non-obese adolescents. *Postgrad. Med.* 51: 99.
50. Stefanik, P. A., et al. 1959. Caloric intake in relation to energy output of obese and non-obese adolescent boys. *Amer. J. Clin. Nutr.* 12: 55.
51. Wolley, S. C., et al. 1979. Theoretical, practical, and social issues in behavioral treatments of obesity. *J. Appl. Behav. Anal.* 12: 3.
52. Mayer, J. 1968. *Overweight, Causes, Cost and Control.* Englewood Cliffs, N.J.: Prentice-Hall.

53. Epstein, L. H. and Wing, R. R. 1980. Aerobic exercise and weight. *Addictive Behaviors* 5: 371.
54. Karvonen, M., et al. 1954. Consumption and selection of food in competitive lumber work. *J. Appl. Physiol.* 5: 603.
55. Ward, P., et al. 1978. USA discus camp: preliminary report. *Track & Field Quarterly Rev.* 76: 29.
56. Wilmore, J. H. and Brown, C. H. 1974. Physiological profiles of women distance runners. *Med. Sci. Sports* 6: 178.
57. Dempsey, J. A. 1964. Anthropological observations on obese and non-obese adolescent girls appraised by motion picture sampling. *Res. Quart.* 37: 275.
58. Jankowski, L. and Foss, M. 1972. The energy intake of sedentary men after moderate exercise. *Med. Sci. Sports* 4: 11.
59. Katch, F. I. 1969. Effects of physical training on the body composition and diet of females. *Res. Quart.* 99.
60. Bray, G. 1969. Effect of caloric restriction on energy expenditure in obese subjects. *Lancet* 2: 397.
61. Mayer, J., et al. 1954. Exercise, food intake and body weight in normal rats and genetically obese adult mice. *Am. J. Physiol.* 177: 544.
62. Mayer, J., et al. 1956. Relation between caloric intake, body weight and physical work in an industrial male population in West Bengal. *Am. J. Clin. Nutr.* 9: 169.
63. Johnson, R. E., et al. 1972. Exercise, dietary intake and body composition. *J. Am. Dietetic Assoc.* 61: 399.
64. Leon, A. S., et al. 1979. Effects of a vigorous walking program on body composition, and carbohydrate and lipid metabolism of obese young men. *Am. J. Clin. Nutr.* 32: 1776.
65. Passmore, R. and Durnin, J. V. G. A. 1955. Human energy expenditure. *Physiol. Rev.* 35: 801.
66. Katch, F. I. and McArdle, W. D. 1977. *Nutrition, Weight Control and Exercise.* Boston: Houghton Mifflin.
67. McArdle, W. D. and Magel, J. R. 1970. Physical work capacity and maximum oxygen uptake in treadmill and bicycle exercise. *Med. Sci. Sports* 2: 118.
68. Moody, D. L., et al. 1969. The effect of a moderate exercise program on body weight and skinfold thickness in overweight college women. *Med. Sci. Sports.* 17: 75.
69. Boileau, R. A. 1971. Body composition changes in obese and lean men during physical conditioning. *Med. Sci. Sports* 3: 183.
70. Gettman, L. R., et al. 1976. Physiological responses of young men to 1, 3, and 5 day per week training programs. *Res. Quart.* 47: 638.
71. Milesis, C. A., et al. 1976. Effects of different durations of physical training on cardiorespiratory function, body composition and serum lipids. *Res. Quart.* 47: 716.
72. Amsterdam, E. A., et al., eds. 1977. *Exercise in Cardiovascular Health and Disease.* New York: Yorke Medical Books.
73. Pollock, M. L. and Schmidt, D. H., eds. 1979. *Heart Disease and Rehabilitation.* Boston: Houghton Mifflin.
74. Ehsani, A. A., et al. 1981. Effects of 12 months of intense exercise training on ischemic ST-segment degression in patients with coronary artery disease. *Circulation* 64: 1116.
75. Pollock, M. L., et al. 1975. Effects of mode of training on cardiovascular function and body composition of adult men. *Med. Sci. Sports* 7: 139.

76. Gwinup, G. 1975. Effect of exercise alone on the weight loss of obese women. *Arch. Int. Med.* 135: 676.
77. Pollock, M. L. 1973. The quantification of endurance training programs. In: *Exercise and Sport Sciences Reviews.* vol 1., J. H. Wilmore, ed. New York: Academic Press.
78. Foss, M. L., et al. 1977. Physical training program for rehabilitating extremely obese patients. *Arch. Int. Med.* 137: 1381.
79. Carter, J. E. L. and Phillips, W. H. 1969. Structural changes in exercising middle-aged males during a 2-year period. *J. Appl. Physiol.* 27: 787.
80. Pollock, M. L., et al. 1975. Frequency of training as a determinant for improvement in cardiovascular function and body composition of middle-aged men. *Arch. Phys. Med. Rehabil.* 56: 141.
81. Pollock, M. L., et al. 1978. *Health and Fitness Through Physical Activity.* New York: John Wiley & Sons.
82. American College of Sports Medicine. 1978. The recommended quantity and quality of exercise for developing and maintaining fitness in healthy adults. *Med. Sci. Sports* 10: VII.
83. Wilmore, J. H. 1974. Alterations in strength, body composition and anthropometric measurements consequent to a 10-week weight training program. *Med. Sci. Sports* 6: 133.
84. Mayhew, J. L. and Gross, P. M. 1974. Body composition changes in young women with high resistance weight training. *Res. Quart.* 45: 433.
85. McArdle, W. D. and Foglia, G. F. 1969. Energy cost and cardiorespiratory stress of isometric and weight training exercises. *J. Sports Med. and Phys. Fitness* 9: 23.
86. Gettman, L. R. and Pollock, M. L. 1981. Circuit weight training: a critical review of its physiological benefits. *Physician Sportsmed.* 9: 44.
87. Wilmore, J. H., et al. 1978. Energy cost of circuit weight training. *Med. Sci. Sports* 10: 75.
88. Wilmore, J. H., et al. 1978. Physiological alterations consequent to circuit weight training. *Med. Sci. Sports* 10: 79.
89. Gettman, L. R., et al. 1978. The effects of circuit weight training on strength, cardiorespiratory function, and body composition of adult men. *Med. Sci. Sports* 10: 171.
90. Gettman, L. R., et al. 1982. A comparison of combined running and weight training with circuit weight training. *Med. Sci. Sports Exercise* 14: 229.
91. Moody, D. L., et al. 1972. The effect of a jogging program on the body composition of normal and obese high school girls. *Med. Sci. Sports* 4: 210.
92. Stalonas, P. M., et al. 1978. Behavior modification for obesity: the evaluation of exercise, contingency management and program adherence. *J. Consult. Clin. Psychol.* 46: 463.
93. Dahlkoetler, J., et al. 1979. Obesity and the unbalanced energy equation: Exercise versus eating habit change. *J. Consult. Clin. Psychol.* 47: 898.
94. Oscai, L. B. and Holloszy, J. O. 1969. Effects of weight changes produced by exercise, food restriction, or overeating on body composition. *J. Clin. Invest.* 48: 2124.
95. Benoit, B. L., et al. 1965. Changes in body composition during weight reduction in obesity. *Ann. Int. Med.* 63: 604.

96. Franklin, B. A., et al. 1979. Effects of physical conditioning on cardio-respiratory function, body composition, and serum lipids in relatively normal weight and obese middle-aged women. *Int. J. Obes.* 3: 97.
97. Gilder, H., et al. 1967. Components of weight loss in obese patients subjected to prolonged starvation. *J. Appl. Physiol.* 23: 304.
98. Paul, P. and Holmes, W. L. 1975. Free fatty acid and glucose metabolism during increased energy expenditure and after training. *Med. Sci. Sports* 7: 176.
99. Goldberg, A. L., et al. 1975. Mechanism of work-induced hypertrophy of skeletal muscle. *Med. Sci. Sports* 7: 185.
100. Felig, P. and Wahren, J. 1971. Amino acid metabolism in exercising man. *J. Clin. Invest.* 50: 2703.
101. Felig, P. and Wahren, J. 1975. Fuel homeostasis in exercise. *New Engl. J. Med.* 293: 1078.
102. Gwinup, G., et al. 1971. Thickness of subcutaneous fat and activity of underlying muscles. *Ann. Int. Med.* 74: 408.
103. Carns, M., et al. 1960. Semental volume reduction by localized versus generalized exercise. *Human Biol.* 32: 370.
104. Schade, F. A., et al., 1962. Spot reducing in overweight college women. *Res. Quart.* 33: 461.
105. Noland, M. and Kearney, J. T. 1978. Anthropometric and densitometric responses of women to specific and general exercise. *Res. Quart.* 49: 322.

6

PHYSIOLOGICAL DIFFERENCES
BETWEEN STARCHES AND SUGARS

SHELDON REISER, PH.D.

Introduction

CARBOHYDRATES are composed primarily of carbon, hydrogen and oxygen in the proportion of CH_2O, hence the name carbohydrate. Carbohydrates are classified as either simple or complex, depending on the number of monosaccharide units in the molecule. Simple carbohydrates are usually composed of mono- or disaccharides. They are also referred to as sugars, although to the nonscientific public the term sugar is usually reserved for the disaccharide sucrose. Complex carbohydrates such as starches may contain thousands of monosaccharide units.

Dietary carbohydrate supplies a large proportion of the caloric requirements of man. In the developing countries (i.e., not Western Europe, North America, Japan, Israel, Australia or South Africa) as much as 80 percent of the total calories consumed is carbohydrate. In societies described as developed (i.e., the more industrialized countries), carbohydrate supplies about 50 percent of the total caloric intake. The commonest forms of dietary carbohydrate are starch and sucrose. Changes in the pattern of dietary carbohydrate intake appear to be characteristic of societies as they become more industrialized. In the United States, the percent of total dietary carbohydrate provided by sugars (predominantly sucrose) as compared to starch has increased from 32 percent to more than 50 percent between 1910 and 1972.[1] Sucrose is believed to contribute 15 to 20 percent of the calories in the present American diet.[2,3] The combined average fructose intake in the United States is probably about 70 g/day. With increased intake

133

of high fructose corn sweeteners in the American diet, the proportion of this sugar can be expected to increase.

The impact on health of this pattern of carbohydrate consumption in developed societies has become the object of concern. Dietary factors are believed to influence the characteristics and prevalence of diseases.[4] In societies such as ours in the United States where degenerative diseases such as heart disease and diabetes are common, a diet typically high in total and saturated fat, cholesterol, sucrose and salt and low in starch and fiber is consumed. Suggested modifications of this diet have included a decrease in the consumption of refined and processed sugar and replacement of the sugar by carbohydrates rich in starch.[4,5]

This chapter will describe some of the metabolic and physiologic effects observed after feeding starch as compared to sugars such as sucrose, fructose and glucose to experimental animals and humans. Major emphasis will be placed on the effects that influence those metabolic parameters considered to be risk factors associated with degenerative diseases such as heart disease and diabetes. In addition, differences in metabolic effects observed after feeding sugars such as sucrose, fructose and glucose will be described. The influences of other environmental factors and of genetic factors in assessing the metabolic effects of the carbohydrates will be evaluated. Mechanisms proposed to explain observed differences in metabolic effects will be discussed.

Intestinal Events

Digestion

Starch is the major dietary polysaccharide ingested by man. Glycogen may also contribute somewhat to the total intake of digestible polysaccharide. The process of starch digestion is facilitated by cooking food, a process that ruptures the starch granules and facilitates subsequent enzyme hydrolysis. Despite the presence of α-amylase in the saliva, the major digestion of dietary polysaccharide occurs in the small intestine by the action of pancreatic α-amylase. Pancreatic amylase initially splits the interior α-1,4 glucose linkages of starch and glycogen, producing oligosaccharides. The final products of the action of α-amylase on amylose are maltose and maltotriose.[6] Since α-amylase is unable to hydrolyze the α-1,6 branching points and α-1,4 linkages adjacent to the branching points,[6] the end products of amylopectin and glycogen hydrolysis by α-amylase also include low molecular weight branched oligosaccharides.[7] The final digestion of the oligosaccharides and disaccharides formed from the action of α-amylase on polysaccharides is mediated by enzymes found in the brush border membrane of the intestinal epithelial cell.

The digestion of the major dietary sugar, sucrose, is mediated by sucrase, an enzyme present at the external surface of the brush border membrane of intestinal epithelial cells.[8] It appears that the small intestines of animals and humans can adapt to various nutritional and physiologic stresses with changes in digestive and absorptive activities. The feeding of diets containing high levels of sucrose has been shown to produce an adaptive increase in sucrase activity in both experimental animals and humans. Rats starved for three days and then refed a diet containing 70 percent sucrose for twenty-four hours showed greater levels of sucrase activity than did rats refed a sucrose-free, high casein diet.[9] Rats starved for three days and then refed a diet containing 68 percent sucrose for twenty-four hours had significantly greater levels of sucrase activity than did rats refed a diet different only in that maltose replaced sucrose.[10] Sucrase activity in rats fed diets containing 70 percent carbohydrate was greater with sucrose than with either maltose or glucose.[11] Feeding diets containing 40–80 percent of the calories as sucrose or fructose, compared with glucose, increased the activity of sucrase and maltase, but not of lactase, in human small intestine.[12,13] The increase in maltase activity due to sucrose or fructose feeding can be attributed to the maltolytic activity of intestinal sucrase.[14]

From these intestinal events it can be concluded that the digestion of the high molecular weight starch is a much slower process than is the digestion of the sugar sucrose. It would, therefore, be expected that the carbohydrate components of a diet containing sucrose would become available for absorption much more quickly than those from a diet containing starch.

Absorption

The absorption of glucose and galactose liberated from dietary carbohydrates or found as such in the diet is mediated by a structurally specific binding site or carrier located on the brush border of the intestinal epithelial cell. This site also has affinity for Na^+. The process is energized by the maintenance of a disequilibrium between intracellular and extracellular Na^+ at the expense of ATP.[15] Fructose absorption in mammalian intestine is mediated by a relatively specific carrier mechanism with properties distinct from those of the carrier utilized by other monosaccharides.[16,17] In general, fructose absorption has been found to be a Na^+-independent process that is not inhibited by phlorizin or glucose. There is also evidence for the existence of a specific absorption process, different from that used by monosaccharides, for the transport of monosaccharides derived from disaccharides such as sucrose and maltose.[18,19]

These intestinal absorption processes also appear to be influenced by the nature of the dietary carbohydrate. Rats accustomed to being fed a 65 percent sucrose diet showed significant increases in the intestinal transport of glucose, fructose and sucrose as compared with rats fed a stock diet.[20] The ad libitum or meal-feeding of diets containing 54 percent sucrose as compared to 54 percent starch to rats for eight to twelve weeks produced similar increases in sugar absorption.[21] Sucrose, however, produced greater increases in sugar absorption when compared to a natural stock diet[20] than when compared to a starch-containing synthetic diet.[21] The difference in the magnitude of the increase in transport after sucrose feeding in these two studies was due to the higher levels of sugar absorption found in the starch-fed than in the stock-fed rats. The synthetic diets contained 4 percent cellulose, as compared to the 6 percent mixed fiber in the natural diet. The well-documented modulating action of dietary fiber on sugar absorption[22] could be responsible for the lower sugar transport in rats fed the stock diet. In a study utilizing baboons, the absorption capability for fructose, and to a lesser extent glucose, following a sucrose meal was greater after adaptation to a 75 percent sucrose diet for nine weeks.[23]

A possible mechanism by which sucrose feeding can produce the observed increases in the intestinal absorption of sucrose and its component monosaccharides is based on the relationships between sucrase and the sugar transport systems. The translocation of sucrose across an artificial lipid membrane was much faster when the membrane also contained the sucrase-isomaltase enzyme complex.[24] This finding suggests that the sucrase-isomaltase complex, which is shown to be increased due to sucrose feeding, has the property of a transport carrier specific for sucrose or its constituent monosaccharides. Added support for a role of sucrase in the absorptive process comes from the findings that not only is sucrase activated by Na^+,[25] but the kinetic properties of the Na^+ activation resemble the kinetic properties of the interaction of Na^+ with the glucose absorption carrier.[26]

The process mediating the absorption of fructose appears to be particularly responsive to dietary adaptation. A twofold increase in fructose absorption was demonstrated after only three days in rats fed a 60 percent fructose diet as compared to rats fed a stock diet.[27] The feeding of diets containing either 70 percent sucrose or fructose, but not glucose, increased the intestinal absorption of fructose in rats.[28] In this study, glucose absorption was not affected by the type of dietary carbohydrate.

Gastrointestinal hormones

An enteric factor is involved in carbohydrate metabolism since a dose of glucose given orally elicits a significantly greater insulin secretory response than does the same dose of glucose given intravenously.[29] The term "entero-insular axis" has been used to describe the influence of intestinal hormones on the insulin-secreting activity of the pancreas.[30] It has been suggested that defects in the entero-insular axis may contribute to the pathogenesis of diabetes.[30,31] Gastric inhibitory polypeptide (GIP), a hormone secreted from the upper small intestine[32] after ingestion of various dietary components, is considered to play an important role in the entero-insular axis.[33] GIP has been found to enhance pancreatic insulin secretion during states of relative hyperglycemia (e.g., in response to a carbohydrate meal).[34] It was found that the GIP response of humans after a sucrose load (2 g/kg body weight) was significantly greater after they consumed a diet containing 30 percent sucrose as compared to 30 percent wheat starch for six weeks.[35] Since glucose absorbed in the proximal intestine is a more efficient secretagogue for GIP than is glucose absorbed more distally in the intestine,[36] the more rapid absorption of glucose after a sucrose load in sucrose-adapted as compared to starch-adapted mammals might partially explain the enhanced levels of GIP in the sucrose-adapted subjects. It was also found that the magnitude of the GIP response to the oral sucrose load was more than double that reported after an oral glucose load.[35,37] The greater GIP response after the ingestion of sucrose could not be explained on the basis of differing amounts of glucose given in the tolerance tests.

Disaccharide effect

The finding that sucrose is a much more efficient secretagogue for GIP than is glucose might explain some of the metabolic differences observed after feeding sucrose and other carbohydrates. For example, there are a number of studies with both rats and humans indicating that the metabolic effects of disaccharides such as sucrose and maltose are different from those of their component monosaccharides. Michaelis and Szepesi have referred to this response as a "disaccharide effect."[38] The activities of various hepatic lipogenic enzymes were greater in rats starved for two days and then refed diets containing 31 percent or 40 percent sucrose as compared to invert sugar.[38,39] Rats meal-fed diets containing 45 percent sucrose or maltose as compared to an equivalent amount of the constituent monosaccharides for two weeks showed significant increases in fasting serum insulin and food efficiency.[40] Rats fed diets containing 60 percent sucrose *ad libitum* for two weeks showed differences in the activities of hepatic aromatic hydroxylases and of cytochrome P-450 as compared to rats fed the same amount of invert sugar.[41] The insulinogenic index (Σ Insulin/Σ Glucose, 0-180 minutes) of obese women with mild glucose intolerance was significantly higher after an oral load of sucrose than after a load of equal amounts of invert sugar.[42] The mean twenty-four-hour integrated concentration of plasma triglyceride was significantly greater after normal young male volunteers had consumed for ten days a liquid diet in which sucrose, rather than an equivalent amount of glucose and fructose, provided 22.5 percent of the calories.[43] These findings indicate that the effects observed after sucrose feeding cannot be attributed entirely to the metabolic effects of the component monosaccharides. Since the disaccharides are believed to be hydrolyzed prior to or during their intestinal absorption, these findings indicate that the disaccharides have a specific effect at the intestinal level not shared by the monosaccharides. It is possible that the disaccharides and monosaccharides differ in their capacity to act at an enteric receptor site as a secretagogue for intestinal hormones such as GIP. An increased insulin response to dietary disaccharide mediated through GIP would explain many of the metabolic differences noted in the studies described in this section.

Physiological implications

The intestinal events described suggest the following:

a) The liberation of glucose and fructose from sucrose and the subsequent absorption of these monosaccharides are much more rapid and efficient processes than are the liberation and absorption of glucose from starch.

b) Adaptation to sucrose feeding would further increase the digestive and absorptive efficiency of the small intestine for sucrose and its component monosaccharides and increase the activity of at least one enteric hormone involved in mediating pancreatic insulin secretion (i.e., GIP).

The resultant steep increases in postprandial blood glucose with the associated strong stimulation of the insulin response following sucrose feeding might produce a chronic hyperinsulinism, which would decrease insulin sensitivity and eventually might impair the insulin-producing system and lead to symptoms of diabetes.

The initial period of hyperinsulinism could signal a pattern of enzyme inductions that would direct the pathway of carbohydrate metabolism toward increased lipogenesis. Many of the experimental findings to be presented in subsequent sections of this chapter appear to be consistent with such a series of events.

Glucose Tolerance

Although diagnosis of clinical glucose intolerance and diabetes is based on elevations in fasting and postprandial blood glucose levels, blood insulin levels may be a more sensitive indicator of impairment of glucose tolerance. Elevated insulin levels in response to a glycemic stress have been associated with mild maturity-onset diabetes and are considered to be one of the earliest detectable signs of diabetes.[44,45] Recent population studies in Finland[46] and Australia[47] have shown that hyperinsulinism is an independent risk factor for coronary heart disease. These epidemiological observations are in accord with experimental evidence showing that the arterial wall is an insulin sensitive tissue and responds to high levels of insulin with the development of lipid-filled lesions.[48] The findings of increased incidence of atherosclerotic disease in patients with impaired glucose tolerance[49] and abnormal glucose tolerance in many patients with cardiovascular disease[50] suggest a relationship between these diseases which may be due to hyperinsulinism. Reduced insulin sensitivity has been postulated to be the primary step that leads to hyperinsulinemia and then hypertriglyceridemia.[51] In this section the effects of dietary carbohydrates on blood insulin and glucose and on insulin sensitivity will be described and the implications of these effects discussed as they pertain to the relevant disease states.

Responses to different carbohydrates

In accordance with the material presented in the section on intestinal events, the acute intake of sucrose, as compared to starch, in both experimental animals and humans has generally resulted in more rapid and greater responses of blood insulin and, to a lesser extent, blood glucose. Naismith and Rana[52] measured changes in the concentration of reducing sugars in the blood over a period of thirty minutes following the feeding of 2 grams of synthetic diets containing 60 percent carbohydrate to rats adapted to these diets. After both five and ten minutes the blood sugar of the rats fed a sucrose diet had risen about twice as fast as in rats fed the starch diet. Serum insulin responses of rats thirty minutes and four hours after a meal of a diet containing 54 percent sucrose was significantly higher than after a meal of a diet containing 54 percent starch.[53] Glucose response was not determined in this study. In a similar study in which insulin and glucose responses of rats to high fat diets containing either 30 percent sucrose or starch were determined, insulin levels were significantly greater thirty minutes and three hours after sucrose was fed than after starch was fed.[54] Serum glucose levels were not affected by the diet. These results indicate that there was a decrease in insulin sensitivity when the rats consumed the sucrose diet. The effects of sucrose, glucose and starch on plasma insulin and glucose responses were determined in nineteen normal human volunteers after ingestion of drinks or meals calculated to contain 50 grams of glucose.[55] It was found that at all sampling times up to sixty minutes after the drink or meal, glucose and insulin responses were 35–65 percent lower when starch was the carbohydrate source than when either glucose or sucrose was the carbohydrate source. The plasma insulin curve was about 20 percent higher after the sucrose drink than after the glucose drink with significant differences at thirty and 120 minutes. Similar findings were observed 120 and 180 minutes following the sucrose and glucose meals. These results suggest that sucrose produces a greater insulin response than does glucose on a molar basis. Although a greater insulin response to sucrose as compared to glucose was reported in rats,[56] results from other human studies have shown greater insulin responses following the feeding of glucose[57] or corn syrup with a dextrose equivalent of forty-two[58] than after the feeding of sucrose.

Rat feeding studies

Many studies with rats have shown that the feeding of high levels of sucrose, as compared to starch, produces an impairment of glucose tolerance, an increase in fasting blood insulin levels and a decrease in the tissue sensitivity to insulin. These metabolic changes are characteristic of the symptomology found in maturity-onset diabetes. Rats fed diets containing 67 percent sucrose, as compared to 67 percent starch, for twenty-one days showed increased levels of blood glucose thirty, sixty, and ninety minutes following an intragastric glucose load.[59] Increases in blood glucose were also observed after forty days of feeding a 40 percent sucrose diet and after fifty to one hundred days of feeding a 33 percent sucrose diet. Rats fed diets containing 70 percent sucrose, as compared to 70 percent starch, for fifty days exhibited a decreased adipose tissue sensitivity to insulin without increased levels of blood insulin.[60] Rats fed diets containing 65 percent[20] and 68 percent[61] sucrose for four to eleven weeks showed increased levels of fasting serum insulin when compared to rats fed a stock diet. In the latter study, a decreased insulin sensitivity of adipose tissue and diaphragm was also noted in the sucrose-fed rats. The *ad libitum* or meal-feeding of diets containing 54 percent sucrose, as compared to 54 percent starch, for twelve to seventeen weeks resulted in increased levels of fasting serum insulin and decreased insulin sensitivity of adipose tissue.[62] Meal-fed rats consuming a diet containing 56 percent sucrose, as compared to 56 percent glucose, for twenty-four days showed increased blood glucose levels sixty, ninety and one hundred and twenty minutes following a glucose tolerance test.[63] Feeding rats sucrose, as compared to starch, has been reported to have a distinct stimulatory action on the secretion of insulin by isolated pancreas perfused with glucose.[64] Both the glucose and insulin responses to an oral glucose tolerance test were significantly greater after rats had been fed a diet containing 70 percent sucrose as compared to 70 percent starch for four to six weeks.[65] Serum glucose levels following an intraperitoneal glucose tolerance test were significantly higher in rats adapted to a 54 percent sucrose diet than in rats adapted to a 54 percent starch diet for eleven to thirteen weeks.[53] The sucrose-fed rats also exhibited a relative insensitivity to exogenous insulin. The insulin response, but not the glucose response, to an oral glucose tolerance test was significantly higher in rats fed a high-fat diet containing 30 percent sucrose, as compared to 30 percent starch, for eight to nine weeks.[54]

The strongest experimental evidence that sucrose is an etiological factor in diabetes has come from the work of Aharon Cohen using genetically selected rats.[66] Rats were bred on the basis of blood glucose levels following an intragastric glucose tolerance test. Animals with the greatest increase in blood glucose (Upward selection) were mated and those with the smallest increase (Downward selection) were mated. In succeeding generations of the Upward selection fed a diet containing 72 percent sucrose, the rats developed diabetes-like symptoms including high fasting blood sugar, hyperinsulinemia, peripheral insulin resistance and retinal and renal vascular complications. This effect could be demonstrated with as little as 25 percent dietary sucrose fed over more extended time periods. In contrast, sibling rats of the Upward selection fed a diet containing 72 percent starch did not show these symptoms. In the offspring of the Downward selection, the diabetes-like symptoms did not appear in rats fed either the 72 percent sucrose or starch diets. These results show that in these rats the interaction between genetic and dietary factors was required for the expression of the metabolic defects characteristic of diabetes and suggest that similar interactions might influence the expression of such defects in humans.

Effects of fructose on glucose tolerance

The undesirable effects of sucrose on parameters of glucose tolerance appear to be due, at least partly, to the metabolic properties of the fructose moiety. The feeding of either sucrose[67,68] or fructose,[69] as compared to glucose or glucose polymers, has been shown to increase the activity of glucose-6-phosphatase in the liver of rats. The increased activity of glucose-6-phosphatase is not compatible with the efficient utilization of glucose via tissue phosphorylation. The activities of other gluconeogenic enzymes were also reported to be increased in rats fed fructose as compared to starch.[70] There also appears to be a depressed metabolism of glucose by the liver of rats adapted to the feeding of sucrose or fructose as compared with starch.[71] This depression is probably the result of the enhancement of the activity of fructokinase[72,73] and the impairment of glucokinase[74,75] by dietary sucrose or fructose. Enhancement of fructokinase activity would be expected to decrease the levels of hepatic ATP required for the phosphorylation of circulating glucose.

The hyperinsulinism associated with the feeding of sucrose as compared to starch may be due to an increased insulin requirement to compensate for a decreased insulin binding. Fructose infusion in humans[76] and in rats[77,78] has been shown to produce large decreases in the ATP content of the liver. Fructose may then contribute to a decrease in the cellular binding of insulin by decreasing cellular levels of cyclic AMP which have been shown to increase the concentration of insulin receptors in cultured cells.[79] Inadequate insulin binding could also be due to a decreased protein synthesis caused by the depletion of ATP.

These metabolic properties of fructose may explain findings from a number of recent studies which show that the feeding of fructose, as compared to starch or glucose, produces undesirable effects on parameters of glucose tolerance in both experimental animals and humans. Rats genetically susceptible to diabetes[66] showed a diabetic response to a glucose tolerance test and diffuse glomerulosclerosis when fed a diet containing 72 percent fructose for two months.[80] Siblings of these rats fed an identical diet containing 72 percent cornstarch did not develop these metabolic and histopathological defects. Plasma insulin levels six hours after removal of food from rats fed 66 percent of calories from fructose for one week were significantly higher than insulin levels of rats fed an identical diet containing 66 percent of calories from glucose.[81]

No differences in plasma glucose concentrations due to dietary carbohydrate were found. In a subsequent study from the same laboratory,[82] the rats fed 66 percent fructose also exhibited significantly higher insulin responses during an oral glucose tolerance test than did rats fed a standard rat chow diet. A decrease in insulin-sensitivity of rats fed either 33 percent or 66 percent fructose as compared to the chow diet was also reported. In a study of the prolonged effects of moderate fructose levels on parameters of glucose tolerance, rats were fed diets containing either 54 percent cornstarch or 39 percent cornstarch plus 15 percent fructose for 15 months.[70] Fasting insulin, glucose and the insulin response to an oral glucose tolerance test were significantly greater in the fructose-fed rats after three, five, seven, nine and fifteen months. The glucose response to the tolerance test was not consistently affected by diet. These results suggest a decreased insulin sensitivity in the fructose-fed rats. Normal human volunteers fed their usual diet plus 1,000 Kcal of fructose per day for one week showed a significant reduction of both insulin binding to isolated monocytes and insulin sensitivity.[83] In contrast, the feeding of 1,000 Kcal per day of glucose under the same experimental conditions did not significantly change insulin binding or sensitivity. These findings that fructose adversely affects parameters of glucose tolerance are of particular importance since fructose is considered to belong to a group of polyols (e.g., sorbitol and xylitol) that can be safely consumed by diabetics. The major advantages of fructose over glucose intake by diabetics are that fructose is more slowly absorbed in the intestine and its uptake by the tissues is insulin independent. Fructose alone also appears to be a poor stimulus for insulin release.[84] However, acute loading studies have revealed the existence of a synergism between glucose and fructose with regard to insulin secretion. Neither fructose nor glucose, when given as the sole monosaccharide, stimulates insulin secretion as potently as glucose and fructose combined.[85,86] Since diets rarely contain fructose in the absence of glucose or glucose polymers, small amounts of fructose reaching the general circulation postprandially could greatly affect insulin secretion. On the basis of the findings reported in this section, the consumption of fructose by maturity-onset diabetics should be carefully controlled.

Human feeding studies

In many, but not all, studies in which humans were fed diets containing sucrose as compared to starch, indices of glucose tolerance were reported to be impaired. The glucose response to an

oral glucose tolerance test was significantly higher in fifteen normal humans who had consumed for five weeks a diet in which
most of the 66 percent of carbohydrate calories was supplied by
sucrose as compared to starch from bread.[87] Human volunteers
receiving 52 to 64 percent of the calories from sucrose, as compared to starch, for seven days had increased levels of insulin two
to eight minutes after the intravenous administration of 25 grams
of glucose. [88] Insulin levels sixty minutes after a glucose load were
significantly higher after young women had consumed for four
weeks a diet containing 42 percent of the calories as sucrose as
compared to glucose.[89] A synergistic effect appears to exist between the action of dietary sucrose on indices of glucose tolerance
and the use of oral contraceptives by women. Young women
taking oral contraceptives had significantly higher glucose and
insulin responses to a sucrose load after consuming for three
weeks a diet containing 43 percent of calories as sucrose as
compared to wheat starch.[90] Young women who had never taken
oral contraceptives did not show these dietary effects. Reiser et
al[91] reported that fasting serum insulin and glucose levels were
significantly higher when nineteen adult volunteers consumed
natural diets containing 30 percent of the calories as sucrose as
compared to wheat starch for six weeks. The insulin response one
hour after a sucrose load was significantly greater in the subjects
adapted to sucrose. No significant differences in glucose response
to the sucrose load as a function of dietary carbohydrate were
seen. Dunnigan et al[92] found that the isocaloric exchange of 32
percent of calories as starch by sucrose for four weeks produced
significant elevation in fasting blood glucose but had no effect on
insulin levels. The differences in insulin response to sucrose
feeding in the last two studies performed under similar experimental conditions may be due to the meal patterns employed. Reiser
et al[91] fed their diets in a gorging pattern (i.e., two meals per
day) while Dunnigan et al[92] fed their diets in three meals and
three snacks daily. Consumption of total calories in a few meals
(gorging) as compared to more numerous meals has been reported
to adversely affect glucose tolerance in humans.[93,94] A significant
reduction in both insulin binding to isolated monocytes and insulin sensitivity was found when twenty-four young volunteers
consumed their usual diets plus 1,000 kcal per day from sucrose
for two weeks.[95]

In contrast to these findings, glucose tolerance was not altered
in three subjects consuming carbohydrate either as sucrose or as
uncooked maize starch.[96] The isocaloric exchange of dietary sucrose and starch from potato and rice at 23 percent of the total

calories did not significantly alter fasting serum insulin or the insulin response to a meal in five volunteers.[97] Human volunteers changed from a solid control diet containing 40 percent calories as carbohydrate, 43 percent as fat and 17 percent as protein to a liquid diet containing 80 percent of calories as sucrose and 15 percent as protein showed significant improvement in the glycemic response to an oral glucose tolerance test.[98] The improvement in glucose tolerance was associated with a slight reduction in plasma insulin values. Since high fat diets have been reported to impair glucose tolerance parameters,[95,99,100] it is difficult to attribute the improvement of glucose tolerance to an increase in sucrose rather than a decrease in fat.

Genetic predisposition; carbohydrate sensitivity

The human dietary studies described above have attempted to utilize subjects representative of the general population. Due to the heterogeneity of the population, it is common to observe large differences in the response of subjects to a given dietary variable. For example, the intake of a self-selected diet in which the approximately 60 percent of calories from carbohydrates was mainly in the form of sucrose, as compared to starch, significantly increased fasting insulin and the insulin response to a glucose tolerance test in six of nineteen human volunteers.[101] The finding that a finite portion of the population is more sensitive to sucrose than is the general population is compatible with studies using rats that demonstrated that an interaction between genetic factors and sucrose intake was necessary for the expression of the metabolic defects characteristic of diabetes to become evident.[66] Members of one segment of the population appear to have a genetic predisposition that results in a large and nonadaptable increase in blood triglycerides when they consume diets that are high in carbohydrate, especially sucrose.[102] Those individuals have been called carbohydrate-sensitive because their lipemia appears to be carbohydrate induced.[102] This genetic predisposition is also associated with abnormal glucose tolerance.[103]

Previous studies on the effects of the intake of sucrose or fructose as compared to starch in subjects described as having carbohydrate-induced hyperlipemia or being carbohydrate-sensitive have concentrated on the effects on blood lipid, rather than on indices of glucose tolerance. Nine out of nineteen human subjects, defined as potentially carbohydrate-sensitive on the basis of fasting triglyceride levels above the normal range, were found to have insulin responses to a sucrose load that were 2.2 to 3.8 times greater than the insulin responses of ten noncarbohydrate-sensitive subjects.[91] The feeding of 30 percent sucrose, as compared to 30 percent wheat starch, produced increases in fasting insulin and in the insulin: glucose ratios that were of greater magnitude and level of significance in potentially carbohydrate-sensitive subjects than in the noncarbohydrate-sensitive subjects. The increase in the insulin response to a sucrose load found in the entire group of nineteen subjects fed the sucrose, as compared to starch, was entirely due to the response of the nine potentially carbohydrate-sensitive subjects. In a subsequent study,[104] twenty-four subjects classified as carbohydrate-sensitive on the basis of an exaggerated insulin response to a sucrose load showed significantly greater levels of fasting insulin and glucose and of the insulin response to a sucrose load after adaptation to diets containing either 18 percent or 33 percent of the calories as sucrose as compared to diets containing 5 percent of the calories as sucrose. The sucrose in this study was replaced isocalorically with purified wheat starch. These results indicate that the present level of sucrose consumption in this country may produce undesirable effects on parameters of glucose tolerance in carbohydrate-sensitive individuals. Nikkila[105] observed small increases in fasting blood glucose in subjects with mild-onset diabetes with and without hypertriglyceridemia when 80 to 100 grams per day of either sucrose or fructose replaced starch. Turner et al[106] reported no differences in either basal or response levels of plasma insulin and glucose after triglyceridemic men were fed fat-containing and fat-free formula diets in which studies difficult. Both sucrose and maltose have been shown to produce metabolic effects, including increases in fasting serum insulin[40] and the insulin response to a glucose tolerance test,[65] different from those of their component monosaccharides.

Physiological implications

Despite the numerous studies that have implicated the feeding of sucrose, as compared to starch, with impairment of indices of glucose tolerance, the present level of sucrose consumption is not generally accepted as a primary or significant factor in the incidence of diabetes in this country.[3,107,108] In some of the human studies, serious experimental defects have prevented clear-cut interpretation of the results. Generally, sucrose at levels greatly in excess of those presently consumed was fed for relatively short time periods. The question of how much sucrose to use in a finite study to simulate metabolic effects produced by exposure to sucrose over long time periods is difficult to answer. It appears that the feeding of up to 35 percent of calories as sucrose for time periods up to six weeks is reasonable and should give meaningful results considering the present level of sucrose consumption in this country. In addition, the premise that high levels of any dietary component could produce adverse effects and that, therefore, these adverse effects do not reflect a true dietary hazard is not necessarily valid. Studies with sucrose are comparative; the effects of a large amount of sucrose are compared to the effects of an equally large amount of another carbohydrate, usually starch. In addition, some individuals consume much more sucrose than the average.[1,3] Other experimental criticisms of some of the human studies have included comparison of the effects of sucrose to those of starch present in natural foods[22] and the consumption of self-selected instead of standardized diets.[102] Published data, nevertheless, when evaluated overall, support the contention that the substitution of complex dietary carbohydrates, such as starch, for simple sugars, such as sucrose, will improve glucose tolerance. For the 9 to 17 percent of the adult American population that may be carbohydrate-sensitive,[102,109,110] sucrose consumption appears to constitute a greater environmental hazard than for the general population and the present level of sucrose intake in this country may produce undesirable changes in metabolic parameters associated with glucose tolerance.

Lipid Metabolism

In man and rat, the liver appears to be a primary site of the synthesis of lipid from carbohydrate. Hepatic triglyceride synthesis and secretion are believed to be the major sources of endogenous hypertriglyceridemia in man.[51,111] Insulin appears to play an important role in hepatic lipogenesis. Numerous studies have shown a relationship between insulin levels, both fasting and in response to a glycemic stress, and blood triglyceride levels.[111] An elevated level of fasting blood triglycerides is generally considered to be a risk factor in the etiology of heart disease.[112–114] The important role of insulin in the formation of blood triglycerides is further evidence for the relationship between insulin and heart disease alluded to in the section on glucose tolerance. There is almost unanimous agreement among scientists that a correlation exists between cholesterol levels and the development of heart disease.[114] Elevation in the blood cholesterol associated with LDL and VLDL is considered to be a risk factor for heart disease.[115] Elevation of cholesterol associated with HDL is considered to be a protective factor against heart disease.[115] In this section, the effects of dietary carbohydrates on hepatic lipogenesis, blood triglycerides and blood cholesterol will be described and discussed in relation to the disease states involved.

Hepatic lipogenesis

The activities of various hepatic enzymes involved in the conversion of carbohydrate to lipid have been reported to be increased in rats fed sucrose as compared to an equivalent amount of glucose or glucose polymers. The increased activities of the lipogenic enzymes produced by sucrose feeding appear to be associated with an increased deposition of liver lipid.

Liver lipid was increased in rats fed diets containing approximately 80 percent sucrose as compared to diets containing an equivalent amount of either dextrin,[116] liquid glucose or dextrose,[117] or various starches.[118] The incorporation of radioactive acetate into total lipid and cholesterol was markedly greater in the liver of rats after twenty weeks of the *ad libitum* or meal-feeding of diets containing 70 percent sucrose as compared to 70 percent starch.[119] Weanling rats fed diets containing 58 percent sucrose as compared to starch for ten weeks had significantly higher incorporation of glucose-^{14}C and acetate-1-^{14}C into the cholesterol and neutral lipid fraction of liver.[120] Incorporation of acetate-2-^{14}C and ^3H_2O into liver fatty acids and palmitate-1-^{14}C into hepatic triglycerides was significantly greater in rats fed for two to three weeks a 70 percent sucrose diet than either a 70 percent glucose diet or a chow diet.[121] The activity of hepatic fatty acid synthase was reported to be quadrupled after only three days in rats changed from a starch diet to one containing 50 percent sucrose.[122] The activity of hepatic glucose-6-phosphate dehydrogenase,[20,52,68,69,123,124] malic enzyme,[20,69,123,124] pyruvic kinase[52,69,124] and total liver lipid[20,68,123] was increased in rats fed diets containing 50 to 72 percent sucrose as compared to diets containing an equivalent amount of starch or glucose. The increase in liver lipid[68] and hepatic lipogenic metabolites[125] due to sucrose feeding was greater in the carbohydrate-sensitive BHE strain of rat than in the Wistar strain. Hepatocytes isolated from rats fed a diet containing 30 percent sucrose as compared to a chow diet showed significant 4-fold increases in the incorporation of ^3H glycerol into VLDL triglycerides and significant 1.6-fold increases in the net secretion of VLDL triglyceride.[126] Since this effect could be demonstrated in hepatocytes cultured for as long as three days, these results show that the nutritional state of the animal can have long lasting effects on hepatic VLDL secretion. The need for the transport of greater amounts of lipid from the liver to adipose tissue may partially explain the higher levels of blood triglycerides observed in animals fed sucrose (see below).

Extensive studies using rats have shown that the feeding of diets containing at least 40 percent of the calories from fructose, as compared to equivalent amounts of glucose polymers or glucose, increases the levels of hepatic lipogenic enzymes[39,52,73,127–129] and liver lipid.[52,117,129–131] The similarity between these findings and those from sucrose diets indicates that the fructose moiety of sucrose may be primarily responsible for sucrose-induced hepatic lipogenesis. The hepatic metabolism of fructose favors a lipogenic pathway. Fructose is converted to fructose-1-phosphate by a fructokinase that has greater activity than either hexokinase or glucokinase[75] and shows an adaptive increase in activity after fructose-feeding.[72,73] Fructose-1-phosphate is then cleaved to dihydroxyacetone phosphate and glyceraldehyde by fructose-1-phosphate aldolase. Further metabolism of glyceraldehyde requires either phosphorylation to glyceraldehyde-3-phosphate, oxidative conversion to glyceric acid followed by phosphorylation, or reduction to glycerol followed by phosphorylation by glycerokinase to α-glycerophosphate, a direct precursor of triglyceride. This metabolic sequence effectively produces substrates required for lipogenesis and circumvents two important control mechanisms in hepatic glycolysis: the reactions catalyzed by hexokinase and phosphofructokinase. An enhanced hepatic lipogenic metabolism of fructose would also be compatible with the finding that high levels of fructose decrease hepatic glycogen synthesis.[132]

Studies in both rats and humans have demonstrated that fructose is more readily converted into lipogenic substrate than is glucose. Rats fed a diet containing 70 percent fructose for two days following a two-day fast had higher levels of liver pyruvate and acyl CoA derivatives than did rats refed a diet containing an equivalent amount of glucose.[75] Liver slices from rats fed a chow diet converted three to nineteen times more uniformly labeled fructose than uniformly labeled glucose into lactic acid, pyruvic acid, carbon dioxide, fatty acid and glyceride glycerol.[133] The infusion of fructose, but not glucose, into the livers of rats increased both the secretion of VLDL-triglycerides and the incorporation of free fatty acids from the perfusate into VLDL-lipid.[134] Human liver biopsy samples metabolized radioactive fructose to fatty acids, carbon dioxide and glyceride-glycerol at rates three to twenty-four times greater than those of an equivalent concentration of radioactive glucose.[135]

Adipose fat deposition

There has been considerable speculation that the high incidence of human obesity observed in affluent or Westernized societies is due, in part, to high intakes of sucrose.[136] Although diets containing sucrose or fructose have been shown to produce larger increases in hepatic lipogenic enzyme activity and more liver lipid than diets containing an equivalent amount of glucose or glucose polymers, a greater deposition of body fat in animals fed sucrose, as compared to starch, has not been consistently observed.[137] However, a number of studies measuring the removable fat tissue in the abdominal and retroperitoneal cavities have shown that the feeding of sucrose produced greater adiposity than did the feeding of starch. Male baboons fed a diet containing 76 percent of the calories from sucrose for twenty-six weeks had 60 percent and 300 percent more omental, pericardial and retroperitoneal fat than did baboons fed equivalent amounts of a partial starch hydrolysate and starch, respectively.[138] There was a greater amount of removable adipose tissue in the abdominal and retroperitoneal cavities in rats fed for fifteen weeks a diet containing 68 percent sucrose as compared to 68 percent starch.[139] The *ad libitum* or meal-feeding of diets containing 54 percent sucrose, as compared to 54 percent starch, for eleven to seventeen weeks resulted in a greater relative deposition of epididymal and perirenal fat.[53,62] Replacement of 55 percent dietary starch with sucrose resulted in a 16 percent to 26 percent increase in the perirenal fat content of rats after two weeks.[140] In that study, the complexities that may be introduced by interactions among dietary components were illustrated by the finding that perirenal fat did not increase due to the replacement of starch by sucrose when the dietary fat was increased from 5 percent to 20 percent. Since obesity has been generally regarded as an important risk factor in the etiology of both diabetes and heart disease, an enhancement of fat deposition as the result of sucrose feeding would be undesirable.

Blood triglycerides

Studies with both experimental animals and humans have established that diets containing high levels of sucrose or fructose produce larger increases in endogenous blood triglycerides than do diets containing an equivalent amount of glucose or glucose polymers. These findings are compatible with the higher hepatic lipogenic capacity of animals fed sucrose and the necessity of transporting larger amounts of neutral fat from the liver to the adipose tissue.

In the rat, the feeding of sucrose, as compared to either starch[52,53,73,128,141–144] or glucose,[127,144] has been shown to result in large increases in endogenous blood triglycerides under a variety of experimental conditions. Similar results have been obtained when rats are fed fructose, as compared to starch[80,128,144–147] or glucose,[127,128,131,144–150] indicating that the fructose moiety is at least partly responsible for sucrose-induced hypertriglyceridemia. The failure of some animal species to show increased levels of blood triglycerides when fed sucrose, as compared to starch or glucose, may be due to differences in the intestinal metabolism of fructose. In the rat, as in man, fructose is poorly metabolized during intestinal absorption and appears primarily unchanged in the portal blood.[27,151] In contrast, in the small intestine of the guinea pig fructose is mainly converted to glucose.[152] The acute or prolonged feeding of fructose, as compared to glucose, did not increase serum triglyceride levels in the guinea pig.[149] It may, therefore, be possible to associate the hypertriglyceridemic effect of sucrose in various species with the postabsorptive appearance of nonmetabolized fructose in the circulation.

As might be expected on the basis of its more lipogenic metabolism, fructose appears to be incorporated into blood triglycerides more rapidly than is glucose. Fructose intragastricly instilled into rats adapted to a diet containing 72 percent fructose was more rapidly converted to serum glycerides than was glucose instilled into glucose-adapted rats.[150] More radioactivity from uniformly labeled[14] C fructose than from uniformly labeled[14] C glucose was found in serum triglycerides one hour after the intravenous injection of these sugars.[149] Rats refed a diet containing 70 percent fructose for two days following a two-day fast had greater concentrations of serum triglycerides than did rats refed a diet containing an equivalent amount of glucose.[75] It has been suggested that sucrose (or fructose) induced hypertriglyceridemia in rats is due to a combination of metabolic changes in the liver and adipose tissue that result in a futile cycling of endogenous triglycerides between these two tissues.[153]

Studies utilizing nonhuman primates have not given definitive results as to the effect of the feeding of sucrose or fructose, as compared to glucose polymers, on fasting triglyceride levels. Among the factors that might be responsible for differences in the reported results are interspecies variation, the sex of the animal and the nature of the dietary fat. Male baboons incorporated a greater amount of radioactivity into serum glycerides after consuming radioactive sucrose than after either a radioactive starch hydrolysate or radioactive glucose.[154] Fasting serum triglycerides were higher in male, but not female, baboons fed a 75 percent sucrose, fat-free diet for seventeen weeks.[155] After adaptation to the high-sucrose diet, there was an increase in the incorporation of radioactive sucrose into serum triglycerides, the increase being greater in male than in female baboons. Kritchevsky et al[156,157] studied the effects of various dietary carbohydrates on lipid metabolism in equal numbers of male and female baboons fed diets containing 14 percent saturated fat for twelve to seventeen months. In one study,[157] 0.1 percent cholesterol was also added to the diet. In both studies, the feeding of 40 percent fructose produced higher levels of fasting triglycerides than did feeding an equivalent amount of sucrose, glucose or starch. In these studies, female baboons tended to have higher levels of blood triglycerides than did male baboons, but fructose appeared to be more effective in raising the triglyceride level in the males. Male monkeys of three species, *Macaca mulatta, Macaca arctoides* and *Cebus albifrons,* were fed diets containing 66 percent of either sucrose or dextrin for sixteen months.[158] The P/S ratio of the diets was .48. Only in the *Cebus albifrons* were serum triglycerides significantly higher when the monkeys consumed the sucrose as compared to the dextrin diet. Similar species' differences in response to dietary carbohydrate were found when squirrel monkeys of mixed sex, but not spider monkeys, showed significant increases in fasting serum triglycerides after consuming a diet containing 69 percent sucrose and 5 percent saturated fat (P/S ratio of .03) for six weeks.[159] The addition of 0.1-1 mg cholesterol per kcal to the diet negated the effect of sucrose. In contrast, spider monkeys of both sexes fed a 40 percent sucrose diet for forty-eight weeks showed significant increases in plasma triglycerides as compared to monkeys fed a 40 percent dextrose diet.[160] When the 9 percent coconut oil used in the diet was replaced by safflower oil, the sucrose effect was eliminated, suggesting that an interaction between dietary sucrose and saturated fat is required to increase triglyceride levels in some species.

In human studies in which the intake of sucrose has been either eliminated[161] or reduced[162,163] significant decreases in fasting serum triglycerides occurred. The decreases were greater in subjects having the highest initial blood triglyceride levels.[161,163] In two of the studies,[162,163] the reduction in sucrose intake produced decreases in body weight, which may have contributed to the decrease in blood triglycerides. However, it has been reported that weight gain induced in humans by the intake of excess calories increased serum triglycerides when sucrose, but not starch, consumption was also increased.[164]

The feeding of at least 30 percent of the calories as sucrose, as compared to an equivalent amount of starch, for periods of time up to six weeks, has consistently produced large and significant increases in endogenous blood triglycerides in groups of subjects that were ostensibly normal and mostly male.[88,96,101,102,164–170]

Similar studies in which diets contained less than 30 percent of the calories as sucrose, as compared to starch, have not shown differences in fasting serum triglyceride levels.[92,97,171] The effect of sucrose on blood triglycerides appears to depend on the age and sex of the subject. In contrast to men and postmenopausal women,[172,173] fasting blood triglycerides of young women did not increase after they consumed diets containing as much as 70 percent of the total calories as sucrose.[173,174] The elevation of fasting blood triglycerides generally observed when the carbohydrate content of the diet is increased at the expense of fat similarly appears to be absent in young females.[175] The magnitude of the increase of blood triglycerides by sucrose is also affected by the nature of the dietary fat. When 75 percent of the fat of a diet typical of that consumed in industrialized societies was replaced by unsaturated fat, the increase in endogenous blood triglycerides produced by 34 percent sucrose calories in the diet was prevented.[169] Young men consuming a diet containing 60 percent sucrose, 30 percent fat, and 9 percent protein for five days showed significantly increased fasting blood triglycerides when the fat was saturated (cream) and not when it was unsaturated (sunflower oil).[176] These results indicate that the usual diet consumed in industrialized societies with a low polyunsaturated/saturated fatty acid ratio is conducive to a large increase in serum triglycerides when high amounts of sucrose are also ingested. The pattern of diet intake may also play a role in the expression of the effect of sucrose on blood triglycerides. In two studies in which approximately 30 percent sucrose, as compared to starch, was fed to a similar population group, significant increases in serum triglycerides were found when the diet was consumed in a gorging pattern[102] but not when the diet was consumed in a nibbling pattern.[92] These experimental variables may explain apparent contradictions in the literature regarding the magnitude of the effect of dietary sucrose on blood triglycerides.

The human studies described above have generally utilized normal subjects. Subjects described as having carbohydrate-induced hyperlipemia or a type IV lipoprotein pattern have shown increases of 23 to 300 percent in fasting blood triglycerides when fed diets containing sucrose as compared to equivalent amounts of starch.[102,105, 173,177–180] Blood triglycerides were increased significantly in these subjects with sucrose levels as low as 20 to 25 percent,[105] 18 percent[173] and 14 percent[179] of the total caloric intake. Although the levels of blood triglycerides were lower with diets containing unsaturated as compared to saturated fats, the magnitude of the increase of blood triglycerides by sucrose was unaffected by the nature of the dietary fat in these individuals.[179,180] Subjects with known coronary-artery disease had significantly greater increases in fasting plasma triglycerides after being fed diets containing 3 g sucrose per kg of body weight per day than did subjects without known coronary-artery disease.[181] Adaptation to carbohydrate-induced increases in blood triglyceride levels was not observed in hypertriglyceridemic subjects after ten weeks of feeding.[182] It therefore appears that sucrose consumption constitutes a greater environmental hazard in the segment of the population that has a genetic predisposition toward carbohydrate-induced hyperlipemia than in the general population.

The feeding of sucrose also appears to produce greater increases in blood triglycerides than does the feeding of glucose or partial starch hydrolysates. Fasting blood triglycerides were significantly higher after young adults consumed diets containing 6 g sucrose per kg body weight per day for nineteen days than after they consumed an equivalent amount of glucose.[183] The integrated twenty-four-hour concentration of plasma triglycerides, but not fasting triglycerides, was significantly higher when sucrose rather than corn syrup supplied either 45 percent or 65 percent of the total energy of young males for ten days.[184]

Relatively few human studies have compared the effects of dietary fructose and glucose-based carbohydrates on blood triglycerides. Men and postmenopausal women, but not premenopausal women, showed significantly higher levels of fasting triglycerides after consuming, for five days, a diet containing 3 g of fructose per kg body weight than when consuming a diet containing an equivalent amount of glucose.[172] The extent of the contribution of the fructose moiety of sucrose to the triglyceridemia found in subjects with type IV hyperlipoproteinemia or carbohydrate-induced hyperlipemia is still not clear. Patients with carbohydrate-induced hypertriglyceridemia generally showed larger increases in serum triglycerides when they consumed 300 g per day of fructose than when an equivalent amount of glucose or starch was consumed.[185] In contrast, in subjects with type IV hyperlipoproteinemia, 20 to 25 percent of the calories as sucrose produced significantly higher triglycerides than the same amount of starch or fructose.[105] The replacement of 9 to 17 percent of calories supplied by dextromaltose with fructose failed to increase fasting plasma triglycerides in hypertriglyceridemic men.[106] In hypertriglyceridemic patients with known coronary-artery disease, however, fructose (2 g per kg of body weight per day) appeared to be at least as effective as sucrose (3 g per kg of body weight per day) and more effective than glucose (2 g per kg of body weight per day) in raising blood triglycerides.[181] Comparisons between these studies are complicated by differences in the nature of the diets employed (e.g., solid vs. liquid, amount and type of dietary fat).

Blood cholesterol

In studies with rats, the feeding of sucrose or fructose, as compared to glucose or glucose polymers, has given apparently conflicting results pertaining to effects on blood cholesterol levels. Differences in the strain and age of rats used, the level of dietary carbohydrate fed, and the length of time on the study may in part explain these conflicting results. In the Wistar rat, the feeding of diets containing either 30 percent,[54] 39 percent,[142] 54 percent (unpublished results) or 65 percent[186] sucrose, as compared to starch, failed to significantly increase serum cholesterol. However, blood cholesterol levels were significantly higher when a Wistar CF strain of rat was fed a diet containing 75 percent fructose than when fed identical diets containing 72 percent of either starch or glucose.[187] Serum cholesterol levels were significantly higher when BHE rats were fed a diet containing 65 percent sucrose as compared to starch[186] but not different when the carbohydrates were fed at 39 percent of the diet.[142] No differences in serum cholesterol were observed in Holtzman strain rats after a forty-eight-hour starvation and refeeding of a diet containing 70 percent fructose as compared to 70 percent glucose.[75] Similarly, no differences in plasma cholesterol were found in Sprague Dawley rats fed diets containing 68 percent of either glucose, fructose or sucrose for twenty-four days.[127] In rats of a Medical Research Council Wistar-derived strain, however, diets containing 81 percent of either sucrose or fructose significantly increased plasma cholesterol after twenty-six weeks as compared to rats fed an equivalent amount of partially hydrolyzed starch.[117] Increased blood cholesterol has also been reported in CDRI Lucknow,[144] Haffkine,[120] Sprague Dawley[52] and Hebrew University[80] strains of rats when fed diets containing 12 percent,[144] 58 percent[120] and 68 percent[52] sucrose or 72 percent fructose[80] as compared to diets containing equivalent amounts of starch.

Dietary cholesterol appears to act synergistically with dietary sucrose, but not dietary starch, to increase blood cholesterol levels in experimental animals. As early as 1956, it was reported that feeding rats diets containing 56 percent sucrose, as compared to 56 percent starch, elevated serum cholesterol when 5 percent cholesterol was also added in the diet.[188] In the absence of dietary cholesterol, the increase in serum cholesterol due to sucrose was markedly reduced. Rats fed diets containing 55 percent carbohydrate as either sucrose, glucose or pregelatinized potato starch for four weeks showed no difference in serum cholesterol.[189] When 1 percent cholesterol was added to the diets, the sucrose-fed rats showed large and significant increases in serum cholesterol as compared to the rats fed glucose or starch. Rats fed diets containing 1 percent[141] and 1.5 percent[190] cholesterol had higher levels of serum cholesterol when consuming diets containing 40 to 60 percent sucrose than when consuming diets containing equivalent amounts of starch over experimental periods as long as 180 days. In rats fed diets containing 2 percent cholesterol and 60 percent carbohydrate for four months, serum cholesterol was higher when the carbohydrate was sucrose than when it was glucose or starch from ragi, jowar, tapioca and bajra.[191] However, in these studies, rice and wheat starch were about as cholesterolemic as was sucrose. In contrast to these results, lower serum cholesterol was found in rats fed diets containing 1 percent cholesterol and 68 percent sucrose than in rats fed diets containing 1 percent cholesterol and various forms of modified starch.[192] Chicks fed a diet containing 60 percent sucrose as compared to glucose for four weeks showed no difference in plasma cholesterol.[193] When the diets also contained 3 percent cholesterol the sucrose-fed chicks showed 50 to 100 percent increases in plasma cholesterol. Similarly, diets containing 3 percent cholesterol produced much greater increases in serum cholesterol in both conventional and germ-free chickens when the 54 percent carbohydrate was supplied by sucrose than when it was supplied by either glucose or starch.[194] Serum cholesterol levels of rabbits fed a cholesterol diet containing 50 percent sucrose for sixty days were 50 percent higher than those of rabbits fed a diet containing 50 percent glucose.[193] In contrast, dietary cholesterol appears to interact with other dietary carbohydrates in addition to sucrose in raising blood cholesterol levels in nonhuman primates. Three species of monkeys fed diets containing 0.5 percent cholesterol for sixteen months showed no difference in serum cholesterol when the carbohydrate was 66 percent sucrose as compared to 66 percent dextrin.[158] In spider monkeys[159,160] and squirrel monkeys,[159] there were no differences in the increase in blood cholesterol when cholesterol was included in diets containing 49–69 percent of the carbohydrate as either sucrose or dextrin. The spider monkeys fed the diet containing sucrose-cholesterol but not dextrin-cholesterol showed significant increases in plasma cholesterol when coconut oil replaced safflower oil as the dietary fat[160] suggesting a synergism between saturated fat, sucrose and cholesterol. The feeding of diets containing 40 percent carbohydrate as either fructose, sucrose, starch or glucose to baboons for twelve to seventeen months did not significantly affect serum cholesterol either in the absence[156] or presence[157] of dietary cholesterol.

Significant increases in total blood cholesterol have not been consistently observed in humans consuming diets containing sucrose as compared to starch. The effect of dietary sucrose on cholesterol metabolism appears to be complex and is apparently governed to a great extent by the nature of other dietary constituents as well as by genetic factors. Comparisons between the studies to be described therefore become difficult. In general, it appears that sucrose is more cholesterolemic than starch when fed in diets high in cholesterol and saturated fat, and low in fiber. It also appears that men, older women and subjects with carbohydrate-induced hyperlipemia may be more susceptible to the effects of sucrose. Since sucrose-induced increases in blood triglycerides are also more pronounced in these population groups, the increase in blood cholesterol due to sucrose feeding may in part be attributable to the cholesterol present in the elevated levels of VLDL produced in response to the high triglyceride levels.

Male subjects fed a chemically defined diet composed of amino acids, vitamins, minerals, ethyl linoleate and 90 percent of the calories from glucose showed a decrease in serum cholesterol from 227 mg percent on their usual diet to 160 mg percent in four weeks.[195] When 25 percent of the glucose was replaced by sucrose, the serum cholesterol rose an average of 48 mg percent in three weeks. Cholesterol levels fell again when the glucose diet alone was fed. Although the diets fed in this study are not of practical nutritional importance, these results illustrate that blood cholesterol levels can be dramatically influenced by the nature of the dietary carbohydrate. When natural dietary components were fed, sucrose had been reported to either have no effect,[196,197] or slightly increase[183] blood cholesterol levels in comparison with glucose.

The nature of the dietary fat appears to influence the effect of sucrose on blood cholesterol levels. Serum cholesterol was significantly increased in men when the sucrose content of a diet typical of that consumed in affluent societies was doubled at the expense of complex carbohydrate to provide 34 percent of the total calories.[169] However, this increase was prevented by the replacement of 75 percent of the total fats by unsaturated fats. Patients (predominantly males) with types II, III and IV hyperlipoproteinemia showed significant increases in serum total cholesterol after consuming diets containing 20 to 40 percent of the calories as sucrose, as compared to starch, for twenty-eight days only when most of the dietary fat was saturated[180] but not when it was mainly unsaturated.[179]

A number of studies have compared the effects on blood cholesterol between sucrose and that of starch present in natural foods, such as cereals and vegetables. Humans fed a diet containing 35 percent of the calories from sucrose, as compared to starch from bread, showed increases in serum that were not significant after two weeks (13 mg percent) but were significant after four to five weeks (24 mg percent).[198] The exchange of 16 percent of calories of starch from mixed vegetables, but not wheat flour, for an equivalent amount of sucrose significantly increased serum cholesterol levels in humans after two weeks.[199] Humans consuming diets containing 17 to 23 percent of the calories as sucrose showed significant increases in serum cholesterol (8 to 18 mg percent) over those observed when they were consuming diets containing equicaloric amounts of starch from vegetables and legumes[200,201] and from cereals and potatoes.[171] Replacement of 200 g of starch from self-selected foods with sucrose for fourteen days significantly increased plasma cholesterol in male students.[164] In contrast, no significant increases in serum cholesterol were observed when starch from cereals and potatoes,[92,97] bread and potatoes,[201] or rice[202] was replaced by equivalent amounts of sucrose. Under these experimental conditions, observed differences in blood cholesterol cannot be attributed entirely to sucrose rather than to the differences in the levels of other dietary components present in the foods such as unsaturated fat[169,179,180] and fiber.[203]

Studies in which blood cholesterol levels have been determined in response to diets containing sucrose as compared to purified sources of starch have also given inconsistent results. Serum cholesterol levels were higher in men after they consumed, for twenty-five days, a diet providing 500 g of sucrose daily than after they consumed an identical diet providing 500 g of raw cornstarch daily.[96] The differences were due to a decrease in cholesterol levels on the starch diet. There appears to be a difference in the ability of large amounts of sucrose, as compared to starch, to elevate cholesterol levels in young and postmenopausal women. Women aged twenty-one to twenty-five years did not show any difference in serum cholesterol levels when fed diets providing 450 g of either sucrose or purified cornstarch daily for twenty-five days.[174] Twenty young women (average age, thirty-one years) showed no differences in plasma cholesterol after being fed for one week each diets containing 45 percent of the calories as either sucrose or starch.[170] Women aged nineteen to twenty-five years showed no differences in serum cholesterol levels after consuming, for four weeks, diets containing 43 percent of the calories from either sucrose or wheat starch.[204] However, women aged fifty-four to sixty-eight years showed an average 30 mg percent higher level of serum cholesterol twenty-five days after consuming diets containing 7.5 g per kg body weight of sucrose daily than after consuming diets having an equivalent amount of purified wheat starch.[205] Serum cholesterol levels in a group of ten men and nine women, aged thirty-five to fifty-five years, were significantly higher during the six weeks when they consumed a typical American diet containing 30 percent of the calories as sucrose as compared to wheat starch in a gorging pattern.[102] In this study the men and women showed similar increases in serum cholesterol due to sucrose. Studies with hyperlipemic subjects have generally shown an increase in blood cholesterol when sucrose, as compared to starch, is fed. The importance of the nature of the dietary fat in the expression of this difference has already been discussed (see above and[179,180]). In patients with hypertriglyceridemia, diets containing large amounts of sucrose, up to 60 percent of calories[178] and 70 percent to 80 percent of calories,[177] increased serum cholesterol. An equivalent amount of starch from natural sources decreased serum cholesterol. Lower levels of sucrose appear to be effective in increasing blood cholesterol in carbohydrate-sensitive individuals. Serum cholesterol levels in twelve men and twelve women diagnosed as carbohydrate-sensitive, on the basis of an exaggerated insulin response to a sucrose load, showed significant increases in total cholesterol when the sucrose content of a typical American diet was increased from 5 percent to either 18 percent or 33 percent at the expense of wheat starch.[173] In this study the men showed larger increases in cholesterol due to sucrose than did the women.

Significant negative correlations between HDL cholesterol and either blood triglycerides or VLDL have been observed in a number of studies.[173,206-210] Large inverse relationships between VLDL cholesterol and HDL cholesterol have been demonstrated after the feeding of diets containing 80 percent to 90 percent of the calories as carbohydrate in humans.[211,212] A reduction in the hypertriglyceridemia associated with type IV hyperlipoproteinemia resulted in an increased concentration of cholesterol in LDL and HDL fractions and a fall in the VLDL fraction.[213] If, as these results suggest, an increase in VLDL to carry excess triglyceride is associated with a concurrent decrease in HDL cholesterol, then sucrose would be expected to lower HDL cholesterol to a greater extent than would either glucose or glucose polymers. There are indications that sucrose consumption does decrease the relative concentration of HDL cholesterol in the blood. Subjects (predominantly young males) showed a significant decrease in the ratio of HDL cholesterol to total cholesterol when consuming self-selected diets containing 6 g per kg body weight daily of sucrose, but not of glucose, for nineteen days.[183] Carbohydrate-sensitive males, but not females, had a significantly decreased ratio of HDL cholesterol to LDL + VLDL cholesterol six weeks after consuming a diet typical of the present American diet and containing 33 percent, as compared to 5 percent, of the calories as sucrose.[173]

Physiological implications

The present level of sucrose consumption in this country is not generally accepted as an important factor in the incidence of heart disease. [107,108] Some of the experimental defects in the human studies that have prevented definitive interpretation of the positive results have already been discussed (see above under glucose tolerance). In addition, with the exception of the rabbit[214] and possibly the BHE rat,[186] sucrose feeding has not produced definitive signs of atherosclerosis in experimental animals. However, there appears to be little doubt that the feeding of sucrose as compared to starch produces increases in the production of endogenous triglycerides. That effect is reflected in an increase in blood triglycerides, especially in carbohydrate-sensitive or type IV hyperlipoproteinemic individuals in whom intakes of sucrose at levels approximating those that are common in the United States produced significant increases. Endogenous hypertriglyceridemia is commonly associated with premature atherosclerosis.[113]

In contrast to the effect on endogenous blood triglycerides, the effect of dietary carbohydrate on blood cholesterol is small and mainly determined by the nature of the dietary fat. However, there are relationships between the metabolism of triglycerides and cholesterol that favor higher levels of blood cholesterol after the feeding of sucrose as compared with starch. The VLDL produced in the liver in response to increased triglyceride synthesis contains 10 percent to 20 percent cholesterol.[215] The removal of triglycerides from VLDL by adipose tissue results in the formation of cholesterol-rich LDL.[216] The increase in cholesterol by sucrose feeding may therefore be attributed in part to the elevated levels of VLDL produced in response to high triglycerides. An increase in endogenous cholesterol synthesis by dietary sucrose, as mediated through increased insulin production,[48] may also partially explain increases in blood cholesterol due to sucrose feeding. Even though the effect of sucrose might be either indirect, due to increased production of VLDL triglyceride, or secondary to and small in comparison with the effects of dietary cholesterol and fat, the increase in blood cholesterol that is associated with the substitution of dietary sucrose for starch could contribute to the numerous environmental factors producing the high levels of blood cholesterol that are common in industrialized societies.

Other Effects

Blood uric acid

Blood uric acid has been reported to be elevated in patients with heart disease.[217,218] Although blood uric acid has been found to be valuable in prediction of cardiovascular mortality,[219] there is no known basis for a causative role of uric acid in cardiovascular disease. A number of studies indicate that the feeding of sucrose as compared to starch produces increases in blood uric acid. Serum uric acid was found to be significantly higher in twelve young women when they consumed a diet containing 43 percent of calories from sucrose as compared to wheat starch.[220] Also using a cross-over, isocaloric exchange pattern, ten men and nine women showed significantly higher fasting serum uric acid when they consumed a diet containing 30 percent of the calories from sucrose as compared to wheat starch.[221] In this study, uric acid levels in response to a sucrose load of 2 g per kg body weight were significantly higher in men than in women and increased as a function of time up to two hours following the sucrose load. In carbohydrate-sensitive subjects of both sexes, serum uric acid, both fasting and in response to a sucrose load, was greater when the subjects consumed 18 percent and 33 percent sucrose than when they consumed 5 percent sucrose; the men again had higher levels than the women.[222] No difference in serum uric acid were observed after men consumed, for twenty-one days, a diet containing 35 percent sucrose as compared to 49 percent dextromaltose.[223]

The fructose moiety of sucrose appears to be responsible for the increase in blood uric acid. The feeding of 250 to 290 g per day of fructose for seven days produced hyperuricemia and increased urinary urate excretion in humans while glucose fed at the same level did not.[224] Fructose administered intravenously at the rate of more than 0.5 g per kg body weight per hour increased both blood and urinary urate.[225-228] Glucose and galactose administration at the same level as fructose failed to produce comparable increases in blood uric acid.[227]

The hyperuricemia observed after the administration of fructose or feeding of high levels of sucrose may be explained on the basis of fructose metabolism in the liver.[229] The phosphorylation of fructose has been shown to produce a rapid decrease of both hepatic ATP and inorganic phosphate. Since ATP inhibits 5' nucleotidase and inorganic phosphate inhibits AMP deaminase, the AMP formed in the liver is readily converted to IMP and then to inosine. Inosine is then oxidized to uric acid which appears in the blood as the major product of hepatic adenine nucleotide degradation. The higher levels of uric acid found in subjects fed sucrose as compared to starch may also be explained on the basis of increased synthesis.[221]

Blood pressure

Hypertension has been identified as one of the most significant risk factors in heart disease.[230,231] There is some evidence from studies using experimental animals that sucrose, especially in combination with salt, may produce larger increases in blood pressure than do other dietary carbohydrates. Rats ingesting a solution containing 5 percent sucrose and 1 percent sodium chloride were reported to have higher blood pressure than rats ingesting a solution of 5 percent glucose and 1 percent sodium chloride.[232] Rats fed a diet high in sucrose for ten weeks exhibited higher levels of systolic blood pressure than did rats fed a natural grain ration or diets high in fat or cornstarch.[233] The increases were greater when 1 to 2 percent sodium chloride was added to the drinking water. The replacement of 10 to 20 percent of starch by sucrose produced significant increases in the systolic blood pressure of rats after fourteen weeks on diet.[234] The diets in this study contained 0.035 percent sodium. Systolic blood pressure of normotensive WKY and spontaneously hypertensive SHR rats were significantly higher after they consumed, for fourteen weeks, diets containing 54 percent of either sucrose, invert sugar or glucose than after an equivalent amount of starch.[235] Within each genotype, blood pressure was not significantly different between rats fed the three sugars.

In a study using spider monkeys, the effects of salt and sucrose on the development of hypertension were investigated.[236] The monkeys were fed either a chow-based diet high in complex carbohydrate containing no added sodium chloride (control), the control diet with 3 percent sodium chloride or the control diet with sodium chloride in which 38 percent of the calories were supplied by sucrose. There were no significant differences in body weights after eight weeks on diet. Blood pressure was significantly higher in monkeys fed the salt containing diets than in monkeys fed the control diet. However, the monkeys fed the sucrose-containing diet had significantly greater increases in both systolic and distolic blood pressure as compared to the monkeys fed the salt-containing diet without sucrose.

Cariogenicity

In the United States, approximately 95 percent of children have some form of tooth decay and about 55 percent of the population have lost their teeth by the age of fifty-five. It is clear from studies using both experimental animals[237-240] and humans[241-243] that sucrose is among the most cariogenic of the sugars occurring in the diet. Since sucrose is the cariogenic substance which is most extensively ingested, it is considered to be the primary dietary culprit in the causation of caries.[3,108] Sucrose appears to be converted by cariogenic microorganisms to polymers that favor their adherence to the teeth.[108] The severity of sucrose-induced cariogenicity is complex and depends on genetic factors, frequency of consumption, duration of the exposure, the form in which the sucrose is eaten (e.g., sticky vs granular foods) and the nature of other dietary constituents ingested. Individuals with hereditary fructose intolerance who must avoid all forms of dietary fructose and sucrose have substantially fewer dental caries than the general population,[244] but are not caries-free.[245]

Summary and Conclusions

The studies described in this section show that the feeding of sucrose, as compared to starch, increases many of the risk factors associated with degenerative diseases. The implication of these findings on human health is still controversial. In many of the studies the nature of the experimental protocol employed prevented definitive interpretation of the results. An overall evaluation of these results, however, supports the following conclusions:

1) Regardless of the experimental conditions used, the feeding of sucrose, as compared to starch, either had no effect or produced undesirable effects on metabolic parameters associated with degenerative diseases; a beneficial effect of sucrose was rarely observed.
2) In the context of the diet presently consumed in more affluent or industrializd societies (e.g., high levels of saturated fat, cholesterol, salt; low level of fiber), dietary sucrose can act synergistically with other dietary ingredients and thus contribute to the many environmental factors producing the high level of degenerative diseases in these societies.
3) A finite segment of the population that may be described as carbohydrate-sensitive is at a substantially higher risk than is the

general population from the intake of sucrose and these individuals should be identified and encouraged to reduce their sucrose intake.

REFERENCES

1. Page, L. and Friend, B. 1974. In: *Sugars in Nutrition*. H. L. Sipple and K. W. McNutt, eds. New York: Academic Press.
2. Friend, B. and Marston, R., eds. 1974. Nutritional review. *Natl. Food Situation* 150: 26.
3. SCOGS, -69. 1976. *Evaluation of the Health Aspects of Sucrose as a Food Ingredient*. Contract No. FDA 223-75-2004. Bethesda, MD: Life Sciences Research Office, FASEB.
4. Select Committee on Nutrition and Human Needs, United States Senate. 1977. *Dietary Goals for the United States*. 2nd Edition, U.S. Government Printing Office, Washington, D.C.
5. Wretlind, A. 1974. In: *Sugars in Nutrition*. H. L. Sipple and K. W. McNutt, eds. New York: Academic Press.
6. Roberts, P. J. P. and Whelan, W. J. 1960. The mechanism of carbohydrase action. 5. Action of human salivary α-amylase on amylopectin and glycogen. *Biochem. J*. 76: 246.
7. Gray, G. M. 1971. In: *Annual Review of Medicine*. A. C. Degraff, ed. vol. 22, Annual Reviews, Inc. Palo Alto, CA.
8. Johnson, C. F. 1969. Hamster intestinal brush-border surface particles and their function. *Fed. Proc*. 28: 26.
9. Blair, D. G., Yakimets, W. and Tuba, J. 1963. Rat intestinal sucrase. II. The effects of rat age and sex and of diet on sucrase activity. *Can. J. Biochem. Physiol*. 41: 917.
10. Deren, J. J., Broitman, S. A. and Zamcheck, N. 1967. Effect of diet upon intestinal disaccharidases and disaccharide absorption. *J. Clin. Invest*. 46: 186.
11. Reddy, B. S., Pleasants, J. R. and Wostmann, B. S. 1968. Effect of dietary carbohydrates on intestinal disaccharidases in germ free and conventional rats. *J. Nutr*. 95: 413.
12. Rosensweig, N. S. and Herman. R. H. 1968. Control of jejunal sucrase and maltase activity by dietary sucrose or fructose in man: a model for the study of enzyme regulation in man. *J. Clin. Invest*. 47: 2253.
13. Rosensweig, N. S. and Herman, R. H. 1970. Dose response of jejunal sucrase and maltase activities to isocaloric high and low carbohydrate diets in man. *Amer. J. Clin. Nutr*. 23: 1373.
14. Kolínská, J. and Kraml, J. 1972. Separation and characterization of sucrase-isomaltase and of glucoamylase of rat intestine. *Biochim. Biophys. Acta* 284: 235.
15. Crane, R. K. 1968. *Alimentary Canal*. vol. III, C. F. Code, ed. Washington, D.C.: American Physiological Society.
16. Honegger, P. and Semenza, G. 1973. Multiplicity of carriers for free glucalogues in hamster small intestine. *Biochim. Biophys. Acta* 318: 390.
17. Sigrist-Nelson, K. and Hopfer, U. 1974. A distinct D-fructose transport system in isolated brush-border membrane. *Biochim. Biophys. Acta* 367: 247.

18. Malathi, P., Ramaswamy, K., Caspary, W. F. and Crane, R. K. 1973. Studies on the transport of glucose from disaccharides by hamster small intestine in vitro. I. Evidence for a disaccharide-related transport system. *Biochim. Biophys. Acta* 307: 613.

19. Ramaswamy, K., Malathi, P., Capsary, W. F. and Crane, R. K. 1974. Studies on the transport of glucose from disaccharides by hamster small intestine in vitro. II. Characteristics of the disaccharide-related transport system. *Biochim. Biophys. Acta*. 345: 39.

20. Reiser, S., Michaelis IV, O., Putney, J. and Hallfrisch, J. 1975. Effect of sucrose feeding on the intestinal transport of sugars in two strains of rats. *J. Nutr.* 105: 894.

21. Reiser, S., Hallfrisch, J., Putney, J. and Lev, F. 1977. Enhancement of intestinal transport sugar by rats fed sucrose as compared to starch. *Nutr. Metabol.* 20: 461.

22. Reiser, S. 1979. In: *Dietary Fibers—Chemistry and Nutrition*. G. E. Inglett and S. I. Falkehag, eds. New York: Academic Press.

23. Crossley, J. N. and Macdonald, I. 1970. The influence in male baboons, of a high sucrose diet on the portal and arterial levels of glucose and fructose following a sucrose meal. *Nutr. Metabol.* 12: 171.

24. Storelli, C., Vögeli, H. and Semenza, G. 1972. Reconstitution of a sucrase-mediated sugar transport system in lipid membranes. *FEBS Lett.* 24: 287.

25. Semenza, G., Tosi, R., Valloton-Delachaux, M. C. and Mühlhaupt, E. 1964. Sodium activation of human intestinal sucrase and its possible significance in the enzymic organization of brush borders. *Biochim. Biophys. Acta* 89: 109.

26. Semenza, G. 1968. In: *Modern Problems in Pediatrics*. A. Hottinger and H. Berger, eds. Basel: Karger.

27. Mavrias, D. A. and Mayer, R. J. 1973. Metabolism of fructose in the small intestine. I. The effect of fructose feeding on fructose transport and metabolism in rat small intestine. *Biochim. Biophys. Acta* 291: 531.

28. Vráná, A., Fábry, P. and Kazdová, L. 1977. Diet-induced adaptation of intestinal fructose absorption in the rat. *Physiol. Bohemoslov.* 26: 225.

29. McIntyre, N., Holdsworth, C. D. and Turner, D. S. 1965. Intestinal factors in the control of insulin secretion. *J. Clin. Endocrin.* 25: 1317.

30. Unger, R. H. and Eisentraut, A. M. 1969. Entero-insular axis. *Arch. Intern. Med.* 123: 261.

31. Kipnis, D. M. 1972. Nutrient regulation of insulin secretion in human subjects. *Diabetes* 21: suppl. 2, 606.

32. Buffa, R., Polak, J. M. Pearse, A. G. E., Solcia, E., Grimelius, L. and Capella, C. 1975. Identification of the intestinal cell storing gastric inhibitory polypeptide. *Histochemistry* 43: 249.

33. Creutzfeldt, W. 1979. The incretin concept today. *Diabetologia* 16: 75.

34. Dupre, J., Ross, S. A., Watson, D. and Brown, J. C. 1973. Stimulation of insulin secretion by gastric inhibitory polypeptide in man. *J. Clin. Endocrin. Metabol.* 37: 286.

35. Reiser, S., Michaelis IV., O. E., Cataland, S. and O'Dorisio, T. M. 1980. Effect of isocaloric exchange of dietary starch and sucrose in humans on the gastric inhibitory polypeptide response to a sucrose load. *Am. J. Clin. Nutr.* 33: 1907.

36. Thomas, F. B., Shook, D. F., O'Dorisio, T. M., Cataland, S. Mekhjian, H. S., Caldwell, J. H. and Mazzaferri, E. L. 1977. Localization of

gastric inhibitory polypeptide release by intestinal glucose perfusion in man. *Gasteroenterology* 72: 49.

37. Cataland, S., Crockett, S. E., Brown, J. C. and Mazzaferri, E. L. 1974. Gastric inhibitory polypeptide (GIP) stimulation by oral glucose in man. *J. Clin. Endocrinol. Metabol.* 39: 223.

38. Michaelis IV, O. E. and Szepesi, B. 1974. The mechanism of a specific metabolic effect of sucrose in the rat. *J. Nutr.* 104: 1597.

39. Michaelis IV, O. E., Nace, C. S. and Szepesi, B. 1975. Demonstration of a specific metabolic effect of dietary disaccharides in the rat. *J. Nutr.* 105: 1186.

40. Michaelis IV, O. E., Scholfield, D. J., Nace, C. S. and Reiser, S. 1978. Demonstration of the disaccharide effect in nutritionally stressed rats. *J. Nutr.* 108: 919.

41. Basu. T. K., Dickenson, J. W. T. and Parke, D. V. 1975. Effect of dietary substitution of sucrose and its constituent monosaccharides on the activity of aromatic hydroxylase and the level of cytochrome p-450 in hepatic microsomes of growing rats. *Nutr. Metabol.* 18: 302.

42. Shreeve, W. W., Hoshi, M. and Kikkawa, R. 1971. Insulin responses to ingested sucrose or glucose-fructose in obese patients. *Diabetes* 20: suppl. 1, 377.

43. Thompson, R. G., Hayford, J. T. and Hendrix, J. A. 1979. Triglyceride concentrations: the disaccharide effect. *Science* 206: 838.

44. Jackson, W. P. U., van Mieghem, W. and Keller, P. 1972. Insulin excess as the initial lesion in diabetes. *Lancet* 1: 1040.

45. Kraft, J. R. and Nosal, R. A. 1975. Insulin values and diagnosis of diabetes. *Lancet* 1: 637.

46. Pyörälä, K. 1979. Relationship of glucose tolerance and plasma insulin to the incidence of coronary heart disease: results from two population studies in Finland. *Diabetes Care* 2: 131.

47. Welborn, T. A. and Wearne, K. 1979. Coronary heart disease incidence and cardiovascular mortality in Busselton with reference to glucose and insulin concentrations. *Diabetes Care* 2: 154.

48. Stout, R. S. 1977. The relationship of abnormal circulating insulin levels to atherosclerosis. *Atherosclerosis* 27: 1.

49. Ostrander, L. D., Neff, B. J., Block, W. D., Francis, T. and Epstein, F. H. 1967. Hyperglycemia and hypertriglyceridemia among persons with coronary heart disease. *Ann. Internal Med.* 67: 34.

50. Wahlberg, F. and Thomasson, B. 1968. Glucose tolerance in ischaemic cardiovascular disease In: *Carbohydrate Metabolism and its Disorders*. vol. 2, chap. 8. F. Dickens, P. J. Randle and W. J. Whelan, eds. New York: Academic Press.

51. Olefsky, J. M., Farquhar, J. W. and Reaven, G. M. 1974. Reappraisal of the role of insulin in hypertriglyceridemia. *Am. J. Med.* 57: 551.

52. Naismith, D. J. and Rana, I. A. 1974. Sucrose and hyperlipidaemia. *Nutr. Metabol.* 16: 285.

53. Hallfrisch, J., Lazar, F., Jorgensen, C. and Reiser, S. 1979. Insulin and glucose responses in rats fed sucrose or starch. *Am. J. Clin. Nutr.* 32: 787.

54. Hallfrisch, J., Cohen, L. and Reiser, S. 1981. Effects of feeding rats sucrose in a high fat diet. *J. Nutr.* 111:531.

55. Crapo, P. A., Reaven, G. and Olefsky, J. 1976. Plasma glucose and insulin responses to orally administered simple and complex carbohydrates. *Diabetes* 25: 741.

56. Norden, D. A. and Davison, A. N. 1971. The effect of oral sugars and glycerol on the release of insulin and the utilization of blood glucose for lipid synthesis. *So. Afr. J. Med. Sci.* 36: 77.
57. Macdonald, I., Keyser, A. and Pacy, D. 1978. Some effects, in man, of varying the load of glucose, sucrose, fructose, or sorbitol on various metabolites in blood. *Am. J. Clin. Nutr.* 31: 1305.
58. Thompson, R. G., Hayford, J. T. and Danney, M. M. 1978. Glucose and insulin responses to diet. Effect of variations in source and amount of carbohydrates. *Diabetes* 27: 1020.
59. Cohen, A. M. and Teitelbaum, A. 1964. Effect of dietary sucrose and starch on oral glucose tolerance and insulin-like activity. *Am. J. Physiol.* 206: 105.
60. Vrána, A., Slabochová, Z., Kazdová, L. and Fábry, P. 1971. Insulin sensitivity of adipose tissue and serum insulin concentration in rats fed sucrose or starch diets. *Nutr. Rep. Int.* 3: 31.
61. Blazquez, E. and Quijada, C. L. 1969. The effect of high-carbohydrate diet on glucose, insulin sensitivity and plasma insulin in rats. *J. Endocrinol.* 44: 107.
62. Reiser, S. and Hallfrisch, J. 1977. Insulin sensitivity and adipose tissue weight of rats fed starch or sucrose diets ad libitum or in meals. *J. Nutr.* 107: 147.
63. Romsos, D. R. and Leveille, G. A. 1974. Effect of meal frequency and diet composition on glucose tolerance in the rat. *J. Nutr.* 104: 1503.
64. Pfeiffer, E. F. 1974. In: *Lipid Metabolism, Obesity and Diabetes Mellitus: Impact upon Atherosclerosis.* H. Greten. R. Levine, E. F. Pfeiffer and A. E. Renold, eds. Stuttgart: George Thieme.
65. Laube, H. Wojcikowski, C., Schatz, H. and Pfeiffer, E. F. 1978. The effect of high maltose and sucrose feeding on glucose tolerance. *Horm. Metabol. Res.* 10: 192.
66. Cohen, A. M., Teitelbaum, A., Briller, S., Yanko, L., Rosenmann, E. and Shafrir, E. 1974. In: *Sugars in Nutrition.* H. L. Sipple and K. W. McNutt, eds. New York: Academic Press.
67. Freedland, R. A. and Harper, A. E. 1966. Initiation of glucose 6-phosphatase adaptation in the rat. *J. Nutr.* 89: 429.
68. Chang, M. L. W., Lee, J. A., Schuster, E. M. and Trout, D. L. 1971. Metabolic adaptation to dietary carbohydrate in two strains of rats at three ages. *J. Nutr.* 101: 323.
69. Cohen, A. M., Briller, S. and Shafrir, E. 1972. Effect of long term sucrose feeding on the activity of some enzymes regulating glycolysis, lipogenesis and gluconeogenesis in rat liver and adipose tissue. *Biochim. Biophys. Acta* 279: 129.
70. Blakely, S. R., Hallfrisch, J. Reiser, S. and Prather, E. S. 1981. Long-term effects of moderate fructose feeding on glucose tolerance parameters in rats. *J. Nutr.* 111: 307.
71. Touvinen, C. G. R. and Bender, A. E. 1975. Some metabolic effects of prolonged feeding of starch, sucrose, fructose and carbohydrate free diets in rats. *Nutr. Metabol.* 19: 1.
72. Adelman, R. A., Spolter, P. D. and Weinhouse, S. 1966. Dietary and hormonal regulation of enzymes of fructose metabolism in rat liver. *J. Biol. Chem.* 241: 5467.
73. Chevalier, M. M., Wiley, J. H. and Leveille, G. A. 1972. Effect of dietary fructose on fatty acid synthesis in adipose tissue and liver of the rat. *J. Nutr.* 102: 337.

74. Hill, R., Baker, N. and Chaikoff, I. L. 1954. Altered metabolic patterns induced in the normal rat by feeding an adequate diet containing fructose as sole carbohydrate. *J. Biol. Chem.* 209: 705.
75. Zakim, D., Pardini, R. S., Herman, R. H. and Sauberlich, H. E. 1967. Mechanism for the differential effects of high carbohydrate diets on lipogenesis in rat liver. *Biochim. Biophys. Acta* 144: 242.
76. Bode, C., Schumacher, H., Goebell, H., Zelder, O. and Pelzel, H. 1971. Fructose induced depletion of liver adenine nucleotides in man. *Horm. Metabol. Res.* 3: 289.
77. Woods, H. F., Eggleston, L. V. and Krebs, H. A. 1970. The cause of hepatic accumulation of fructose 1-phosphate on fructose loading. *Biochem. J.* 119: 501.
78. Burch, H. B., Lowry, O. H., Meinhardt, L., Max, Jr., P. and Chyu, K. 1970. Effect of fructose dihydroxyacetone, glycerol, and glucose on metabolites and related compounds in liver and kidney. *J. Biol. Chem.* 245: 2092.
79. Thomopoulos, P., Kosmakos, F. C., Pastan, I. and Lovelace, E. 1977. Cyclic AMP increases the concentration of insulin receptors in cultured fibroblasts and lymphocytes. *Biochem. Biophys. Res. Commun.* 75: 246.
80. Cohen, A. M., Teitelbaum, A. and Rosenmann, E. 1977. Diabetes induced by a high fructose diet. *Metabolism* 26: 17.
81. Sleder, J., Chen, Y-D I., Cully, M. D. and Reaven, G. M. 1980. Hyperinsulinemia in fructose-induced hypertriglyceridemia in the rat. *Metabolism* 29: 303.
82. Zavaroni, I., Sander, S., Scott, S. and Reaven, G. M. 1980. Effect of fructose feeding on insulin secretion and insulin action in the rat. *Metabolism* 29: 970.
83. Beck-Neilsen, H., Pedersen, O. and Lindskov, H. O. 1980. Impaired cellular insulin binding and insulin sensitivity induced by high-fructose feeding in normal subjects. *Am. J. Clin. Nutr.* 33: 273.
84. Grodsky, G. M., Batts, A. A., Bennett, L. L. Voella, C., McWilliams, W. B. and Smith, D. F. 1963. Effects of carbohydrates on secretion of insulin from isolated rat pancreas. *Am. J. Physiol.* 205: 638.
85. Curry, D. L., Curry, K. P. and Gomez, M. 1972. Fructose potentiation of insulin secretion. *Endocrinology* 91: 1493.
86. Dunnigan, M. G. and Ford, J. A. 1975. The insulin response to intravenous fructose in relation to blood glucose levels. *J. Clin. Endocrinol. Metabol.* 40: 629.
87. Cohen, A. M., Teitelbaum, A., Balogh, M. and Groen, J. J. 1966. Effect of interchanging bread and sucrose as main source of carbohydrate in low fat diet on glucose tolerance curve of healthy volunteer subjects. *Am. J. Clin. Nutr.* 19: 59.
88. Nestel, P. J., Carroll, K. F. and Havenstein, N. 1970. Plasma triglyceride response to carbohydrates, fats and calorie intake. *Metabolism* 19: 1.
89. Kelsay, J. L., Behall, K. M., Holden, J. M. and Prather, E. S. 1974. Diets high in glucose or sucrose and young women. *Am. J. Clin. Res.* 27: 926.
90. Behall, K. M., Moser, P. B., Kelsay, J. L. and Prather, E. S. 1980. The effect of kind of carbohydrate in the diet and use of oral contraceptives on metabolism of young women. III. Serum glucose, insulin and glucagon. *Am. J. Clin. Nutr.* 33: 1041.

91. Reiser, S., Handler, H. B., Gardner, L. B., Hallfrisch, J., Michaelis IV, O. E. and Prather, E. S. 1979. Isocaloric exchange of dietary starch and sucrose in humans. II. Effect on fasting blood insulin, glucose, and glucagon and on insulin and glucose response to a sucrose load. *Am. J. Clin. Nutr.* 32: 2206.

92. Dunnigan, M. G., Fyfe, T., McKiddie, M. T. and Crosbie, S. M. 1970. The effects of isocaloric exchange of dietary starch and sucrose on glucose tolerance, plasma insulin and serum lipids in man. *Clin. Sci.* 38: 1.

93. Gwinup, G., Byron, R. C., Roush, W., Kruger, F. and Hamwi, G. J. 1963. Effect of nibbling versus gorging on glucose tolerance. *Lancet* 2: 165.

94. Pringle, D. J., Wadhwa, P. S. and Elson, C. E. 1976. Influence of frequency of eating low energy diets on insulin response in women during weight reduction. *Nutr. Rept. Intern.* 13: 339.

95. Beck-Nielsen, H., Pedersen, O. and Schwartz Sorensen, N. 1978. Effects of diet on the cellular insulin binding and the insulin sensitivity in young healthy subjects. *Diabetologia* 15: 289.

96. Macdonald, I. and Braithwaite, D. M. 1964. The influence of dietary carbohydrates on the lipid pattern in serum and in adipose tissue. *Clin. Sci.* 27: 23.

97. Mann, J. I. and Truswell, A. S. 1972. Effects of isocaloric exchange of dietary sucrose and starch on fasting serum lipids, postprandial insulin secretion and alimentary lipaemia in human subjects. *Br. J. Nutr.* 27: 395.

98. Anderson, J. W., Herman, R. H. and Zakim, D. 1973. Effect of high glucose and high sucrose diets on glucose tolerance of normal men. *Am. J. Clin. Nutr.* 26: 600.

99. Olefsky, J. M. and Saekow, M. 1978. The effects of dietary carbohydrate content on insulin binding and glucose metabolism by isolated rat adipocytes. *Endocrinology* 103: 2252.

100. Tepperman, H. M., DeWitt, J. and Tepperman, J. 1978. Hormone effects on glycogenolysis, gluconeogenesis, and cyclic AMP production by liver cells from rats fed diets high in glucose or lard. *J. Nutr.* 108: 1924.

101. Szanto, S., and Yudkin, J. 1969. The effect of dietary sucrose on blood lipids, serum insulin, platelet adhesiveness and body weight in human volunteers. *Postgrad. Med. J.* 45: 602.

102. Reiser, S. Hallfrisch, J., Michaelis IV., O. E., Lazar, F., Martin, R. E., and Prather, E. S. 1979. Isocaloric exchange of dietary starch and sucrose in humans. I. Effects on levels of fasting blood lipids. *Am. J. Clin. Nutr.* 32: 1659.

103. Fredrickson, D. S., Levy, R. I. and Lees, R. S. 1967. Fat transport in lipoproteins—an integrated approach to mechanisms and disorders. *New Engl. J. Med.* 276: 273.

104. Reiser, S., Bohn, E., Hallfrisch, J., Michaelis IV, O. E., Keeney, M. and Prather, E. S. 1981. Serum insulin and glucose in hyperinsulinemic subjects fed three different levels of sucrose. *Am. J. Clin. Nutr.* 34: 2348.

105. Nikkila, E. A. 1974. In: *Sugars in Nutrition*. H. L. Sipple and K. W. McNutt, eds. New York: Academic Press.

106. Turner, J. L., Bierman, E. L., Brunzell, J. D. and Chait, A. 1979. Effect of dietary fructose on triglyceride transport and glucoregulatory hormones in hypertriglyceridemic men. *Am. J. Clin. Nutr.* 32: 1043.
107. West, K. M. 1978. In: *Epidemiology of Diabetes and its Vascular Lesions*. New York: Elsevier.
108. Bierman, E. L. 1979. Carbohydrates, sucrose, and human disease. *Am. J. Clin. Nutr.* 32: 2712.
109. Wood, P. D. S., Stern, M. P., Silvers, A., Reaven, G. M. and van der Groeben, J. 1972. Prevalence of plasma lipoprotein abnormalities in a free-living population of the Central Valley, California. *Circulation* 45: 114.
110. Brown, D. F. and Daudiss, K. 1973. Hyperlipoproteinemia prevalence in a free-living population in Albany, New York. *Circulation* 47: 558.
111. Reaven, G. M. and Bernstein, R. M. 1978. Effect of obesity on the relationship between very low density lipoprotein production rate and plasma triglyceride concentration in normal and hypertriglyceridemic subjects. *Metabolism* 27: 1047.
112. Anonymous 1972. Diet and coronary heart disease. A joint statement of the Food and Nutrition Board, Division of Biology and Agriculture, National Academy of Sciences—National Research Council and the Council on Foods and Nutrition, American Medical Association. *Nutr. Rev.* 30: 223.
113. Tzagournis, M. 1978. Triglycerides in clinical medicine. A review. *Am. J. Clin. Nutr.* 31: 1437.
114. Norum, K. R. 1978. Some present concepts concerning diet and prevention of coronary heart disease. *Nutr. Metabol.* 22: 1.
115. Witzum, J. and Schonfeld, G. 1979. High density lipoproteins. *Diabetes* 28: 326.
116. Litwack, G., Hankes, L. V. and Elvehjem, C. A. 1952. Effect of factors other than choline on liver fat deposition. *Proc. Soc. Exp. Biol. Med.* 81: 441.
117. Allen, R. J. L. and Leahy, J. S. 1966. Some effects of dietary dextrose, fructose, liquid glucose and sucrose in the adult male rat. *Br. J. Nutr.* 20: 339.
118. Marshall, M. W. and Womack, M. 1955. Starches, sugars and related factors affecting liver fat and nitrogen balances in adult rats fed low levels of amino acids. *J. Nutr.* 57: 193.
119. Fábry, P., Poledne, R., Kazdová, L. and Braun, T. 1968. The effect of feeding frequency and type of dietary carbohydrates on hepatic lipogenesis in the albino rat. *Nutr. Dieta* 10: 81.
120. Dumaswala, U. J., Dumaswala, R. U. and Venkataraman, A. 1977. In vivo studies on the effect of dietary carbohydrates on the lipid metabolism in rats. *Nutr. Rep. Int.* 16: 719.
121. Holt, P. R., Dominguez, A. A. and Kwartler, J. 1979. Effect of sucrose feeding upon intestinal and hepatic lipid synthesis. *Am. J. Clin. Nutr.* 32: 1792.
122. Veech, R. L. 1975. in *Sweeteners Issues and Uncertainties*. Washington, D. C: National Academy of Sciences.
123. Michaelis IV., O. E. and Szepesi, B. 1973. Effect of various sugars on hepatic glucose-6-phosphate dehydrogenase, malic enzyme and total liver lipid of the rat. *J. Nutr.* 103: 697.

124. Roggeveen, A. E., Geisler, R. W., Peavy, D. E. and Hansen, R. J. 1974, Effects of diet on the activities related to lipogenesis in rat liver and adipose tissue. *Proc. Soc. Exp. Biol. Med.* 147: 467.
125. Berdanier, C. D., Tobin, R. B. and DeVore, V. 1979. Effects of age, strain, and dietary carbohydrate on the hepatic metabolism of male rats. *J. Nutr.* 109: 261.
126. Davis, R. A., Engelhorn, S. C., Pangburn, S. H., Weinstein, D. B. and Steinberg, D. 1979. Very low density lipoprotein synthesis and secretion by cultured rat hepatocytes. *J. Biol. Chem.* 254: 2010.
127. Waterman, R. A., Romsos, D. R., Tsai, A. C., Miller, E. R. and Leveille, G. A. 1975. Effects of dietary carbohydrate source on growth, plasma metabolites and lipogenesis in rats, pigs and chicks. *Proc. Soc. Exp. Biol. Med.* 150: 210.
128. Bruckdorfer, K. R., Kahn, I. H. and Yudkin, J. 1972. Fatty acid synthetase activity in the liver and adipose tissue of rats fed with various carbohydrates. *Biochem. J.* 129: 439.
129. Sugawa-Katayama, Y. and Morita, N. 1975. Effects of a high fructose diet on lipogenic enzyme activities in some organs of rats fed ad libitum. *J. Nutr.* 105: 1377.
130. Maruhama, Y. and Macdonald, I. 1972. Some changes in the triglyceride metabolism of rats on high fructose or glucose diets. *Metabolism* 21: 835.
131. Waddell, M. and Fallon, H. J. 1973. The effect of high carbohydrate diets on liver triglyceride formation in the rat fed 75% fructose or glucose diet. *J. Clin. Invest.* 52: 2725.
132. Regan, Jr., J. J., Dorneweerd, D. D., Gilboe, D. P. and Nuttall, F. Q. 1980. Influence of fructose on the glycogen synthase and phosphorylase systems in rat liver. *Metabolism* 29: 965.
133. Pereira, J. N. and Jangaard, N. O. 1971. Different rates of glucose and fructose metabolism in rat liver tissue *in Vitro. Metabolism* 20: 392.
134. Topping, D. L. and Mayes, P. A. 1976. Comparative effects of fructose and glucose on the lipid and carbohydrate metabolism of perfused rat liver. *Br. J. Nutr.* 36: 113.
135. Zakim, D., Herman, R. H. and Gordon, Jr., W. C. 1969. The conversion of glucose and fructose to fatty acids in the human liver. *Biochem. Med.* 2: 427.
136. Cleave, T. L., Campbell, G. C. and Painter, W. S. 1969. In: *Diabetes, Coronary Thrombosis and the Saccharine Disease.* 2nd ed. Bristol: John Wright & Sons.
137. Bender, A. E. and Damji, K. B. 1971. In: *Sugar, Chemical, Biological and Nutritional Aspects of Sucrose.* J. Yudkin, J. Edelman and L. Hough, eds. London: Butterworth's.
138. Brook, M. and Noel, P. 1969. Influence of dietary liquid glucose, sucrose and fructose on body fat formation. *Nature* 222: 562.
139. Laube, H., Klör, H. U., Fussgänger, R. and Pfeiffer, E. F. 1973. The effect of starch, sucrose, glucose and fructose on lipid metabolism in rats. *Nutr. Metabol.* 15: 273.
140. Chang, M. L. W. and Johnson, M. A. 1976. Influence of fat level and type of carbohydrate on the capacity of pectin in lowering serum and liver lipids of young rats. *J. Nutr.* 106: 1562.
141. Qureshi, P., Akinyanju, P. A. and Yudkin, J. 1970. The effect of an "atherogenic" diet containing starch or sucrose upon carcass composition and plasma lipids in the rat. *Nutr. Metabol.* 12: 347.

142. Taylor, D. D., Conway, E. S., Schuster, E. M. and Adams, M. 1967. Influence of dietary carbohydrates on liver content and on serum lipids in relation to age and strain of rat. *J. Nutr.* 91: 275.

143. Bruckdorfer, K. R., Kari-Kari, B. P. B., Khan, I. H. and Yudkin, J. 1972. Activity of lipogenic enzymes and plasma triglyceride levels in the rat and the chicken as determined by the nature of the dietary fat and dietary carbohydrate. *Nutr. Metabol.* 14: 228.

144. Mukherjee, S., Basu, M. and Trivedi, K. 1969. Effect of low dietary levels of glucose, fructose and sucrose on rat lipid metabolism. *J. Atheroscler. Res.* 10: 261.

145. Chevalier, M. M., Wiley. J. H. and Leveille, G. A. 1972. The age-dependent response of serum triglycerides to dietary fructose. *Proc. Soc. Exp. Biol. Med.* 139.

146. Heller, G., Fürster, H. and Fortmeyer, H. P. 1977. Influence of the various dietary carbohydrates on the concentration of metabolites and the activity of enzymes in the liver of diabetic rats. *Nutr. Metabol.* 21: (suppl. 1) 177.

147. Merkens, L. S., Tepperman, H. M. and Tepperman, J. 1980. Effects of short-term dietary glucose and fructose on rat serum triglyceride concentration. *J. Nutr.* 110: 982.

148. Nikkila, E. A. and Ojala, K. 1965. Induction of hypertriglyceridemia by fructose in the rat. *Life Sci.* 4: 937.

149. Bar-On, H. and Stein, Y. 1968. Effect of glucose and fructose administration on lipid metabolism in the rat. *J. Nutr.* 94: 95.

150. Macdonald, I. and Roberts, J. B. 1965. The incorporation of various C^{14} dietary carbohydrates into serum and liver lipids. *Metabolism* 14: 991.

151. Cook, G. C. 1971. Absorption and metabolism of D(-) fructose in man. *Am. J. Clin. Nutr.* 24: 1302.

152. Mavrias, D. A. and Mayer, R. J.: 1973. Metabolism of fructose in the small intestine. II. The effect of fructose feeding on fructose transport and metabolism in guinea pig small intestine. *Biochim. Biophys. Acta* 291: 538.

153. Molaparast-Shahidsaless, F., Shrago, E. and Elson, C. E. 1979. Glycerophosphate and dihydroxyacetone phosphate metabolism in rats fed high-fat or high-sucrose diets. *J. Nutr.* 109: 1560.

154. Macdonald, I. and Roberts, J. B. 1967. The serum lipid response of baboons to various carbohydrate meals. *Metabolism* 16: 572.

155. Coltart, T. M. and Macdonald, I. 1971. Effect of sex hormones on fasting serum triglycerides in baboons given high sucrose diets. *Br. J. Nutr.* 25: 323.

156. Kritchevsky, D., Davidson, L. M., Shapiro, I. L., Kim, H. K., Kitagawa, M., Malhotra, S., Nair, P. P., Clarkson, T. B., Bersohn, I. and Winter, P. A. D. 1974. Lipid metabolism and experimental atherosclerosis in baboons: influence of cholesterol-free, semi-synthetic diets. *Am. J. Clin. Nutr.* 27: 29.

157. Kritchevsky, D., Davidson, L. M., Kim, H. K., Krendel, D. A., Malhotra, S., Mendelsohn, D., van der Watt, J. J., du Plessis, J. P. and Winter, P. A. D. 1980. Influence of type of carbohydrate on atherosclerosis in baboons fed semipurified diets plus 0.1% cholesterol. *Am. J. Clin. Nutr.* 33: 1869.

158. Lang, C. M. and Barthel, C. H. 1972. Effects of simple and complex carbohydrates on serum lipids and atherosclerosis in nonhuman primates. *Am. J. Clin. Nutr.* 25: 470.

159. Srinivasan, S. R., Radhakrishnamurthy, B., Webber, L. S., Dalferes Jr., E. R., Kokatnur, M. G. and Berenson, G. S., 1978. Synergistic effects of dietary carbohydrate and cholesterol on serum lipids and lipoproteins in squirrel and spider monkeys. *Am. J. Clin. Nutr.* 31: 603.

160. Corey, J. E., Hayes, K. C., Dorr, B. and Hegsted, D. M. 1974. Comparative lipid response of four primate species to dietary changes in fat and carbohydrates. *Atherosclerosis* 19: 119.

161. Roberts, A. M. 1973. Effects of a sucrose-free diet on the serum-lipid levels of men in Antarctica. *Lancet* 1: 1201.

162. Rifkind, B. M., Lawson, D. H. and Gale, M. 1966. Effect of short term sucrose restriction on serum-lipid levels. *Lancet* 2: 1379.

163. Mann, J. I., Hendricks, D. A., Truswell, A. S. and Manning, E. 1970. Effects of serum-lipids in normal men of reducing dietary sucrose or starch for five months. *Lancet* 1: 870.

164. Naismith, D. J., Stock, A. L. and Yudkin, J. 1974. Effect of changes in the proportions of the dietary carbohydrates and in energy intake on the plasma lipid concentrations in healthy young men. *Nutr. Metabol.* 16: 295.

165. Antar, M. A. and Ohlson, M. A. 1965. Effect of simple and complex carbohydrates upon total lipids, nonphospholipids and different fractions of phospholipids of serum in young men and women. *J. Nutr.* 85: 329.

166. Hodges, R. E. and Krehl, W. A. 1965. The role of carbohydrates in lipid metabolism, *Am. J. Clin. Nutr.* 18: 334.

167. Hodges, R. E., Krehl, W. A., Stone, D. B. and Lopez, A. 1967. Dietary carbohydrates and low cholesterol diet: effects on serum lipids in man. *Am. J. Clin. Nutr.* 20: 198.

168. Akinyanju, P. A., Qureshi, R. U., Salter, A. J. and Yudkin, J. 1968. Effect of an "atherogenic" diet containing starch or sucrose on the blood lipids of young men. *Nature* 218: 975.

169. Mann, J. I., Watermeyer, G. S., Manning, E. B., Randles, J. and Truswell, A. S. 1973. Effects on serum lipids of different dietary fats associated with a high sucrose diet. *Clin. Sci.* 44: 601.

170. Wu, C-H., Hoshi, M. and Shreeve, W. W. 1974, Human plasma triglyceride labeling after high-sucrose feeding. I. Incorporation of sucrose-U-^{14}C. *Metabolism* 23: 1125.

171. McGandy, R. B., Hegsted, D. M., Myers, M. L. and Stare, F. J. 1966. Dietary carbohydrates and serum cholesterol levels in man. *Am. J. Clin. Nutr.* 18: 237.

172. Macdonald, I. 1966. Influences of fructose and glucose on serum lipid levels in men and pre- and post-menopausal women. *Am. J. Clin. Nutr.* 18: 369.

173. Reiser, S., Bickard, M. C., Hallfrisch, J., Michaelis IV, O. E. and Prather, E. S. 1981. Blood lipids and their distribution in lipoproteins in hyperinsulinemic subjects fed three different levels of sucrose. *J. Nutr.* 111: 1045.

174. Macdonald, I. 1965. The lipid response of young women to dietary carbohydrates. *Am. J. Clin. Nutr.* 16: 458.

175. Beveridge, J. M. R., Jagannathan, S. N. and Connell, W. F. 1964. The effect of the type and amount of dietary fat on the level of plasma triglycerides in human subjects in the postabsorptive state. *Can. J. Biochem.* 42: 999.

176. Macdonald, I. 1967. Inter-relationship between the influences of dietary carbohydrates and fats on fasting serum lipids. *Am. J. Clin. Nutr.* 20: 345.

177. Kaufmann. N. A., Poznanski, R., Blondheim, S. H. and Stein, Y. 1966. Changes in serum lipid levels of hyperlipemic patients following the feeding of starch, sucrose and glucose. *Am. J. Clin. Nutr.* 18: 261.

178. Kuo, P. T., Feng, L., Cohen, N. N. Fitts, Jr., W. T. and Miller, L. D. 1967. Dietary carbohydrates in hyperlipemia (hyperglyceridemia); hepatic and adipose tissue lipogenic activities. *Am. J. Clin. Nutr.* 20: 116.

179. Little, J. A., Birchwood, B. L., Simmons, D. A., Antar, M. A., Kallos, A., Buckley, G. C. and Csima, A. 1970. Interrelationship between the kinds of dietary carbohydrate and fat in hyperlipoproteinemic patients. I. Sucrose and starch with polyunsaturated fat. *Atherosclerosis.* 11: 173.

180. Antar, M. A., Little, J. A., Lucas, C., Buckley, G. C. and Csima, A. 1970. Interrelationship between the kinds of dietary carbohydrate and fat in hyperlipoproteinemic patients. III. Synergistic effect of sucrose and animal fat on serum lipids. *Atherosclerosis* 11: 191.

181. Palumbo, P. J., Briones, E. R., Nelson, R. A. and Kottke, B. A. 1977. Sucrose sensitivity of patients with coronary-artery disease. *Am. J. Clin. Nutr.* 30: 394.

182. Mancini, M., Mattock, M., Rabaya, E., Chait, A. and Lewis, B. 1973. Studies of the mechanisms of carbohydrate-induced lipaemia in normal men. *Atherosclerosis* 17: 445.

183. Macdonald, I. 1978. The effects of dietary carbohydrate on high density lipoprotein levels in serum. *Nutr. Rep. Int.* 17: 663.

184. Hayford, J. T., Danney, M. M., Wiebe, D., Roberts, S. and Thompson, R. G. 1979. Triglyceride integrated concentrations: effect of variation of source and amount of dietary carbohydrate. *Am. J. Clin. Nutr.* 32: 1670.

185. Kaufmann, W. A., Poznanski, R., Blondheim, S. H. and Stein, Y. 1966. Effect of fructose, glucose, sucrose and starch on serum lipids in carbohydrate induced hypertriglyceridemia and in normal subjects. *Isr. J. Med. Sci.* 2: 715.

186. Berdanier, C. D. 1974. Metabolic characteristics of the carbohydrate-sensitive BHE strain of rats. *J. Nutr.* 104: 1246.

187. Baron, P., Griffaton, G. and Lowy, R. 1971. Metabolic inductions in the rat after an intraperitoneal injection of fructose and glucose, according to the nature of the dietary carbohydrate. II. Modification after seven months of diet. *Enzyme* 12: 481.

188. Portman, O. W., Lawry, E. Y. and Bruno, D. 1956. Effect of dietary carbohydrate on experimentally induced hypercholesteremia and hyperbetalipoproteinemia in rats. *Proc. Soc. Exp. Biol. Med.* 91: 321.

189. Staub, H. W. and Thiessen, Jr., R. 1968. Dietary carbohydrate and serum cholesterol in rats. *J. Nutr.* 95: 633.

190. Fillios, L. C., Naito, C., Andrus, S. B., Portman, O. W. and Martin, R. S. 1958. Variations in cardiovascular sudanophilia with changes in the dietary levels of protein. *Am. J. Physiol.* 194: 275.

191. Vijayagopalan, P. and Kurup, P. A. 1972. Effect of dietary starches on the serum, aorta and hepatic lipid levels in high fat cholesterol-fed rats. 2. Nature of the starch and hypolipidaemic activity. *Atherosclerosis* 16: 247.

192. Anderson, T. A. 1969. Effect of carbohydrate source on serum and hepatic cholesterol levels in the cholesterol-fed rat. *Proc. Soc. Exp. Biol. Med.* 130: 884.

193. Grant, W. C. and Fahrenbach, M. J. 1959. Effect of dietary sucrose and glucose on plasma cholesterol in chicks and rabbits. *Proc. Soc. Exp. Biol. Med.* 100: 250.

194. Kritchevsky, D., Kolman, R. R., Guttmacher, R. M. and Forbes, M. 1959. Influence of dietary carbohydrate and protein on serum and liver cholesterol in germ-free chicken. *Arch. Biochem. Biophys.* 85: 444.

195. Winitz, M., Graff, J. and Seedman, D. A. 1964. Effect of dietary carbohydrate on serum cholesterol levels. *Arch. Biochem. Biophys.* 108: 576.

196. Anderson, J. T., Grande, F., Matsumoto, Y. and Keys, A. 1963: Glucose, sucrose and lactose in the diet and blood lipids in man. *J. Nutr.* 79: 349.

197. Shammaá, M. and Al-Khalidi, U. 1963. Dietary carbohydrates and serum cholesterol in man. *Am. J. Clin. Nutr.* 13: 194.

198. Groen, J. J., Balogh, M., Yaron, E. and Cohen, A. M. 1966. Effect of interchanging bread and sucrose as main source of carbohydrate in a low fat diet on the serum cholesterol levels of healthy volunteer subjects. *Am. J. Clin. Nutr.* 19: 46.

199. Anderson, J. T., Grande, F., Foster, N. and Keys, A. Different dietary carbohydrates and blood lipids in man. 1972. *Proc. 9th Int. Congr. Nutr.* p. 64. Cited by Grande, F. 1974. In: *Sugars in Nutrition*. H. L. Sipple and K. W. McNutt eds. New York: Academic Press.

200. Keys, A., Anderson, J. T. and Grande, F. 1960. Diet-type (fat constant) and blood lipids in man. *J. Nutr.* 70: 257.

201. Grande, F., Anderson, J. T. and Keys, A. 1965. Effects of carbohydrates of leguminous seeds, wheat and potatoes on serum cholesterol concentration in man. *J. Nutr.* 86: 313.

202. Irwin, M. I., Taylor, D. D. and Feeley, R. M. 1964. Serum lipid levels, fat, nitrogen, and mineral metabolism of young men associated with kind of dietary carbohydrate. *J. Nutr.* 82: 338.

203. Jenkins, D. J. A., Leeds, A. R., Newton, C. and Cummings, J. H. 1975. Effects of pectin, guar gum, and wheat fibre on serum-cholesterol. *Lancet* 1: 1116.

204. Behall, K. M., Moser, P. B., Kelsay, J. L. and Prather, E. S. 1980. The effect of kind of carbohydrate in the diet and use of oral contraceptives on metabolism of young women. II. Serum lipid levels. *Am. J. Clin. Nutr.* 33: 825.

205. Macdonald, I. 1966. The lipid response of postmenopausal women to dietary carbohydrates. *Am. J. Clin. Nutr.* 18: 86.

206. Miller, G. J. and Miller, N. E. 1975. Plasma-high-density-lipoprotein concentration and development of ischaemic heart-disease. *Lancet* 1: 16.

207. Srinivasan, S. R., Frerichs, R. R., Webber, L. S. and Berenson, G. S. 1976. Serum lipoprotein profile in children from a biracial community. The Bogalusa heart study. *Circulation* 54: 309.

208. Castelli, W. P., Doyle, J. T., Gordon, T., Hames, C. G., Hjortland, M. C., Hulley, S. B., Kagan, A. and Zukel, W. J. 1977. HDL cholesterol and other lipids in coronary heart disease. The cooperative lipoprotein phenotyping study. Circulation, 55: 767.
209. Gordon, T., Castelli, W. P., Hjortland, M. C., Kannel, W. B. and Dawber, T. R. 1977. High density lipoprotein as a protective factor against coronary heart disease. Am. J. Med. 62: 707.
210. Mattock, B., Fuller, J. H., Maude, P. S. and Keen, H. 1979. Lipoproteins and plasma cholesterol esterification in normal and diabetic subjects. Atherosclerosis 34: 437.
211. Wilson, D. E. and Lees, R. S. 1972. Metabolic relationships among the plasma lipoproteins. Reciprocal changes in the concentrations of very low and low density lipoproteins in man. J. Clin. Invest. 51: 1051.
212. Schonfeld, G., Weidman, S. W., Witztum, J. L. and Bowen, R. M. 1976. Alterations in levels and interrelations of plasma apolipoproteins induced by diet. Metabolism 25: 261.
213. Carlson, L. A., Olsson, A. G. and Ballantyne, D. 1977. On the rise in low density and high density lipoproteins in response to the treatment of hypertriglyceridaemia in type IV and type V hyperlipoproteinaemics. Atherosclerosis. 26: 603.
214. Ross, A. C., Minick, C. R. and Zilversmit, D. B. 1978. Equal atherosclerosis in rabbits fed cholesterol-free low-fat diet or cholesterol-supplemented diet. Atherosclerosis 29: 301.
215. Fredrickson, D. S., Levy, R. I. and Lees, R. S. 1967. Fat transport in lipoproteins—an integrated approach to mechanisms and disorders. New Engl. J. Med. 276: 94.
216. Goldstein, J. L. and Brown, M. S. 1977. Atherosclerosis: the low-density lipoprotein receptor hypothesis. Metabolism 26: 1257.
217. Jacobs, D. 1972. Hyperuricaemia and myocardial infarction. S. Afr. Med. J. 46: 367.
218. Srivastava, B. N., Om, H., Deshmankar, B. S. and Gupta, R. K. 1974. Serum uric acid in coronary disease. Indian Heart J. 26: 24.
219. Takkunen, H. and Reunanen, A. 1977. Hyperuricemia and other cardiovascular risk factors. Adv. Exp. Med. Biol. 76B: 238.
220. Kelsay, J. L., Behall, K. M., Moser, P. B. and Prather, E. S. 1977. The effect of kind of carbohydrate in the diet and use of oral contraceptives on metabolism of young women. I. Blood and urinary lactate, uric acid and phosphorus. Am. J. Clin. Nutr. 30: 2016.
221. Solyst, J. T., Michaelis IV. O. E., Reiser, S., Ellwood, K. C. and Prather, E. S. 1980. Effect of dietary sucrose in humans on blood uric acid, phosphorus, fructose, and lactic acid responses to a sucrose load. Nutr. Metabol. 24: 182.
222. Israel, K. D., Michaelis IV O. E., Reiser, S. and Keeney, M. 1982. Serum uric acid, inorganic phosphorus and glutamic-oxalacetic transaminase and blood pressure in carbohydrate-sensitive adults consuming three different levels of sucrose. Nutr. Metabol. In progress.
223. Richardson, D. P., Scrimshaw, N. S. and Young, V. R. 1980. The effect of dietary sucrose on protein utilization in healthy young men. Am. J. Clin. Nutr. 33: 264.
224. Emmerson, B. T. 1974, Effect of oral fructose on urate production. Ann. Rheum. Dis. 33: 276.
225. Perheentupa, J. and Raivio, K. 1967. Fructose-induced hyperuricaemia. Lancet 2: 528.

226. Heuckenkamp, P.-U. and Zöllner, N. 1971. Fructose-induced hyperuricaemia. *Lancet* 1: 808.
227. Narins, R. G., Weisberg, J. S. and Myers, A. R. 1974. Effects of carbohydrates on uric acid metabolism. *Metabolism* 23: 455.
228. Raivio, K. O., Becker, M. A., Meyer, L. J., Greene, M. L., Nuki, G. and Seegmiller, J. E. 1975. Stimulation of human purine synthesis de novo by fructose infusion. *Metabolism* 24: 861.
229. Wood, H. F. and Alberti, K. G. M. M. 1972. Dangers of intravenous fructose. *Lancet* 2: 1354.
230. Hollander, W. 1973. Hypertension, antihypertensive drugs and atherosclerosis. *Circulation* 48: 1112.
231. Kannel, W. B. 1974. Role of blood pressure in cardiovascular morbidity and mortality. *Prog. Cardiovasc. Disease.* 17: 5.
232. Hall, C. E. and Hall, O. 1966. Comparative effectiveness of glucose and sucrose in enhancement of hypersalimentation and salt hypertension. *Proc. Soc. Exp. Biol. Med.* 123: 370.
233. Beebe, C. G., Schemmel, R. and Mickelsen, O. 1976. Blood pressure of rats as affected by diet and concentration of NaCl in drinking water. *Proc. Soc. Exp. Biol. Med.* 151: 395.
234. Ahrens, R. A., Demuth, P., Lee, M. K. and Majkowski, J. W. 1980. Moderate sucrose ingestion and blood pressure in the rat. *J. Nutr.* 110: 725.
235. Michaelis IV, O. E., Martin, R. E., Gardner, L. B. and Ellwood, K. L. 1981. Effect of dietary carbohydrate on systolic blood pressure of normotensive and hypertensive rats. *Nutr. Rep. Int.* 23: 261.
236. Srinivasan, S. R., Berenson, G. S., Radhakrishnamurthy, B., Dalferes Jr., E. R., Underwood, D. and Foster, T. A. 1980. Effects of dietary sodium and sucrose on the induction of hypertension in spider monkeys. *Am. J. Clin. Nutr.* 33: 561.
237. Schafer, W. G. 1949. The caries-producing capacity of starch, glucose, and sucrose diets in the Syrian hamster. *Science* 110: 143.
238. Haldi, J., Wynn, W., Shaw, J. H. and Sognnaes, R. F. 1953. The relative cariogenicity of sucrose when ingested in the solid form and in solution by the albino rat. *J. Nutr.* 49: 295.
239. Grenby, T. H. 1967. Investigations in experimental animals on the cariogenicity of diets containing sucrose and/or starch. *Caries Res.* 1: 208.
240. Frostell, G., Keyes, P. H. and Larson, R. H. 1967. Effect of various sugars and sugar substitutes on dental caries in hamsters and rats. *J. Nutr.* 93: 65.
241. Gustafsson, B. E., Quensel, C.-E., Lanke, L. S. Lundqvist, C., Grahnen, H., Bonow, B. E. and Krasse, B. 1954. The Vipeholm dental caries study. *Acta Odontol. Scand.* 11: 23.
242. Knoll, R. G. and Stone, J.H. 1967. Nocturnal bottle-feeding as a contributory cause of rampant dental caries in the infant and young child. *J. Dent. Child.* 30: 454.
243. Bibb, B. G. 1975. The cariogenicity of snack foods and confections. *J. Am. Dent. Assoc.* 90: 121.
244. Newbrun, E. 1969. Sucrose, the arch criminal of dental caries. *J. Dent. Child.* 36: 239.
245. Marthaler, T. M. and Froesch, E. R. 1967. Hereditary fructose intolerance. Dental status of eight patients. *Br. Dent. J.* 123: 597.

7
NUTRITION AND PATHOGENESIS OF THE BLOOD
VESSEL WALL

HERBERT K. NAITO, PH.D.
AND
HENRY F. HOFF, PH.D.

ACKNOWLEDGMENTS

This study was supported by Grant No. HL-6835 from NHLBI, Grant No. 8557 from the Bleeksma Fund of the Cleveland Clinic Foundation and Grant No. USPHS NIH NS 09287.

Introduction

HEART AND BLOOD vessel diseases are the major causes of death in this country. They account for over 50 percent of all deaths annually, nearly three times the death rate from cancer, the next highest cause. Cardiovascular diseases cause over 60 percent of all deaths among people over sixty-five years of age and over 150,000 deaths per year in individuals below age sixty-five. An estimated 30 million persons in the United States have diseases of the heart and blood vessels; this results in a huge burden of acute and chronic illness and disability. About 27 million of these victims of cardiovascular disorders suffer from hypertension, 4 million from coronary heart disease, and 1.8 million from rheumatic heart disease. Approximately eight out of every one thousand children are born with congenital heart disease and half of these do not survive past one year of age.

However, during the last twenty-five years there has been over a 30 percent decrease (Figure 7.1) in cardiovascular death rate (age adjusted).

178

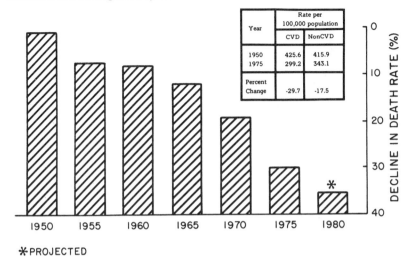

	Rate per 100,000 population	
Year	CVD	NonCVD
1950	425.6	415.9
1975	299.2	343.1
Percent Change	-29.7	-17.5

*PROJECTED

Figure 7.1

Cardiovascular death rate in the U.S.A. (age adjusted over a twenty-year period (Naito, H.K.,[17] printed with permission of Plenum Corp.).

Atheroma is a disease of tremendous importance in contemporary society, not only because of its associated mortality, but also because of its considerable morbidity. Although intensive research efforts have begun to elucidate various facets of its etiology and pathogenesis, to provide improved early diagnostic procedures and more useful approaches to intervention, long-term objectives must logically continue to be those of disease prevention, based upon a thorough understanding of the origin, development and regression of the atheromatous process.

Intermediate objectives could realistically relate to at least two important areas: first, initiation and evaluation of intensive attempts to induce significant lesion regression in patients with severe diffuse disease; and second, further therapeutic attempts to minimize intravascular thrombosis, a process responsible in many patients for the rapid conversion of latent atheroma to events of overt clinical significance, such as cerebral or myocardial infarction.

In clinical medicine we have been aware of the complications of atherosclerosis for centuries. A good deal of confusion still exists over the word "atherosclerosis," which designates the most prevalent and important form of arterial disease in man.

This chapter highlights selected aspects of the pathology and clinicopathological implications of atheroma and presents, in an overview format, the present status of our understanding of etiologic and pathogenic mechanisms. It is clearly neither possible nor desirable to examine the minutia of atherogenesis in this review.

Pathology of the Human Atherosclerotic Lesion

The precise nature of atherosclerosis is still not fully understood. We are, therefore, forced to resort, by way of definition, to a brief description of the condition emphasizing those features that characterize a "lesion" as being atherosclerotic in nature.

Atherosclerosis affects the large- and medium-sized arteries, with the lesions becoming less numerous and severe as the smaller arteries are reached and disappearing entirely some distance proximal to the arterioles. The essential lesions of atherosclerosis occur in the arterial intima, although secondary changes in the internal elastic lamina (IEL) and media are common. The lesions are usually localized and irregular in their distribution in the intima. However, certain anatomic sites are especially prone to involvement; and often the lesions, originally discrete, irregular and patchy, become so numerous and large that they run together forming large areas of confluent plaques. Individual foci consist of localized intimal thickenings composed of an admixture of fatty deposits, blood-borne elements (i.e., fibrin, fibrinogen), glycosaminoglycan, proliferated fibrous tissue and smooth muscle cells.

The late stages of atherosclerotic process show a narrowing of the arterial lumen, thickened arterial wall, irregular intimal surface (including ulcerations in advanced stages), and gruel-like material deposited primarily in the intima. These advanced lesions contain many lipids (particularly cholesterol esters) as well as fibroelastic tissue, glycosaminoglycan smooth muscle cells, and calcium deposits, as well as necrotic debris.

Histologic features of the atheromatous plaque

The goal of defining the most important sequelae of events leading to the formation of an atherosclerotic plaque has been sought by many investigators ever since it was recognized that most coronary heart disease is a clinical consequence of advancing atherosclerosis. The histologic features of human atheroma are summarized in Figure 7.2. Intimal changes, traditionally regarded as characteristic of the raised or fibrous plaque, include a dense collagenous cap which is covered by endothelium on the luminal surface and which overlies and partially encases a necrotic, pultaceous, lipid-rich core. The cellularity of the intimal plaque may vary considerably. Cells that have some of the morphological criteria of smooth muscle cells are copious. Other cells can be

MEDIA
Thinning

ADVENTITIA
Fibrosis
Increased
vascularity
Lymphocytic
infiltration

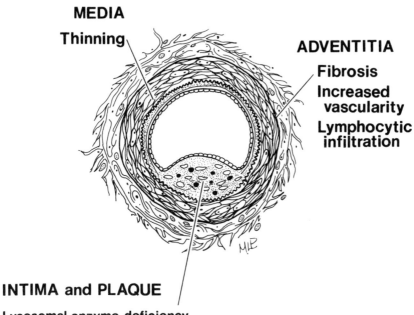

INTIMA and PLAQUE
Lysosomal enzyme deficiency
Lipid lipoprotein accumulation
Central pultaceous lipid core
Smooth muscle cell proliferation
Elastosis
Fibrinogen− fibrin deposits
Thrombosis
Increased glycosaminoglycans
Hemorrhage
Hemosiderin deposits
Disruption of internal elastic lamina
Vascularity
Granulomata
Calcification
Ulceration, rupture
Fibrosis (collagenous cap)
Macrophage penetration

Figure 7.2
Summary of the histologic features of human atheroma.

identified as macrophages, lymphocytes and polymorphonuclear leucocytes.

As might be expected, the identity or origin of some cells remains uncertain, even at the ultrastructural level. Currently, there appears to be considerable interest centered on mononuclear cells and their role in atherogenesis. Lipid-rich macrophages or foam cells occur most consistently around the periphery of the central lipid core but may also be observed toward and on the surface of the collagenous cap, particularly toward the edges of a lesion. The presence of large mononuclear lipid-filled cells in the intimal lesion is one of the most prominent and consistently found features of atherosclerosis both in humans[1] and in experimental animals.[2,3] The source of these cells has long been a point of controversy, with possible origins from the blood[4] tissue macrophages[5] or smooth muscle cells.[1] The studies of O'Neal and co-workers[2,6–10] examined the possibility that foam cells arose from blood lipophages. These workers found that in hypercholesterolemia, circulating monocytes increased in number and that as many as 50 percent of these were lipid-laden. Their implication was that, since foam cells could be observed crossing the endothelium and circulating lipophages contained measurable quantities of lipid, blood lipophages could enter the arterial intima and provide at least one source of foam cells. They pointed out, however, that judging from morphologic comparison of the lipid content of circulating lipophages and tissue foam cells, further lipid accumulation must occur after penetration.

The results of our present study on swine suggest an alternative explanation.[11] Blood mononuclear cells have been shown to adhere to and penetrate the endothelium in large numbers within two weeks after initiation of a hypercholesterolemia-inducing diet, some ten weeks prior to early lesion formation in this model. These cells have been shown to have the ultrastructural appearance and azurophilic granules typical of the circulating monocyte.[12,13] Monocytes adherent to the endothelium or within the intima at prelesion stages contain no visible lipid inclusions. There is, moreover, a greater frequency of intimal monocytes in areas known to exhibit enhanced permeability[14] which the present results show to be the sites of earliest lesion formation. The reduced number of blocks showing adherent monocytes at twelve weeks may be artifactual due to the increased "clustering" of monocytes on the endothelium at this stage. The reason for this clumping is uncertain at this time, but its occurrence would reduce the probability of finding adherent monocytes on random 1-μ sections through these blocks.

The earliest lesion formed is a foam cell lesion in which there is no evidence of migration of medial smooth muscle cells into the intima or of engorgement by smooth muscle cells in the media. Lee et al[15] have previously described "monocyte-like," "undifferentiated," and "smooth muscle-like" cells in the intima of swine fed various diets. In the present study, undifferentiated intimal cells similar to those found by us in normal pigs[14] and by Lee et al[15] were also seen in foam cell lesions but were morphologically distinct from the much larger foam cells, and they contained little or no lipid. Additionally, no evidence of lipid-laden monocytes adhering to or penetrating the endothelium was observed, contrary to the suggestions of earlier studies.[7–9] The results would suggest, therefore, that foam cells of the early fatty lesions in swine arise from monocytes that penetrate the intima at prelesion stages. Medial smooth muscle cells and undifferentiated intimal cells do not appear to contribute significantly to this population. These conclusions are not antithetical to the hypothesis of smooth muscle cell involvement.[16] However, it must be remembered that the current study describes prelesion and very early lesion development and does not exclude the possibility of subsequent involvement of other cell types. It is also possible that these foam cell lesions do not mature into proliferative lesions with smooth muscle cell involvment.

Whether the initial stimulus that activates the adherence of blood monocytes to endothelium in these areas resides in alteration of the endothelial cells or cell surface, as described, or in changes to the intima, or to the monocyte itself, is uncertain. It is of interest, however, that low permeability areas show similar structural changes in the endothelium and (albeit reduced) adherence and intimal penetration by monocytes, but do not develop lesions by twelve weeks. It is tempting to suggest, therefore, that while hyperlipemia somehow activates monocytic adherence and migration in both blue and white areas, the greater permeability and susceptibility to injury of blue areas results in a more rapid and severe response. Over a protracted period of time, the enhanced permeability of blue areas may allow greater lipid influx and subsequent lipid engorgement of phagocytic monocytes, thus predisposing these areas to early foam cell lesion formation.

Fibrous proteins, which include collagen, elastin and fibrin, are important constituents of the plaque. Collagen, predominantly of Types I and III, is the major component of the fibrous cap. Fibrin can be observed both superficially and in the depths of plaques, and may be derived from circulating fibrin or fibrinogen directly, or from the organization and incorporation of mural thrombi. In this context, it is important to recognize the laminated, almost sedimentary structure of many plaques, a structure which in all likelihood results from the successive organization and incorporation of episodically occurring mural thrombi. There is little doubt that mural thrombosis contributes significantly to plaque growth. In so much as thrombosis and atherosclerosis are so closely associated, risk factors for clinical arterial disease usually do not differentiate between atherogenesis and thrombogenesis. CHD risk factors (Table 7.1) may enhance the risk for CHD[17] through thrombogenic mechanism(s).[18]

TABLE 7.1
Coronary Heart Disease Risk Factors

Primary	*Secondary*
1. Genetic predisposition for CHD	1. Overweight
2. High blood lipids	2. No exercise
3. Hypertension	3. Chronic stress
4. Smoking	4. Imbalanced diet
	5. Diabetes mellitus
	6. Hypothyroidism
	7. Renal disease
	8. Birth control pill
	9. Gout

Most atheromatous plaques contain Schiff-positive material and exhibit varying degrees of metachromasia. These staining reactions reflect the glycosaminoglycan content of lesions and in particular the complex sulfated polysaccharides such as chondroitin sulfate A and C, dermatan sulfate, hyaluronic acid and heparan sulfate. While it is too early to establish the relative significance of the recent findings of Camejo, et al[19, 20] it appears that proteoglycans may play a vital role in the initial role of lesion formation. Their work suggests that proteoglycans found in the arterial wall appear to bind the cholesterol rich particle (low-density lipoprotein, LDL), thus trapping the lipoprotein (or a subclass of this family of lipoprotein) in the arterial intima. Furthermore, they found that the amount of LDL-proteoglycan complex correlated strongly with the patients' history of coronary heart disease and/or the presence of atherosclerosis by angiographic studies.

Atherosclerosis has long been considered a disorder of intimal function, and indeed, intimal cell proliferation associated with tissue thickening and fibrosis are the hallmarks of a developing plaque. It should be emphasized that in human atherosclerotic lesions there is lipid accumulation in medial cells (both extracellularly and intracellularly) as well as in the intima during all stages of the pathogenesis of the lesion formation. Numerous studies by Hoff[20-23] and others[24-26] have clearly shown that LDL or LDL-like materials are found in the developing atheromatous lesions. It has been suggested that much of the intimal thickening, collagen formation and lipid accumulation may derive from cells that are normally present in the media that proliferate and then migrate to the intima in response to the lipid deposition. Once there, their further development contributes to intimal thickening, fibrous encapsulation of the lesion, irregular surface area, all characteristics of the developing plaque. Alternatively, medial cells damaged by the presence of excess blood borne factors may contribute to central necrosis of the atheromatous plaque.

Until very recently the evidence linking the arterial medial cell to the formation of the fibroelastic proteins and ground substance in atherosclerosis has been largely neglected. It is now well acknowledged that the smooth muscle plays a pivotal role in the genesis of the lesion. The critical question is what causes these cells (a) to preferentially take up LDL, (b) to migrate to the intima, (c) to proliferate, (d) to greatly increase the synthetic rate of collagen and elastin production? Since the smooth muscle cell is the principal cell found in human atheroma, further studies are necessary to elucidate the factors that regulate the metabolism and function of this ubiquitous cell in the atherosclerotic plaque.

Medial thinning, characteristic of the advanced raised or fibrous plaque, is largely the result of atrophic loss of smooth muscle cells. Adventitial changes associated with fibrous plaque but not with fatty streaks, include fibrosis, an increased vascularity, and in the majority of patients, a mononuclear infiltrate, which is predominantly lymphocytic.

This triad of histologically identifiable changes in the arterial adventitia is consistent with a chronic "inflammatory" reaction which, because of the considerable lymphocytosis, may have an immune or autoimmune basis. These changes are readily apparent to the vascular surgeon and make adventitial dissection of severely diseased arteries relatively difficult because of thickening and adhesions. The ultimate significance of this adventitial lymphocytosis remains uncertain; studies on the possible role of immune mechanisms in both atherogenesis and thrombogenesis are long overdue.

Definitions of atherosclerotic lesions

The term, "raised atherosclerotic lesion," is sometimes used to indicate the sum of fibrous plaques, complicated lesions and calcified lesions. Raised lesions are contrasted with fatty streaks, which typically show little or no elevation above the surrounding intimal surface.

It should be emphasized that the use of the word "atheroma" is not consistent among investigators. Some use it for the lesion described as a plaque with a pool of degenerated or necrotic lipid-rich debris. Others use atheroma to refer to the process of atherosclerosis or arteriosclerosis. Still others have used the term to refer to various lesions—from a fatty streak to a complicated lesion. To avoid ambiguity when one uses the term, it should be qualified or modified so that its meaning is perfectly clear.

Strong et al[27] described working definitions for different types of atherosclerotic lesions detectable (grossly); although this classification implies a pathogenetic sequence, it can be used as a descriptive classification regardless of the ideas of pathogenetic interrelationships among the lesions.

This classification of lesions based on gross examination does not permit distinction between those plaques, with and without a core of degenerated or necrotic lipid-rich debris. Those plaques with necrotic lesions and ulceration of the surface would of course be classified as complicated lesions. The plaques with necrotic centers and intact intimal surfaces ("atheroma" according to some classifications) would be classified as fibrous plaques. Microscopic examination is usually necessary to distinguish various subtypes of fibrous plaques.

Fatty streak: A fatty intimal lesion that is stained distinctly by Sudan IV and shows no other underlying change. Fatty streaks are flat or only slightly elevated and do not significantly narrow the lumina of blood vessels (Fig. 7.3b and 7.4b).

Fibrous plaque: A firm elevated intimal lesion, which in the fresh state is gray-white, glistening, and translucent. The surface of the lesion may be sudanophilic, but usually is not. Human fibrous plaques characteristically contain fat (Fig. 7.3c and 7.4c). Often a thick fibrous connective tissue cap containing varying amounts of lipid covers a more concentrated "core" of lipid. If a lesion also contains hemorrhage, thrombosis, ulceration or calcification, that lesion is classified according to one of the next two categories.

Complicated lesion: An intimal plaque in which there is hemorrhage, ulceration or thrombosis, with or without calcium.

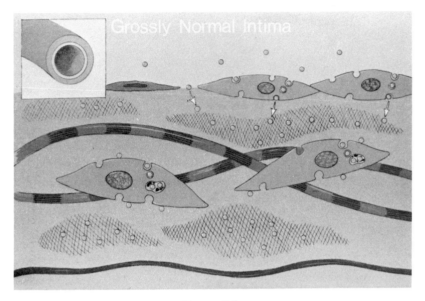

Figure 7.3a
Schematic drawing of a cross-section of the grossly normal intima of a medium- to large-sized human artery. Insert shows the cross-section of the whole vessel illustrating the diffuse intimal thickening (grey regions). Two healthy and one necrotic (on left) endothelial cell can be seen bordering the lumen (at top). Plasma LDL (spheres) can transit the endothelial lining either through a vesicular transport system as seen in the healthy cells or through large gaps between necrotic cells. Some of the LDL particles will pass through the intima, cross the internal elastic membrane (dark wavy line at bottom) and the tunica media (not shown), exit the artery and enter the lymphatics. Other LDL particles will be adsorbed and internalized by the spindle-shaped smooth muscle cells in the intima, enter lysosomes and be degraded. Still others will be trapped by the proteoglycan matrix (cross-hatched areas) in the extracellular space of the intima. Tub-like structures in the intima represent collagen fibers.

Calcified lesion: An intimal plaque in which insoluble mineral salts of calcium are visible or palpable without overlying hemorrhage, ulceration, or thrombosis.

Topographic distribution

The topographic distribution of atherosclerotic lesions has been described qualitatively[28-30] and it appears that lesions occur earliest and most extensively in the aorta. Lesions develop later and less extensively in the coronary and cerebral arteries, and the renal, mesenteric and pulmonary arteries were the least susceptible to atherosclerotic lesions.

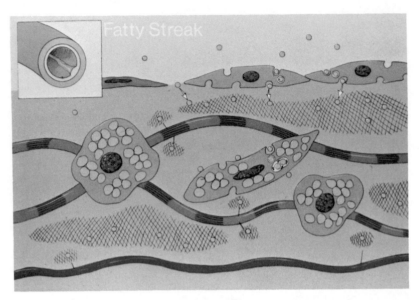

Figure 7.3b

Schematic drawing of a fatty streak lesion in a medium- to large-sized human artery. Insert shows this lesion to be slightly raised in adults and to extend in a longitudinal direction. This lesion is characterized by the presence of both normal and at times spindle-shaped lipid-filtered foam cells. The former are believed to be blood monocytes that have entered the artery at specific sites due to chemotaxis and then take up infiltered LDL by a mechanism still to be elucidated. Intact LDL can be found loosely complexed with proteoglycans (hatched areas) as well as tightly bound to extracellular components of the intima. This is suggested by the coupling of the spheres to the proteoglycan, which itself is associated to insoluble collagen and elastic fibers.

The arteries are involved by atherosclerosis in a definite sequence. The aorta is first involved, beginning in infancy with fatty streaks which increase rapidly during puberty. Fatty streaks begin in the coronary arteries during puberty, but begin to increase significantly and become converted into fibrous plaques in the third decade of life in high risk populations. The carotid arteries begin to be involved with fatty streaks at approximately the same age as the aorta, and the other cerebral arteries begin at approximately the same age as the coronary arteries. Raised lesions develop in the carotid arteries at roughly the same age as in the aorta, but do not develop in the vertebral and intracranial arteries until much later. Detailed quantitative or morphometric

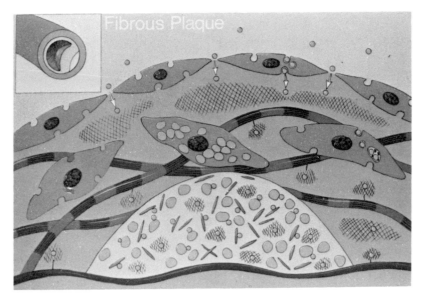

Figure 7.3c

Schematic drawing of a fibrous plaque in a medium- to large-sized human artery. The insert shows how such a lesion could encroach upon the vessel lumen. The lesion is characterized on its lumen side by a fibrous cap in which an intact but possibly more permeable endothelial lining covers a network of collagen fibers and proteoglycans interspersed between smooth muscle cells and macrophages. At the base of the plaque opposing the tunica media is a necrotic core rich in cholesteryl ester droplets and cholesterol crystals. LDL is retained mainly loosely bound to connective tissue in the cap region, but tightly bound in the lipid-rich core.

description on the distribution of lesions within the aorta, coronary arteries and arteries in the brain can be obtained elsewhere.[18]

Sequence of events

Atherosclerosis develops and progresses through stages involving a certain sequence of events.[31,32] The lesions may begin in infancy as one of the three earliest forms, i.e., the fatty dot and streak, microthrombus or gelatinous elevation. In the first two decades of life, only the early lesions are encountered. The second stage of the lesions, i.e., the fibrous atherosclerotic plaque, may develop at the end of the second but is usually established at the beginning of the third decade of life. The so-called complicated third-stage lesions[33,34] develop in the fourth and subsequent decades. Since the clinical manifestations of the disease are pre-

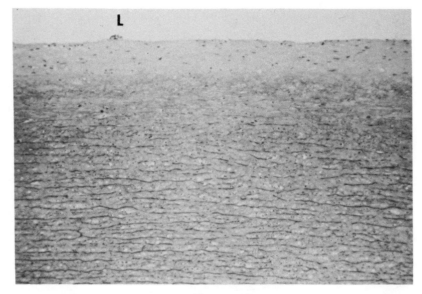

Figure 7.4a

*Light micrograph of a section through a grossly normal human adult aorta.
The intimal lining is subdivided into, (1) the lighter staining area close to the
lumen (L) in which smooth muscle cells are interspersed between collagen
fibers and a proteoglycan matrix; and (2) the darker staining region on the
luminal side of the elastica-rich (dark wavy lines) tunica media.*

ceded by stages in the evolution of the lesion over at least two to
three decades, it is understandable that attention has been di-
rected recently towards early life in the hope of retarding the
conversion of the earliest lesions to the advanced. This conversion
thus becomes important in the study of atheroma, particularly in
view of the fact that at present we are not capable of preventing
the inception of the early lesion, or of treating the advanced
lesions and their sequelae.

In man, the difficulty in unraveling the above problems is
compounded by many factors, which may be minimized or eliminated in experimental animals. One cannot study serially the
evolution of the emerging, complex human lesion at various time
intervals. A given population, no matter how similar the constituent subjects, can never be as homogeneous in a biological sense
as inbred animals of the same litter. The reactions of the highly
individualistic *Homo sapiens* to his environment and to the factors
considered to be important in atherosclerosis, e.g., food, occupation,

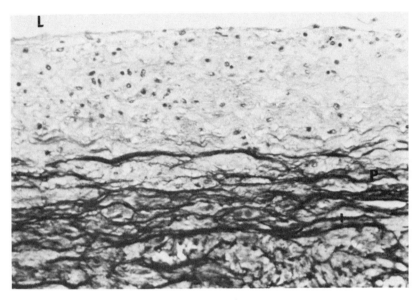

Figure 7.4b
Light micrograph of a fatty streak lesion in a human aorta. The slightly raised lesion is characterized by the presence of blood monocytes and foam cells. Lumen (L) is the top.

stress, genetic predisposition to CHD, cultural background, physical activities, other habits and geography, are expected to vary from one person to another, as do the lesions, even of the same type. It is, therefore, doubtful whether it will ever be possible to provide answers to questions and problems raised in the Introduction, at least with respect to the human lesion. Notwithstanding these limitations, and on the basis of our knowledge of general tissue reactions, it is reasonable to postulate the following course of events in the natural history of the atherosclerotic lesion.

Various factors relating to the make-up of the arterial wall, the prevailing hemodynamic conditions, and the status of the circulating blood may be injurious either to the endothelium or to the elements in the underlying intima.[33,35] Injury to the endothelium may be followed by an influx (insudation) of plasma constituents into the intima to form a gelatinous elevation, or by deposition of a microthrombus, or both.[35] Both processes may induce fatty metamorphosis of the smooth muscle in the underlying intima and in addition the insudation may cause mechanical damage to the intimal connective tissues. The failure to remove or organize the

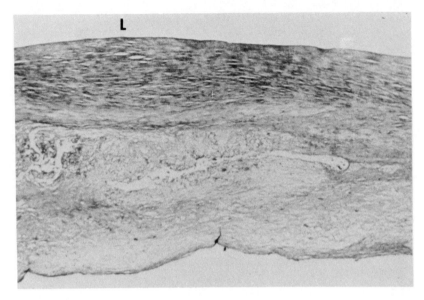

Figure 7.4c

Light micrograph of a fatty-fibrous plaque in a human aorta characterized by the presence of a fibrous cap (darker staining region close to the lumen) filtered with collagen fibers and some smooth muscle cells, and a necrotic core (light staining region) filtered with cholesteryl ester droplets and cholesterol crystals. Lumen is (L) at the top.

insudate and/or the thrombus may furnish substances that induce further lipid accumulation and provide stimuli for smooth muscle cells to proliferate in the area. The latter phenomenon may be enhanced in part by platelet factors[36] and by the nature of the lipoproteins in the insudate.[37]

The native smooth muscle cells accumulating lipid droplets may continue on that course beyond their ability to survive. Necrosis follows and the intracellular lipids, released into the extracellular space, contribute to the lipid component of the lesion. Once established, lesions of any one of the basic types appear to promote the development of some or all features of the two other forms. The tendency to repeated episodes of mural thrombosis and insudation, and the simultaneously ongoing proliferative and reparative phenomenon in the area contribute further to the complexity of the process.

Present knowledge of the morphogenesis of the lesions, while not sufficiently advanced to permit the prevention of their inception, may be considered to be at a stage that provides some basis for rational intervention of their growth, or retardation of their progression to fibrous atherosclerotic plaques and their complicated forms according to Wissler.[38] There are three stages in the reversal of the atherosclerotic process: (a) regression (decreased lipid content, cells, collagen, elastin and calcium), (b) remodeling (condensation and reorientation of collagen and elastin), and (c) healing (decreased evidence of endothelial cell damage, increased cell proliferation, etc.).

Risk factors and atherosclerosis

Epidemiologic investigation of living populations has disclosed characteristics of persons that are associated with increased risk of developing clinically manifest disease due to atherosclerosis—myocardial infarction, sudden death, angina pectoris, stroke or peripheral vascular disease. These characteristics are known as "risk factors," a descriptive but noncommittal term, which avoids

TABLE 7.2.

Degree of CHD Risk Based on Risk Factors

		Risk for CHD	
Risk Factors	*Normal*	*Above Average*	*High*
Total cholesterol (mg/dl)	<200	220–240	>240
Blood Pressure (mm Hg)			
Diastolic	80	90	105
Systolic	120	140	160
Smoking (pks/day)	0	1	2
Family History for CHD	Normal	Mod. high	High
Body weight	Normal	10% above normal	20% above normal
Exercise	Regularly	Infrequently	Never
Chronic stress	Minimal	Mod. exposure	High exposure
Diet	Low cholesterol Low saturated fat High fiber	Mod. cholesterol Moderate saturated fat Moderate fiber	High chol. High saturated fat Low fiber

the question of whether these characteristics are causative agents, intervening variables, early manifestations of disease, or secondary indicators of an underlying disturbance (see Table 7.1).

One can further define the risk factors as high, above average and normal risk as shown in Table 7.2.

While this concept for categorizing risk for CHD into high, above average and normal risk is convenient, it is a simplistic approach to assessing a patient's risk for CHD. For example, it is well established that elevated serum cholesterol concentration is associated with increased risk of atherogenesis and CHD.[39,40,41,42] Persons with disorders characterized by elevated levels of serum cholesterol or low density lipoprotein (LDL) have a strikingly high incidence of CHD, which often is evident at an early age.[43] If the familial β-hyperlipoproteinemic condition is of a homozygote origin, fatal complications of premature atherogenesis occur before age thirty.[44,45] From epidemiological studies and basic and clinical research, there appears to be little doubt that hypercholesterolemia exists as an independent risk factor for coronary artery disease (CAD).[46,47,48] Data from Mainland China show that the mean serum cholesterol level in normal people is 136 mg/dl, while in CHD patients it is 190 mg/dl.[49] Thus, in a country with a low rate of CHD, there also appears to be a positive relationship between CHD and cholesterol levels. The relationship is continuous and, in fact, is exponential as the level of serum cholesterol increases. There are no cut-off points to speak of. Therefore, in assessing a person's risk for CHD, the risk factors should be considered as a continuum.

Another concept that should be remembered when considering CHD risk factors is that statistically valid data obtained on large populations and in prospective epidemiological studies are not necessarily directly applicable to an individual. As discussed by Blackburn,[50] there is a large variation among individuals in these predisposing factors, and within a single individual during his life span. Factors acting throughout the entire period of the developing degenerative disease are difficult, if not impossible, to evaluate. At any one time, primary risk factors (hypertension, smoking, elevated blood cholesterol level, family history for coronary artery disease) and secondary risk factors are simultaneously involved in the pathogenesis.

Still another difficulty is that differences in food habits have not been adequately demonstrated within the United States between people with and without coronary disease, although habitual diet is related to serum cholesterol concentrations in different populations. The Framingham Study seems to suggest that individual genetic, personal and environmental differences may override the small differences in dietary intake within any one culture.[51]

In spite of these possible overriding factors, there can be little doubt that the initiation, development, progression, and regression of atherosclerosis are closely associated with nutritional factors. The evidence accumulated over the last forty years in animal, clinical, and epidemiological studies is impressive and persuasive. Nutrition has an important influence on several of the risk factors, particularly serum lipids, lipoproteins, overweight, hypertension, endocrine imbalance and other metabolic conditions closely associated with atherosclerosis. With appropriate nutritional adjustments, these conditions associated with degenerative vascular disease can be altered and controlled. Whether the modification of these risk factors by diet will ultimately lead to lower mortality and morbidity from CHD is yet to be proved. Four primary prevention studies (Los Angeles Veterans Administration Study, Finnish Diet Study, Oslo Diet-Heart Study and U.S. Diet-Heart Study) using dietary measures have shown a trend toward favorable results.[52,53,54,55] Recently, Frantz[56] from the Minnesota Coronary Survey, reported that in the cholesterol-lowering dietary trial, men fifty years of age showed less mortality and morbidity from CHD events than the control group.

It is now believed that dietary treatment in this country should be initiated when the serum cholesterol level is >220 mg/dl in adults and above 200 mg/dl in children.[57,58] The upper limit of serum triglyceride levels is less clear. Perhaps levels in excess of 130–150 mg/dl can be considered unhealthy.[59] The rationale for initiating dietary therapy when the above limits are exceeded is to prevent or minimize the development of CHD, since atherosclerosis seldom occurs with total cholesterol concentration <200 mg/dl over the life span of an individual,[60] unless other risk factors such as genetics, high blood pressure, smoking and obesity play a dominant role.

While serum lipids are not to be neglected, the influence of other risk factors associated with CHD should also be simultaneously considered. They include smoking, hypertension, obesity, stress, lack of physical activity, hormonal imbalances and other primary disease states directly or indirectly associated with abnormal lipid and lipoprotein metabolism.

The primary risk factors also are associated with more severe and more extensive atherosclerotic lesions as well as with more frequent clinical disease. We have various degrees of knowledge about mechanisms of their effects on atherogenesis, but relatively little knowledge about whether they affect thrombosis as a terminal occlusive episode, and if so, how.

Age

Of all risk factors, age has the strongest and most consistent association with lesions. As with so many chronic diseases, the incidence rates of all atherosclerotic diseases increase with age. The simplest explanation of this association is an accumulation of responses to injury as exposure to injury increases. This explanation may be true in middle-aged and older persons, but the early stages of atherogenesis during adolescence show more specific age-dependent changes. Aortic fatty streaks increase rapidly in extent between eight and eighteen years and fibrous plaques begin to form from fatty streaks in the coronary arteries at about twenty years.[61] These age trends suggest that the artery wall undergoes a systematic change with maturation, that the artery wall is exposed to distinctive atherogenic agents at those ages.

The concept of aging as a degenerative change after attaining adult growth is not yet sufficiently refined to explain progression of the advanced lesions of atherosclerosis in biochemical and physiological terms.[62] The cumulative effect of repeated injuries and the associated scarring seem to account for most of the age effects on lesions in adulthood, but a more precise definition of aging of smooth muscle cells may change this view.

Male sex

Except for age, male sex is one of the best documented and strongest risk factors for *coronary* heart disease, but not for the other forms of atherosclerotic disease. Furthermore, the sex differential in coronary heart disease is most marked in whites and is greatly attenuated or absent in nonwhites. The sex differential also is most attenuated in populations with low overall incidence rates of atherosclerotic disease, and is reduced or eliminated among diabetics. Despite the attractiveness of the hypothesis that the estrogenic hormones of the female are responsble for her protection from coronary atherosclerosis, it has become clear that exogenous estrogens do not add to the natural protection of the female. Females have slightly lower levels of three major risk factors between the menarche and the menopause (serum cholesterol, blood pressure and cigarette smoking), but the lower levels of risk factors do not seem sufficient to account for the differences in coronary heart disease. Male sex in whites remains the most puzzling of all of the risk factors, and the one for which we have the least coherent hypothesis regarding mechanism.

Hypercholesterolemia

Until recently total serum cholesterol concentration was recognized as the strongest and most consistent risk factor for atherosclerotic disease other than age and sex, and reduction in serum cholesterol has received much attention as a means of preventing disease. Serum cholesterol concentration can be elevated in many animal species by feeding a human-like high fat, high cholesterol diet, and these animals develop intimal lipid deposits resembling human fatty streaks. Cholesterolemia maintained in the range of 200–400 mg/dl for several years leads to experimental lesions that are reasonable facsimiles of human fibrous plaques. However, in both humans and animals, there remains a high degree of individual variation in cholesterolemic response to an atherogenic diet; and at any level of serum cholesterol, there is wide variation in the response of the arterial wall in forming atherosclerotic lesions.

Knowledge about the cellular metabolism of LDL, which carries most of the plasma cholesterol, provides an attractive hypothesis for the mechanism by which hypercholesterolemia initiates intimal lipid deposits and causes some of them to progress to fibrous plaques.[20-26,62] Cells (including fibroblasts and smooth muscle cells) possess specific receptors that bind LDL and promote internalization. The uptake of LDL suppresses synthesis of cholesterol in the cell. Internalized LDL is degraded, and the cholesterol is hydrolyzed and re-esterified as cholesteryl oleate. The cell thus obtains cholesterol for membrane structures at lower energy cost than by synthesis. In the presence of excess LDL, lipoprotein is internalized by a nonspecific process that does not suppress cholesterol synthesis, and cholesteryl ester accumulates within the cell in excess. Prolonged accumulation leads to cell death, extravasation of cholesterol esters and other debris, and a consequent chronic inflammatory and reparative reaction which results in the fibrous plaque (Figure 7.2 p. 181).

Since elevated serum cholesterol levels can be lowered by diet modification, by exercise, by weight reduction, and by drugs, a major question now is whether reduction in serum cholesterol slows progression or permits regression of advanced atherosclerosis. Clinical trials of lipid-lowering agents in post-myocardial infarction patients (secondary prevention) have shown no benefit, and early trials of lipid-lowering regimens in relatively small numbers of apparently healthy middle-aged or elderly persons (primary prevention) have yielded suggestive but not conclusive results. Currently, large scale trials are underway.[63] It may never be possible to conduct a controlled trial of maintaining low serum cholesterol levels from childhood, but much circumstantial evidence suggests that control in childhood is likely to be more effective than in adults.

The relationship of serum cholesterol concentration to atherosclerotic disease has been strengthened by the recent demonstration of an inverse association with high density lipoprotein (HDL) cholesterol.[64] This epidemiologic observation is consistent with current hypotheses that the metabolic function of HDL is to transport cholesterol from peripheral tissues to the liver for eventual degradation and excretion. However, it now appears that serum total cholesterol levels do not correlate as well as HDL-cholesterol and LDL-cholesterol when studying CHD prevalence in population studies. The data are suggesting that the virtue of partitioning total cholesterol into various lipoprotein fractions assessing CHD risk appears to be a more reasonable approach for biochemical profiling. If one fraction (HDL-cholesterol) has a negative association with the risk for CHD while the other two (VLDL- and LDL-cholesterol) have positive associations with CHD risk, then the arithmetic sum (i.e., total cholesterol) must be a less sensitive indicator of risk than an appropriately weighted algebraic sum.

In recent studies when the apo-β-containing lipoproteins in buffer homogenates of human aortic plaques and grossly normal intima were isolated into a d 1.006-1.063 density fraction by differential ultracentrifugation and further purified by gel filtration, the chemical composition was found to be very similar to that of plasma LDL (Hoff, unpublished results). However, the electrophoretic mobility was pre-β rather than β, signifying a more electronegative charge. This alteration could be due to chemical modification such as interaction with malonaldehyde, which is released in prostaglandin synthesis from arachidonic acid as well as in auto-oxidation of unsaturated fatty acids. The increased negative charge could also be the result of contamination with negatively charged compounds such as tissue sulfated glycosaminoglycans.

When extracts of aortic plaques were introduced to cultured mouse peritoneal macrophages, a dramatic increase in incorporation of C^{14} oleate into cholesteryl oleate was found. By contrast plasma LDL induced minimal esterification. The uptake of cholesterol from the extracts followed the kinetics characteristic of a high affinity binding system. Degradation of those exogenous cholesterol esters was shown to occur in lysosomes since their re-esterification with C^{14} oleate was inhibited with chloroquine. When permitted to incubate for longer time periods, the macrophages esterified so much exogenous cholesterol that foam cells were formed (unpublished observations). Although most of the esterifying activity was found in non-LDL complexes of lipid and protein in plaques, the LDL separated from the remaining material by affinity chromatography also demonstrated an ability to induce enhanced esterification. Further studies will clarify whether the aorta-derived LDL can induce foam cell formation in macrophages. If a similar mechanism of cholesteryl ester accumulation occurs *in vivo* in blood monocytes that have entered into the LDL-rich arterial intima, triggered by chemotaxis, the evolution of topographically thin focal, foam cell-rich fatty streak lesions will become clarified.

Alternatively, the increased negative charge on the aorta-derived LDL could be due to the preferential retention in the aorta of a subclass of plasma LDL with a greater negative charge. This subclass could represent Lp(a) which also possesses pre-β electrophoretic mobility. Moreover, its characteristic apoprotein, apo(a) could be identified in these lipoproteins extracted from aortas.

Berg[65] discovered this apo-β containing lipoprotein he termed Lp(a) by using adsorbed antisera from rabbits obtained by immunization with a β-lipoprotein fraction from human donors. These human sera, which formed immunoprecipitates with the adsorbed rabbit antisera, were referred to a Lp(a$^+$) and those that did not as Lp(a$^-$). The frequency of Lp(a$^+$) individuals in Caucasian populations was found by Berg to be around 35 percent. However, Kostner,[66] using a more sensitive immunochemical technique, reported that Lp(a) was detectable in 96 percent of the sera from a group of 500 healthy Austrians. Although many investigators have found the inheritance of the Lp(a) antigen to be governed by a single gene,[65] others have interpreted their data to be more compatible with a polygenic mechanism of inheritance.[66,67]

The Lp (a) antigen is typically associated with a population of lipoprotein particles that can be isolated ultracentrifugally in the density range 1.050–1.080 gm/ml.[66,67] The contaminating LDL and HDL$_2$ usually present in this density range can be removed by gel filtration chromatography over BioGel A15M[66]. The purified lipoprotein, Lp(a), exhibits pre-β-mobility upon agarose electrophoresis. The molecular weight of the particle has been determined to be 4.8×10^6 by gel filtration chromatography, 5.6×10^6 by electron microscopy and 5.2×10^6 by analytical ultracentrifugation. Other physical properties reported for this lipoprotein include a hydrated density of 1.0855 gm/ml, a flotation rate of $Sf_{20}1.20 = 24$ and an isoelectric point of 4.9.[66] Chemical analysis has revealed Lp(a) to contain 27.0 percent protein, 8.5 percent carbohydrate, 41.7 percent total cholesterol, 19.2 percent phospholipid, and 2.7 percent triglyceride.[67] The esterified:unesterified cholesterol ratio is approximately 4.2 percent. The distribution of hexose, hexosamine, and sialic acid is about 4.4 percent, 2.3 percent, and 1.8 percent respectively of the total. The principal phospholipids in Lp(a) are phosphatidylcholine and sphingomyelin, which occur in 2:1 ratio. The apoprotein obtained by delipidation of Lp(a) is a heterogeneous mixture containing 65 percent apo-β, 15 percent albumin, and 20 percent apo(a), the last component being found in no other lipoprotein than Lp(a).[68] Apo(a) is a glycoprotein, which contains about 20 percent carbohydrate by weight. Amino acid analysis reveals a composition distinctly different from that of apo-β, and is distinguished by its high content of glutamic acid and absence of tryptophan.[66]

Considerably less is known about the metabolism of Lp(a) than about its structure and genetics. Krempler et al[69] have determined its half-life in serum to be 35–58 hr. Apparently, Lp(a) is not a metabolic product of other lipoproteins containing apo-β as determined by the absence of radioactivity from the Lp(a) density range up to five days after the injection of ^{125}I-VLDL into Lp(a$^+$) individuals.[69] However, this study does not discount the possibility that Lp(a) might be synthesized independently, then catabolized to LDL through the loss of apo(a). Jurgens et al[70] have reported that esterase and protease activity are associated with purified Lp(a) and apo(a), and suggest that this enzymatic activity is related to the high tendency of Lp(a) to aggregate and precipitate.

Dahlen and Uricson[71] reported a positive correlation between angina pectoris and the occurrence of a plasma lipoprotein fraction that exhibited pre-β-electrophoretic mobility on cellulose acetate. Subsequently, they observed a highly significant association ($p<0.001$) between the occurrence of this electrophoretic band and the presence of the Lp(a) antigen as detected by standard double immunodiffusion techniques.[72] Lp(a) detected either electrophoretically or immunochemically has been found to occur more frequently in patients with sustained myocardial infarction than in healty controls.[73] Furthermore, the group found a positive correlation ($p<0.005$) between the level of electrophoretically demonstrable Lp(a) and the degree of coronary atherosclerosis, as determined by coronary angiography.[74] In a small group of patients with intermittent claudication, a significantly higher mean level of Lp(a) was found than in age-matched controls.[75] From these studies it was concluded that high levels of Lp(a) may be associated with early atherosclerosis and early coronary heart disease, although no causal relationship has been established, and the statistical relationship may be due to other associations.

The interaction of Lp(a) and other lipoproteins with glycosaminoglycans (GAG) covalently bound to Sepharose has been studied.[76] Binding of Lp(a) to GAG-Sepharose was minimal at physiological ionic strength, but was considerably enhanced by the addition of calcium ions.[72] When calcium was present, the association of Lp(a) to the solid-supported glycosaminoglycan was significantly stronger than that exhibited by HDL, LDL or VLDL. In a study of the effectiveness of different divalent cations for facilitating lipoprotein binding to GAG-Sepharose, Lp(a) was more sensitive than the other classes to the presence of these ions. Lp(a) was found to be the only lipoprotein that precipitated at physiological ionic strength and calcium ion concentration. These studies suggest that Lp(a) might be more easily bound and precipitated in the GAG-lattice of the intima than other atherogenic lipoproteins such as LDL.[77] From the aforementioned survey of the literature as well as of unpublished observations, it would appear that plasma Lp(a), and the apo-β containing lipoprotein fraction extracted from human aortas, have numerous similar characteristics, leading one to speculate that Lp(a) may be more "atherogenic" than LDL.

Thus, knowledge of lipoprotein metabolism supports the link between serum cholesterol concentration and atherogenesis by suggesting biochemical mechanisms for the relationship. Whether elevation of serum cholesterol or a specific lipoprotein concentration contributes to risk of coronary heart disease by other mechanisms, such as, for example, by predisposing to thrombosis, remains a possibility that may provide additional links.

Hypertension

Like serum cholesterol concentration, increase in blood pressure in all ranges is associated with increased risk of atherosclerotic disease,[78] and particularly cerebrovascular disease.[79] The risk increases progressively with higher levels of blood pressure, and is demonstrable in both systolic and diastolic pressure.[80] When diastolic pressures are in the range from 85 to 94 mm Hg, the incidence of events is significantly increased above that of men whose diastolic pressure falls below 85 mm Hg. There is doubling of incidence if diastolic pressures are in the range of 95 to 104 mm Hg, and a quadrupling of this rate with still higher diastolic pressure. Comparable risks attach to these groupings of diastolic pressure when assessed by death rates for CHD. When hypertension coexists along with hypercholesterolemia or ciga-

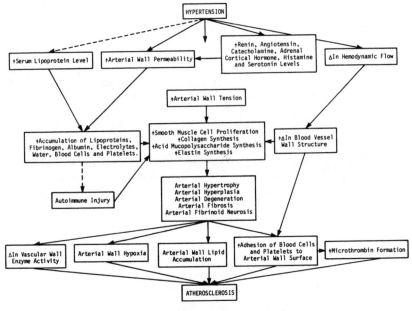

Figure 7.5

A schematic representation of the possible association between elevated blood pressure and pathogenesis of the blood vessel wall from Lewis and Naito,[78] reproduced with permission from Clinical Chemistry.

rette smoking, there is additional risk for first major coronary events. For all levels of diastolic blood pressure, the risk is increased by a factor of two when the persons are also cigarette smokers. In addition to its contribution of risk for CHD, hypertension is an important determinant of the occurrence of other life-threatening illnesses, i.e., renal failure, stroke, and congestive heart failure. Elevation of blood pressure is one of the most commonly occurring physical abnormalities in adults and very probably in adolescents.[81] Hypertension selectively augments cerebral atherosclerosis.[82] The most obvious mechanisms of action of hypertension on atherogenesis are by increasing filtration of lipoprotein-rich plasma through the intima, or by increasing the workload of smooth muscle cells of the artery wall. Less obvious is the potential effect of humoral mediators of blood pressure on the artery wall, as, for example, angiotensin II, norepinephrine, serotonin and bradykinin.[78,83] Figure 7.5 illustrates the complexity of the association of hypertension and atherosclerosis. Since some antihypertensive drugs lead to increased levels of these mediators, such drug regimens may augment rather than ameliorate the atherogenic effect of hypertension. The beneficial effects of antihypertensive drug therapy on stroke and congestive heart failure are not in question, but whether such therapy reduces coronary heart disease incidence is still not clear. Not to be neglected is the fact that hypertension also may affect thrombosis as well as atherogenesis.

Cigarette smoking

As the association between cigarette smoking and atheroslerotic disease was developed in epidemiological studies, there was initial uncertainty whether cigarette smoking accelerated atherogenesis or whether it only predisposed to the terminal episode by precipitating thrombosis or arrhythmia. It now appears certain that cigarette smoking augments atherogenesis in the coronary arteries and the abdominal aorta,[84] and it probably has a similar effect on the peripheral arteries. In essence, the greater the daily usage, the larger the risk. Similarly, the person who characteristically smokes most of each cigarette, and discards but little, increases the hazard of the habit. The age at which cigarette smoking is adopted as a habit is also of importance: the younger the age, the greater the eventual risk of experiencing the clinical manifestations of the disease. The length of the period of habitual smoking in years and the total number of cigarettes smoked are potent determining factors as well. All of these factors seem to pertain only to the use of tobacco in the form of cigarettes. The same risks do not apply to the smoking of a pipe or cigars. Since inhaling of cigarette smoke is a common practice, whereas inhaling of tobacco smoke from cigars or pipes is not, it has been suspected that the process of inhaling is an important determinant.[85]

A number of reports have brought evidence that once the habit of cigarette smoking is discarded, the relative risk of developing manifestations of CHD is reduced. Following an interval of ten or more years of abstinence, the ex-smoker enters a risk category comparable to that of the person who has never smoked.[86-90] The experience of those who stop smoking suggests that it also affects the terminal occlusive episode since the risk of ex-smokers begins to drop more rapidly after cessation than we would expect from regression of advanced atherosclerosis alone.[91]

We do not know what component of cigarette smoke is responsible for the acceleration of atherosclerosis nor the hypothesized effect on thrombosis. Carbon monoxide is widely suspected but its role is not proved. Cigarette smoke contains about 3,000 identified chemicals and probably more unidentified ones, and therefore many possibilities remain.

Of all the risk factors, cigarette smoking seems the most likely to be thrombogenic as well as atherogenic. Scattered reports indicate that it affects several coagulation tests. A promising new lead is that a tobacco glycoprotein activates factor XII.[92]

Becker[93] presented data suggesting that constituents of tobacco might be related to cardiovascular disease through IgE mediated mechanisms, through activation of the clotting cascade, and/or the synergistic action of both.

In these experiments, a glycoprotein of approximately 18,000 daltons was purified from flue-cured Virginia Bright tobacco leaves and from cigarette smoke condensate. Approximately one-third of human volunteers exhibited immediate cutaneous hypersensitivity when inoculated intracutaneously with tobacco glycoprotein (TGP), whether or not they were smokers. The high incidence of hypersensitivity among both groups may be due to either (a) the presence of TGP in cigarette smoke and sensitization of smokers and, vicariously, of nonsmokers, and/or (b) the presence of cross-reacting antigen in commonly eaten members of the family *Solanaceae* to which tobacco belongs.

Neonatal sensitization and subsequent boostering of rabbits with TGP resulted in the selective production of heat labile homocytophilic (hence IgE) antibodies to TGP that could mediate passive cutaneous anaphylaxis reactions when challenged with TGP derived from either cured tobacco leaves or cigarette smoke condensate.[94]

In further experiments TGP was demonstrated to contain rutin, which closely resembles quercetin, a substance known to activate factor XII. The capacity of TGP to activate factor XII was measured and it was observed that addition of TGP to normal human plasma shortened the partial thromboplastin time, activated fibrinolysis, and stimulated generation of bradykinin. These effects were not demonstrable in factor XII deficient plasma.[92]

These experiments taken together suggest that constituents of tobacco can initiate an inflammatory response either through IgE-mediated mechanisms or through activation of factor XII-dependent pathways, and thereby injure blood vessels in both the pulmonary and systemic circulation. The capacity of TGP to activate the intrinsic pathway of coagulation might also contribute to both the growth of arteriosclerotic plaques and to the lethal complications of arteriosclerosis by initiating thrombus formation. In this connection, Theorell et al[95] suggested that large quantities of fibrinopeptide A were found in the blood of human subjects who had been challenged with allergens.

Family history

Familial aggregation of atherosclerotic disease has long been recognized, but only a small beginning has been made in isolating the strictly genetic basis for this aggregation in contrast to the common environment shared by family members. The only specific progress has been in identifying genetic hyperlipidemias. Genetic bases for hypertension and diabetes are suspected. Undoubtedly, a portion of the residual variability in atherosclerosis not explained by the known risk factors lies in unidentified genetic traits, perhaps programmed characteristics of the artery wall. Genetically determined variations in susceptibility to atherosclerosis have been demonstrated in animals and undoubtedly exist in humans as well.

In view of the numerous genetic defects in the coagulation system and the presumed important role of thrombosis in atherosclerotic disease, it is remarkable that no genetic coagulation abnormality has been found associated with atherosclerotic disease.

Obesity

The precise role of obesity in atherosclerotic disease remains uncertain, despite nearly universal recommendations that obesity should be avoided in order to reduce risk of atherosclerotic disease. Obesity appears well established as a risk factor for hypertension, hyperlipidemia, and diabetes, and undoubtedly influences atherosclerosis indirectly through these mechanisms, but in their absence, no clear association of obesity either with atherogenesis or with atherosclerotic disease has been demonstrated.

The Framingham data demonstrate a definite and independent risk for sudden death and the development of angina pectoris in men and a smaller, more indefinite risk in women.[96] In this evaluation, obesity was assessed by assigning a relative weight for each individual derived by comparison of the weight on initial observation with the median weight in the Framingham sample of persons of the same sex and height. Obese persons were defined as having a relative weight of 120 percent or above. The rate of occurrence of angina pectoris was compared in obese and non-obese men who either did or did not have elevation in systolic blood pressure (i.e., 160 mm Hg or above) or serum cholesterol (i.e., 250 mg/dl or greater). The risk of angina was similarly enhanced (by a factor of about 2.7) in obese men, whether or not there was coexisting hypertension or hypercholesterolemia.

However, the existence of one or both of the complicating major risk factors increased the risk for both the nonobese and obese. The morbidity ratio in nonobese men was increased from 0.7, when neither blood pressure nor cholesterol was elevated, to 1.15, when either or both were increased. Comparable ratios in obese men were 1.9 without and 3.29 with these associated major risk factors. The same measures in women show little difference between obese and nonobese when neither blood pressure nor cholesterol was elevated; but with increase in either, the morbidity ratio was increased from 1.13 in nonobese to 1.76 in obese women. Another assessment of the possible effect of obesity was provided by relating gain in body weight after the age of twenty-five years to the rate of development of angina pectoris. The observed increase in risk was proportional to the weight gained. Other evidence indicates that the extent of obesity is an important consideration in assessing risk but that moderate obesity without coexistent hypercholesterolemia, hypertension, or cigarette smoking produces only a modest increase of coronary disease.[86,97]

Physical activity

Many benefits are derived from regular physical activity, and it has been widely recommended for preventing atherosclerotic disease.[98–99] There is some evidence that extreme physical activity is associated with less risk of coronary heart disease, but the level of activity required is difficult to attain in our present society. While exercise directly increases cardiovascular fitness, increased physical activity is known to lower total serum cholesterol,[98,100] LDL-cholesterol, yet raise HDL-cholesterol.[100]

Part of the "anti-coronary effect" of exercise might be through relationships between physical activity and other risk factors. Certainly, relative inactivity and characteristic sedentary modes of living contribute importantly to the occurrence of obesity. Although, as noted above, obesity is not in itself a major risk factor, loss of weight is often accompanied by lessening of other risks, i.e., reduction in serum cholesterol and blood pressure and improvement in glucose tolerance. An important part of effective programs of weight reduction of obese persons is planned and on-going exercise to achieve increased and moderate energy expenditure. Animal experiments have found that exercise may suppress rather than increase appetite.[98,101] Moreover, the physical training brings physiologic and metabolic adaptations that may improve cardiovascular and other organ system function.

Fasting plasma lipids (especially elevated triglycerides) are responsive to physical activity. They are lower in physically trained men as contrasted to others who are sedentary, and these levels are reduced by programs of planned exercise.[102,103] A bout of vigorous activity will reduce elevated levels of triglycerides in plasma. In contrast, the total cholesterol content of plasma is not as responsive to increased physical activity, especially if the concentration is already normal or low-normal, or the exercise program is of not sufficient intensity, duration and frequency. It is likely that reports of reduced cholesterol levels with exercise have been influenced by modification of diet and loss of body weight. A fact of potential significance, however, is the recent demonstration that the cholesterol content of plasma lipoproteins is quite different in very active men when compared to a randomly selected control group of comparable age.[101] Specifically, HDL cholesterol concentration was greater and LDL less in the active group, a situation previously reported as favorable for reduced risk of CHD.

Renal failure patients on chronic hemodialysis

It is well known that patients with renal failure on chronic hemodialysis die of premature CHD. According to Lindner et al[104] more than 60 percent of hemodialysis patients died of arteriosclerotic cardiovascular complications. The mechanism by which this occurs has not been resolved. There is sufficient documentation that hyperlipidemia and dyslipoproteinemia occur in this group of subjects.[105-107] More specifically, 58 percent of the hemodialysis patients have elevated levels of intermediate-density lipoprotein (IDL), which suggests a defect in VLDL catabolism due to a decreased post-heparin lipoprotein lipase activity.[105]

Diabetes mellitus

Cardiovascular disease, particularly atherosclerotic disease, remains the major health hazard for the diabetic. According to the study done by Palumbo et al,[108] 39 percent of the diabetic patients died because of CHD, a rate 1.7 times that expected. Forty percent of the patients were obese and with relative weight of 125 percent or more. The rates of occurrence of other CHD risk factors such as hypercholesterolemia, hypertriglyceridemia, hypertension, and smoking were not given. A comparable mortality experience was reported for a group of 21,447 diabetic patients cared for at the Joslin Clinic in Boston during the period from 1930 to 1960, in which the overall mortality was higher than in the population at large by a factor of 1.93 and the standardized mortality ratio for coronary artery disease was 1.84.[109]

The University Group Diabetes Study (UGDS) was undertaken to determine if use of hypoglycemic agents and the control of blood sugar influenced the rate of occurrence of vascular complications in patients with maturity-onset diabetes.[110] Among the findings of this investigation was the fact that all efforts to control hyperglycemia as measured by fasting blood sugar levels failed to reduce mortality or morbidity from cardiovascular causes. Moreover, the number and proportion of deaths due to myocardial infarction and other cardiovascular diseases were significantly greater among diabetic patients provided treatment with the hypoglycemic agents.

The atherogenic effect of diabetes has not been linked to the capillary basement membrane thickening characteristic of diabetes. Both vascular lesions may have as a common basis a fundamental defect affecting connective tissue, but such a link is speculative. Diabetics have higher serum lipid levels, especially of triglycerides, than do nondiabetics but the differences do not account for the increased risk of atherosclerotic disease. Diabetes reduces greatly the sex differential in mortality from coronary heart disease, but does not change the sex differential in angina pectoris.[111] A diabetic effect on the terminal episode would be consistent with this observation. Neither insulin nor oral hypoglycemic agents protect diabetics from the increased risk of atherosclerotic disease, and the findings of the UGDS indicate that oral hypoglycemic drugs increase the probability of cardiovascular death for the diabetic.[110] As with other complex metabolic diseases, it seems likely that diabetes also may influence thrombosis.

Hypothyroidism

It has long been known from both clinical observations and animal experiments that the metabolism of lipids is influenced by hormones, particularly thyroxine. Among the lipids, serum cholesterol levels show the greatest regularity in response to the circulating level of thyroid hormone, but other lipid components may be affected.[112] Our results indicated that the serum total cholesterol concentration of the hypothyroid patients is higher than the euthyroid group. On the other hand the hyperthyroid patients have slightly lower levels of total cholesterol. The serum triglyceride and phospholipid levels of the hypothyroid group are slightly higher than the euthyroid or hyperthyroid groups, which are in agreement with past reports.

The serum lipoprotein electrophoresis study indicates that there is a higher percentage of β-lipoprotein in the hypothyroid group when compared to the euthyroid patients. This agrees with the elevated serum total cholesterol content seen in the hypothyroid individuals. While there is a reduction in the total cholesterol in the hyperthyroid group, there was no reduction in the distribution of lipoproteins in the β-lipoprotein class. There is, however, less cholesterol (45 ± 3 mg/dl) in the HDL of the hyperthyroid group when compared to the hypothyroid group (53 ± 4 mg/dl). HDL cholesterol concentration for the euthyroid group was 50 ± 4 mg/dl. It is interesting that the slight elevation of serum triglycerides seen in the hypothyroid group did not result in a concomitant rise in pre-β-lipoprotein. Whether the increased proportion of β-lipoprotein in the hypothyroid group resulted in more cholesterol and triglycerides carried in that moiety is not clear. Only when serum triglycerides were markedly elevated (>200 mg/dl) was there a concomitant rise in the pre-β-lipoprotein fraction.

Gout

A common metabolic disorder associated with gout is hyperlipidemia. The high incidence of atherosclerosis as a complication of gout has been recognized for about 100 years. However, the precise relationships of gout or hyperuricemia to coronary artery disease have not been clear. The relationship of primary gout to dysmetabolism of lipids and lipoproteins also is not clear.

A recent review[113] indicated that, although there is much discrepancy in published data on the relationship of increased serum uric acid and blood lipid concentrations, there appears to be a high correlation between the two variables, particularly between hypertriglyceridemia and hyperuricemia. The relationship between serum uric acid and triglyceride concentrations is not always predictable,[114] However, according to Naito and Mackenzie,[115] about 73 percent of the asymptomatic gout patients had hypertriglyceridemia in their study, 1.6-fold the frequency found in the control group. Types IV and IIb lipoprotein electrophoretic patterns were most prevalent in the gout group. Neither alcohol intake nor hyperuricemia, per se, seems to be the cause of the lipid and lipoprotein disorder and cannot be related to liver or kidney dysfunctions. Obesity was the major underlying factor associated with lipidemia. The study suggested that diet and, possibly, defective clearance of triglycerides may be etiologic factors associated with the abnormal serum triglyceride and lipoprotein concentrations in these individuals.

Oral contraceptive agents

The introduction and wide use of oral contraceptive agents has brought significant health and social advantages for women. However, it has become increasingly apparent that there are health hazards involved in their use. Most important among these are morbidity and mortality from cardiovascular diseases. The physiologic and metabolic effects of these agents are dependent on the type and quantity of steroid contained, whether synthetic estrogens or derivatives of nortestosterone and progesterone. These effects cannot be examined in detail here, but a comprehensive review of the subject is available.[116]

Metabolic side effects of the contraceptive steroids include changes in plasma cholesterol and triglyceride concentrations, which are related to the specific steroids used, dosage and duration of treatment.[117] In general, the effects are small and nortestosterone derivatives counteract the triglyceride-increasing effect of synthetic estrogens. The effects on triglycerides are greater than those on cholesterol and persist through the middle fifties. These hormones generally modify the age-related changes in plasma cholesterol and triglyceride levels. There appears to be a small increase in hypercholesterolemia among hormone users up to age forty-nine, after which there was decreased risk among users.[118] Similar analysis of the triglyceride data demonstrated a 5-fold increase in hypertriglyceridemia in the youngest women, ages fifteen to nineteen, on contraceptive steroids, with persistently higher rates up through the forty-five to forty-nine year-old group, when the risk of developing the hyperlipidemia was twice that of nonusers. The significance of the elevation in plasma triglyceride levels is uncertain, since the relation of this hyperlipidemia and VLDL with CHD is inconclusive. Other reports have demonstrated that in postmenopausal women synthetic estrogens increase HDL cholesterol content and decrease the LDL cholesterol,[119,120] effects which should reduce risk.

Oral contraceptives have been reported to produce elevation of blood pressure in hypertensive women.[121] In other instances, hypertensive blood pressures have been observed to fall when women discontinued using the hormones.[122] The frequency and extent of blood pressure elevation has been studied in 13,358 women who were currently using, had discontinued use, or had never used oral contraceptives.[123] Mean systolic and diastolic blood pressures were given by age in these three groups of women. In all age groups, mean values for both systolic and diastolic pressures were greatest in women who were current users. The overall contribution of the oral contraceptive was to increase systolic pressure by 5 to 6 mm Hg and diastolic pressure by 1 to 2 mm Hg. There was an increased proportion of women users with elevated blood pressure, with this risk greatest for women older than 35 years but independent of relative weight.

An increased risk of fatal myocardial infarction in older women using oral contraceptives has been reported.[124] The use of oral contraceptives has been shown to increase the risk of stroke, independent of the effects of smoking and hypertension.[125] This may result from the thrombogenic activity of the contraceptive steroids. The search for the responsible mechanism has been undertaken, and a decrease in plasma of activated factor X inhibitory activity has been reported by Wessler and his associates.[126]

Stress

The term "stress" means many different things to different individuals. Thus, there is no common denominator that unequivocally links stress to CHD.

There is a large body of literature that has sought to examine and describe the various psychologic, social, cultural and behavioral characteristics of individuals and their relationship with the incidence of CHD. A review of this area has recently been published.[127] The interest in the area derives from the fact that only a portion of the total risk for CHD can be ascribed to the major risk factors. In addition, there is a widely held notion that certain individuals are coronary prone because of behavioral and psychologic factors. Such characteristics are also seen to be important determinants of whether an individual smokes cigarettes, selects foods appropriate to health or responds to external stimulus in a way in which blood pressure is increased. Accordingly, psychosocial factors may be of such potency as to determine whether major risk factors exist in the individual and whether they can be dealt with effectively in programs of risk-factor reduction.

Much attention has been given to the claim that persons are at higher risk if they have type A "coronary-prone behavior patterns."[128] This is described as a style of behavior that includes some of the following characteristics: intense striving for achievement, competitiveness, easily provoked impatience, time urgency, abruptness of gesture and speech, overcommitment to vocation and profession and excess of hostility and drive. In contrast, type B behavior is relaxed, calm, and unhurried. Most investigations utilizing this characterization of behavior have found higher CHD morbidity and mortality associated with type A persons. The significance of this finding and its relationship to other risk variables needs further elaboration.

Etiology and pathogenesis

In reviewing the complex subject of the etiology and pathogenesis of atheroma we shall endeavor to adopt a synthetic or holistic approach, rather than subscribe preferentially to one or more of the mutually exclusive hypotheses. We hope it will become apparent that the etiology of atheroma is not the sole domain of the platelet, lipoproteins, high blood pressure, the lysosome or the smooth cell, but rather that each of these factors is an essential piece for the sequential assembly of an exceedingly complex mosaic to which we ascribe the term atherogenesis.

Initiating factors. It is not unreasonable to make the basic and probably correct assumption that the essential event or *sine qua non* of atherogenesis is enhanced transendothelial transport of macromolecules, resulting either from frank endothelial injury or, alternatively, from more subtle modifications in endothelial structure and function. The factors that enhance this transendothelial permeability to macromolecules, including low density lipoprotein, which results in a net influx or retention within the subendothelium and media, may be conveniently considered as initiating factors. Retention may result not only from an enhanced influx but also from a decreased efflux. Decreased efflux may reflect binding of the macromolecules to components of the arterial wall or, alternatively, molecular modifications that occur within the arterial wall and render the molecules less able to traverse the endothelium to the lumen.

Focal hemodynamically-induced endothelial injury with enhanced permeability is the probable determinant of the consistent and discrete localization of the atheromatous process. Hemodynamic effects may be mediated by shear, stretch, vibration or pressure. Additional initiating factors, other than those associated with focal hemodynamics, include the release of platelet constituents, hypertension, carbon monoxide, antigen-antibody complexes and hyperlipidemia. Cigarette smoking may prove to be an important initiating factor, which exerts its effects either directly through an immune mechanism, or indirectly through released platelet constituents or carbon monoxide.

Accelerating factors. Factors that influence the nature or rate of lesion development at all subsequent stages are conveniently classified under the generic term, "accelerating factors." Accelerating factors of note include hypercholesterolemia with an associated excess of low density lipoprotein and disturbances in platelet function, hemostasis and thrombosis. These accelerating factors, namely low density lipoprotein and platelet factors, may influence the nature and rate of plaque development by stimulating the proliferation of smooth muscle cells and, by stimulating to varying degrees, the synthesis by smooth muscle cells (SMC) of collagen, elastin and the glycosaminoglycans. In addition, lipoproteins may

significantly influence SMC lipid metabolism, including cholesterol synthesis, and the uptake and accumulation of lipids within
smooth muscle cells.

Interaction between initiating and accelerating factors. As might
be anticipated, there may be several levels of complex interaction,
not only among differing accelerating factors, but also between
accelerating and initiating factors. For example, platelets, through
the release of their constituents, including 5-hydroxytryptamine,
histamine, thromboxane A_2 and lysosomal enzymes, may directly
cause endothelial injury or modify endothelial permeability. This
modification of endothelial permeability will serve to enhance the
entry of accelerating factors such as low density lipoprotein, and
certain platelet proteins, which subsequently stimulate SMC
proliferation.

In addition, platelets may directly contribute to plaque growth
by serving as components of mural thrombi. LDL may directly
induce a spectrum of changes, consistent with endothelial injury.
In Type II hyperlipoproteinemia, LDL has been shown as well to
be associated with modified platelet function, which might influence the risk of thrombus formation.

Other pathogenic processes. Other processes not yet discussed,
which are of importance in pathogenesis, include the concept of a
monoclonal origin of the cells in atheroma, and also the concept
that atheroma is a lysosomal storage disease, with the marked
accumulation of cholesterol esters resulting from an overload of
the lysosomal enzyme systems. Both the monoclonal explanation
for the cellular monotypism, which in essence implies that atheromatous lesions are benign smooth muscle cell tumors, and the
possible role of a lysosomal enzyme deficit in the accumulation of
arterial lipids, are compatible with the overview presented. Just
how important each of these mechanisms is in the pathogenesis of
atheroma has yet to be established.

There remain many unanswered questions and unresolved issues.
For example, the precise relationship between fatty streaks and
fibrous plaques in the evolution of atheroma has still to be clarified.
Furthermore, how does the fibrous atherosclerotic plaque begin
and progress, are the earliest lesions as characteristic of the
disease as is the atherosclerotic plaque, and what extramural
factors directly or indirectly influence the composition of the
precursor lesions and the rate of their progression to the plaque?
Other important questions relate to the time scale for the development or regression of clinically significant disease, the reasons for
the striking sex-associated differences in disease prevalence and

severity, and the mechanisms underlying the consistently greater frequency of clinical disease in patients with diabetes mellitus.

Finally, there may exist risk factors that so far have not been recognized and therefore are not measured. Identification of measurable characteristics associated with probability of atheroma would make possible testing their relationship to coronary heart disease.

The genesis and progression of atherosclerosis involve a complex interplay of metabolic, structural and environmental elements. A few of the elements or factors are well known but most are just beginning to be identified. How these risk factors are involved in the initiation, development, progression and regression of the vascular disease processes are not yet understood. Consequently, the etiology and precise mechanism(s) of the pathology of CHD are still unclear. It is to be hoped that advancing knowledge concerning the nature of the disease will lead to the development of therapeutic and preventive measures that are more effective than those available at present for a disease that is the most potent force of mortality operating in the world today, particularly in affluent societies.

REFERENCES

1. Greer, J. D., McGill, H. C. and Strong, J. P. 1961. The fine structure of human atherosclerotic lesions. *Amer. J. Pathol.* 38: 263.
2. Still, W. J. S. and O'Neal, R. M. 1962. Electron microscopic study of experimental atherosclerosis in the rat. *Amer. J. Pathol.* 40: 21.
3. Stary, H. C. and Strong, J. P. 1976. The fine structure of nonatherosclerotic intimal thickening, of developing, and of regressing atherosclerotic lesions at the bifurcation of the left coronary artery. *Adv. Exp. Med. Biol.* 67: 108.
4. Poole, J. C. F. and Florey, H. W. 1958. Changes in the endothelium of the aorta and the behavior of macrophages in experimental atheroma of rabbits. *J. Pathol. Bacteriol.* 75: 245.
5. Buck, R. C. 1958. The fine structure of the aortic endothelial lesions in experimental cholesterol atherosclerosis of rabbits. *Amer. J. Pathol.* 34: 897.
6. Suzuki, M. and O'Neal, R. M. 1964. Accumulation of lipids in the leukocytes of rats fed atherogenic diets. *J. Lipid Res.* 5: 624.
7. Suzuki, M., Greenberg, S. D., Adams, J. G. and O'Neal, R. M. 1964. Experimental atherosclerosis in the dog: a morphologic study. *Exp. Mol. Pathol.* 3: 455.
8. Marshall, J. R. and O'Neal, R. M. 1966. The lipophage in hyperlipemic rats: an electron microscopic study. *Exp. Mol. Pathol.* 5: 1.
9. Kim, H. S., Suzuki, M. and O'Neal, R. M. 1967. Leukocyte lipids of human blood. *Amer. J. Clin. Pathol.* 48: 314.
10. Suzuki, M. and O'Neal, R. M. 1967. Circulating lipophages, serum lipids and atherosclerosis in rats. *Arch. Pathol. Lab. Med.* 83: 169.

11. Gerrity, R. G., Naito, H. K., Richardson, M. and Schwartz, C. J. 1979. Dietary induced atherosclerosis in swine. *Amer. J. Path.* 95: 775.
12. Bessie, M. and Thiery, J. P. 1961. Electron microscope of human white blood cells and their stem cells. *Int. Rev. Cytol.* 12: 199.
13. Tanaka, Y. and Goodman, J. R. 1972. In: *Electron Microscopy of Human Blood Cells*. New York: Harper & Row.
14. Gerrity, R. G., Richardson, M., Somer, J. B., Bell, F. P. and Schwartz, C. J. 1977. Endothelial cell morphology in areas of in vivo evans blue update in the aorta of young pigs. II. Ultrastructure of the intima in areas of differing permeability to proteins. *Amer. J. Pathol.* 89: 313.
15. Lee, K. T., Lee, K. J., Lee, S. K., Imai, H. and O'Neal, R. M. 1970. Poorly differentiated subendothelial cells in swine aortas. *Exp. Mol. Pathol.* 13: 118.
16. Ross, R. and Glomset, J. A. 1976. The pathogenesis of atherosclerosis. *N. Engl. J. Med.* 295: 369 and 420.
17. Naito, H. K. 1980. In: *Nutritional Elements and Clinical Biochemistry*. M. A. Brewster and H. K. Naito, eds. New York: Plenum Publishing Corp.
18. Schwartz, C., Chandler, A. B., Gerrity, R. G. and Naito, H. K. 1978. In: *The Thrombic Process in Atherogenesis*. A. B. Chandler, K. Eurenivs, G. C. McMillan, C. B. Nelson, C. J. Schwartz and S. Wissler, eds. New York: Plenum Press.
19. Camejo, G., LaLaguna, F., Lopez and Starosta, R. 1980. Characterization and properties of a lipoprotein-complexing proteoglycans from human aorta. *Atherosclerosis* 35: 307.
20. Camejo, G., Acquatella, H. and LaLaguna, F. 1980. The interaction of low density lipoproteins with arterial proteoglycans. An additional risk factor? *Atherosclerosis* 36: 55.
21. Hoff, H. F., Jackson, R. L., Mao, S. J. T. and Gotto, A. M., Jr. 1974. Localization of low-density lipoproteins in atherosclerotic lesions from human normolipemics employing a purified fluorescent-labeled antibody. *Biochim. Biophys. Acta* 351: 407.
22. Hoff, H. J., Heideman, C. L., Gaubatz, J. W., Titus, J. L. and Gotto, A. M., Jr. 1978. Quantitation of apo B in human aortic fatty streaks: a comparison with grossly normal intima and fibrous plaques. *Atherosclerosis* 30: 263.
23. Hoff, H. F., Bradley, W. A., Heideman, C. L., Gaubatz, J. W., Karagas, M.D. and Gotto, A. M., Jr. 1979. Characterization of low density lipoprotein-like particle in the human aorta from grossly normal and atherosclerotic regions. *Biochim. Biophys. Acta* 573:361.
24. Smith, E. B. and Slater, R. S. 1970. The chemical and immunological assay of low-density lipoproteins extracted from human aortic intima. *Atherosclerosis* 11: 417.
25. Hollander, W., Paddock, J. and Columbo, M. 1979. Lipoproteins in human artherosclerotic vessels. I. Biochemical properties of arterial low density lipoproteins, very low density lipoproteins, and high density lipoproteins. *Exp. Mol. Path.* 30: 144.
26. Hollander, W., Colombo, M. and Paddock, J. 1979. Lipoproteins in human atherosclerotic vessels. II. Biochemical properties of the major apolipoproteins of arterial low density and very low density lipoproteins. *Exp. Mol. Pathol.* 30: 1972.
27. Strong, J. P., Eggen, D. A. and Tracy, R. E. 1978. In: *The Thrombotic Process in Atherogenesis*. A. B. Chandler, K. Eurenivs, G. C.

McMillan, C. B. Nelson, C. J. Schwartz and S. Wissler, eds. New York: Plenum Press.

28. Duff, G. L. and McMillan, G. C. 1951. Pathology of atherosclerosis. *Amer. J. Med.* 11: 92.

29. Glagov, S. and Ozoa, A. K. 1968. Significance of the relatively low incidence of atherosclerosis in the pulmonary, renal and mesenteric arteries. *Ann. N. Y. Acad. Sci.* 149: 940.

30. Schwartz, C. J. and Mitchell, J. R. A. 1962. Observations on the localization of arterial plaques. *Circ. Res.* 11: 73.

31. Haust, M. D. 1978. In: *The Thrombic Process in Atherogenesis*. A. B. Chandler, K. Eurenivs, G. C. McMillan, C. B. Nelson, C. J. Schwartz and S. Wissler, eds. New York: Plenum Press.

32. Strong, J. P., Eggen, D. A. and Oalmann, M. C. 1974. In: *The Pathogenesis of Atherosclerosis*. R. W. Wissler and J. C. Geer, eds. Baltimore: Williams and Wilkins Co.

33. Haust, M. D. and More, R. H. 1972. In: *The Pathogenesis of Atherosclerosis*. R. W. Wissler and J. C. Geer, eds. Baltimore: Williams and Wilkins Co.

34. Morgan, A. D. 1956. In: *The Pathogenesis of Coronary Occlusion*. Oxford, England: Blackwell Engl. Scientific Publications.

35. Haust, M. D. 1970. In: *Atherosclerosis*. R. J. Jones, ed. New York: Springer-Verlag.

36. Rutherford, R. B. and Ross, R. 1976. Platelet factors stimulate fibroblasts and smooth muscle cells quiescent in plasma serum to proliferate. *J. Cell Biol.* 69: 196.

37. Fischer-Dzoga, K., Jones, R. M., Vesselinovich, D. and Wissler, R. W. 1974. In: *Atherosclerosis III*. G. Schettler and A. Weizel, eds. Berlin: Springer-Verlag.

38. Wissler, R. W. 1978. In: *The Thrombic Process in Atherogenesis*. A. B. Chandler, K. Eurenivs, G. C. McMillan, C. B. Nelson, C. J. Schwartz and S. Wissler, eds. New York: Plenum Press.

39. Nichols, A. B., Ravenscroft, C., Lamphier, D. E. and Ostrander, L. D. 1977. Daily nutritional intake and serum lipid levels. The Tecumseh study. *J. Clin. Nutr.* 29: 1384.

40. Glueck, C. J. and Connor, W. E. 1978. Diet-coronary heart disease relationships reconnoitered. *Amer. J. Clin. Nutr.* 31: 727.

41. Davis, C. E. and Havlik, R. J. 1977. In: *Hyperlipidemia: Diagnosis and Therapy*. B. M. Rifkind and R. I. Levy, eds. New York: Gruine and Stratton.

42. Grundy, S. M. 1977. Treatment of hypercholesterolemia. *Amer. J. Clin. Nutr.* 30: 985.

43. Stone, N. J. and Levy, R. I. 1972. Hyperlipoproteinemia and coronary heart disease. *Prog. Cardiovasc. Dis.* 14: 341.

44. Fredrickson, D. S., Levy, R. I. and Lees, R. S. 1967. Fat transport in lipoproteins—an integrated approach to mechanisms and disorders. *N. Engl. J. Med.* 276: 34.

45. Fredrickson, D. S. and Levy, R. I. In: *The Metabolic Basis of Inherited Disease*. J. B. Stanburg, J. B. Wyngaarden and D. S. Fredrickson, eds. New York: McGraw-Hill.

46. Medalie, J. H., Kahn, H. A., Newfeld, H. N., Riss, E. and Goldbourt, U. 1973. Five year myocardial infarcation incidence—II. Association of single variables to age and birthplace. *J. Chronic Dis.* 26: 329.

47. Wilhelmsen, L., Wedel, H. and Tibblin, G. 1973. Multivariate analysis of risk factors for coronary heart disease. *Circulation* 48: 950.
48. Gordon, T., Garcia-Palmieri, M. R., Kogan, A., Kannel, W. B. and Schiffman, J. 1974. Differences in coronary heart disease in Framingham, Honolulu and Puerto Rico. *J. Chronic Dis.* 27: 329.
49. Van die Redaskie. 1973. Coronary heart disease in China. *S. African Med. J.* 47: 1485.
50. Blackburn, H. 1974. In: *Progress in Cardiology*. P. Yu and J. Goodwin, eds. Philadelphia: Lea and Febiger.
51. Kannel, W. B., Castelli, W. P., Gordon, T. and McNamara, P. M. 1971. Serum cholesterol, lipoproteins and the risk of coronary heart disease. *Ann. Intern. Med.* 74: 1.
52. Dayton, S., Pearce, M. L., Hashimoto, S., Dixon, W. J. and Tomiyasu, U. 1969. A controlled clinical trial of a diet high in unsaturated fat is preventing complications of atherosclerosis. *Circulation* 40 (Suppl. II): 1.
53. Meittinen, M., Turpeinen, O., Karvonen, M. J., Elosua, R. and Paavilainen, E. 1972. Effect of cholesterol lowering diet on mortality from coronary heart disease and other causes. *Lancet* 2: 835.
54. Laren, P. 1966. The effect of plasma cholesterol lowering diet in male survivors of myocardial infarction. *Acta Med. Scan.* (Suppl.) 466: 1.
55. The National Diet Heart Study Final Report, National Diet Heart Study Research Group. 1968. *Circulation* 37 (Suppl. I): 1.
56. Frantz, I. D., Jr., Dawson, E. A., Kuba, K., Brewer, E. R., Gatewood, L. C. and Bartsch, G. E. 1975. The Minnesota coronary survey: effect of diet on cardiovascular events and deaths. *Circulation* 52 (Suppl. II): II.
57. Food and Nutrition Board, National Academy of Sciences—National Research Council and Council on Foods and Nutrition, American Medical Assoc. 1972. Diet and coronary heart disease—a joint statement. *Prev. Med.* 1: 559. Fourth Report of the Director, NHLBI: 1977 National Heart, Blood Vessel, Lung and Blood Program March 1977, DHEW Publication No. (NIH) 77-1170.
58. Connor, W. E., Brown, H. B., Frederickson, D. S., Steinberg, D., Connor, S. L. and Bickel, J. H. 1973. A maximal approach to the dietary treatment of the hyperlipidemias. Sub-committee on diet and hyperlipidemia, Council on Atherosclerosis, Amer. Heart Assoc.
59. Rhoads, G. G., Gulbrandsen, C. L. and Kagan, A. 1976. Serum lipoproteins and coronary heart disease in a population study of Hawaii Japanese men. *N. Engl. J. Med.* 294, 293.
60. Connor, W. E. and Connor, S. L. 1972. The key role of nutritional factors in the prevention of coronary heart disease. *Prev. Med.* 1: 49.
61. H. C. McGill, Jr., ed. 1968. *The Geographic Pathology of Athero sclerosis*. Baltimore: Williams and Wilkins.
62. Bierman, E. L. and Ross, R. 1977. In: *Atherosclerosis Reviews*. vol. 2. A. M. Gotto and R. Paoletti, eds. New York: Raven Press.
63. Rifkind, B. M. 1977. In: *Atherosclerosis Reviews*. vol. 2. A. M. Gott and R. Paoletti, eds. New York: Raven Press.
64. Gordon, T., Castelli, W. P. Hjortland, M. C., Kannel, W. B. and Dawber, T. B. 1977. High density lipoproteins as a protective factor against coronary heart disease. The Framingham study. *Amer. J. Med.* 62: 707.

65. Berg, K. 1963. A new serum type system in man—the Lp system. *Acta Path. Microbil. Scand.* 59: 369.
66. Kostner, G. M. 1976. In: *Low Density Lipoproteins.* Charles A. Day and Robert Levy, eds. New York: Plenum Press.
67. Albers, J. J. and Hazzard, W. R. 1974. Immunochemical quantification of human plasma Lp (a) lipoprotein. *Lipids* 9: 15.
68. Ehnholm, C., Garoff, H. Renkonen, O., et al. 1972. Protein and carbohydrate composition of Lp (a) lipoprotein from human plasma. *Biochemistry* 11: 3229.
69. Krempler, F., Kostner, G., Bolanzo K. and Sandhofer, F. 1979. Lipoprotein (a) is not a metabolic product of other lipoproteins containing apolipoprotein B. *Biochim. Biophys. Acta.* 575: 63.
70. Jurgen, G., Marth, E., Kostner, G. M. and Halasek, A. 1977. Investigation of the Lp (a) lipoprotein aggregation and enzymatic activity associated with the Lp (a) polypeptide. *Artery* 3: 13.
71. Dahlen, G. and Uricson, C. 1971. A new lipoprotein pattern in patients with angina pectoris. *Scand. J. Clin. Lab. Invest. Suppl.* 27: 54.
72. Dahlen, G. 1975. The prebeta, lipoprotein phenomenon in relation to serum cholesterol and triglyceride levels, the Lp (a) lipoprotein and coronary heart disease. *Acta Med. Scand. Suppl.* 570.
73. Dahlen, G., Berg, K., Gillnas, T. Ericson, C. 1975. Lp (a) lipoprotein/pre-beta$_1$-lipoprotein Swedish middle aged males and patients with coronary heart disease. *Clin. Genet.* 7: 334.
74. Dahlen, G., Frick, M. H., Berg, K., et al. 1976. Lp (a) lipoprotein/prebeta$_1$-lipoprotein, serum lipids and atherosclerotic disease. *Clin. Genet.* 10: 97.
75. Dahlen, G., Gianturco, S. H., Rohde, M. F., Gotto, A.M. Jr. and Norrisett, J. D. 1979. In: *Fifth Int. Symp. Atheroscl. Abst.*
76. Dahlen, G., Ericson, C. and Berg, K. 1978. In vitro studies of the integration of isolated Lp (a) lipoprotein and other serum lipoproteins with glyco aminoglycans. *Clin. Genetics* 14: 36.
77. Dahlen, G., Ericson, C. and Berg, K. 1978. In vitro studies of the interaction of calcium ions and other divalent cations with the Lp (a) lipoprotein and other isolated serum lipoproteins. *Clin. Genetics* 14: 115.
78. Lewis, L. A. and Naito, H. K. 1978. Relation of hypertension, lipids and lipoproteins to atherosclerosis. *Clin. Chem.* 24: 2081.
79. Stemmermann, G. N., Rhoads, G. G. and Hayashi, T. 1980. In: *Atherosclerosis V.* A. J. Gotto, Jr., L. C. Smith and B. Allen, eds. New York: Springer Verlag.
80. Freis, E. D. 1973. Age, race, sex and other indices of risk in hypertension. *Amer. J. Med.* 55: 275.
81. Londe, S. and Golding, D. 1976. High blood pressure in children: problems and guidelines for evaluation and treatment. *Amer. J. Cardiol.* 37.
82. Solberg, L. A. and McGarry, P. A. 1972. Cerebral atherosclerosis in negroes and caucasians. *Atherosclerosis* 16: 141.
83. Hollander, W. 1976. Role of hypertension in atherosclerosis and cardiovascular disease. *Amer. J. Cardiol.* 38: 786.
84. Strong, J. P. and Richards, M. L. 1976. Cigarette smoking and atherosclerosis in autopsied men. *Atherosclerosis* 23: 451.
85. Doll, R. and Hill, A. B. 1964. Mortality in relation to smoking: ten years' observations of British doctors. *Br. Med. J.* 1: 1399.

86. Report of the Intersociety Commission for Heart Disease Resources. 1970. Primary prevention of the atherosclerotic disease. *Circulation* 62: A-55.

87. Rode, A., Ross, R. and Shepard, R. 1972. Smoking withdrawal programme: personality and cardiorespiratory fitness. *Arch. Environ. Health* 24: 27.

88. Rosenman, R. H., Brand, R. J., Jenkins, C. D., Friedman, M., Strauss, R. and Wurm, M. 1975. Coronary Heart disease in the western collaborative group study. *JAMA* 233: 872.

89. Stamler, J. 1973. Epidemiology of coronary heart disease. *Med. Clin. North Amer.* 57: 5.

90. Telecom Health Research Group 1977. Cardiovascular risk factors among Japanese and American telephone executives. *Int. J. Epidemiol.* 6: 7.

91. Kannel, W. B., Sorlie, P., Brand, F., Castelli, W. P., McNamara, P. M. and Gheradi, G. J. 1980. In: *Atherosclerosis V*. A. M. Gotto, Jr., L. C. Smith, and B. Allen, eds. New York: Springer Verlag.

92. Becker, C. G. and Dubin, T. 1977. Activation of Factor XII by tobacco glycoprotein. *J. Exp. Med.* 146: 457.

93. Becker, C. G., Dubin, T. and Wiedemann, H. P. 1976. Hypersensitivity to tobacco antigen. *Proc. Natl. Acad. Sci.* 73: 1712.

94. Becker, C. G., Levi, R. and Zavecz, J. 1977. Introduction of IgE antibodies to antigen isolated from tobacco leaves and from cigarette smoke condensate. *Circulation Suppl.* 3: 169.

95. Theorell, H., Blomback, M. and Kockum, C. 1976. Demonstration of reactivity to airborne and food allergens in cutaneous vasculitis by variations in fibrinopeptide A and other blood coagulation, fibrinolysis and complement parameters. *Thrombos. Haemostas.* 36: 593.

96. Kannel, W. B., LeBauer, E. J., Dawber, T. R. and McNamara, P. M. 1967. Relation of body weight to development of coronary heart disease. *Circulation* 35: 734.

97. Truett, J., Cornfield, J. and Kannel, W. 1967. A multivariate analysis of the risk of cornary heart disease in Framingham. *J. Chronic. Dis.* 20: 511.

98. Naito, H. K. 1976. Effects of physical activity on serum cholesterol metabolism. A review. *Cleveland Clinic Quarterly* 43: 21.

99. Paffenbarger, R. S., Jr. and Hale, W. E. 1975. Work activity and coronary heart mortality. *N. Engl. J. Med.* 292: 545.

100. Wood, P. D., Haskell, W., Klein, H., Lewis, S., Stern, M. P. and Farquhar, J. W. 1976. The distribution of plasma lipoproteins in middle-aged male runners. *Metabolism* 25: 249.

101. Oscai, L. B. and Holloszy, J. O. 1969. Effects of weight changes produced by exercise, food restriction, or overeating on body composition. *J. Clin. Invest.* 48: 2124.

102. Bjoyntoys, P., Fahlen, M., Grimby, G., Gustafson, A., Holms., Renstrom, P. and Schersten, T. 1972. Carbohydrate and lipid metabolism in middle-aged physically well-trained men. *Metabolism* 21: 1037.

103. Scheuer, J. and Tipton, C. M. 1977. Cardiovascular adaptations to physical training. *Annual Rev. Physiol.* 39: 221.

104. Linder, A., Charra, B., Sherrard, D. J. and Scribner, B. H. 1974. Accelerated atherosclerosis in prolonged maintenance hemodialysis. *N. Engl. J. Med.* 290: 697.

105. Miamisono, T., Wada, M., Akamatsu, A., Okabe, M., Handa, Y., Morita, T., Asagami, C., Naito, H. K., Nakamoto, S., Lewis, L.A. and Mise, J. 1978. Dyslipoproteinemia (a remnant lipoprotein disease) in uremic patients on hemodialysis. *Clin. Chem. Acta.* 84: 163.

106. Wada, M. Minamisono, T., Fujii, H., Morita, T., Akamatsu, A., Mise, J., Nakamoto, S. and Naito, H. K. 1975. Studies on the effects of hemodialysis on plasma lipoproteins. *Trans. Amer. Soc., Artif. Int. Organs XXI* 464.

107. Handa, Y. 1978. Studies on a dyslipoproteinemia in hemodialysis patients. *Jap. Heart J.* 19: 362.

108. Palumbo, P. J., Elveback, L. R., Chu, C. P., Connolly, D. C. and Kurland, L. T. 1976. Diabetes mellitus: incidence, prevalence, survivorship, and causes of death in Rochester, Minnesota, 1945–1970. *Diabetes* 25: 566.

109. Kessler, I. I. 1971. Mortality experience of diabetic patients. A twenty-six year follow-up study. *Amer. J. Med.* 51: 715.

110. University group diabetes program. 1970. A study of the effects of hypoglycemic agents on the vascular complications on patients with adult onset diabetes. *J. Amer. Diabetes Assoc.* 19: 747.

111. Gordon, T. and Shurtleff, D. 1973. An epidemiological investigation of cardiovascular disease. Section 29, DHEW Publ. No. (NIH) 74, Washington, D. C.

112. Naito, H. K. and Kumar, M. S. In: *CRC Handbook of Electrophoresis, vol. II: Lipoproteins in Disease*. L. A. Lewis and J. J. Opplt, eds. Boca Raton, Florida: Chemical Rubber Co. Press, Inc.

113. Naito, H. K., McKenzie, A., Willis, C. E. and Olnyk, M. 1980. *CRC Handbook of Electrophoresis, vol. II: Lipoprotein in Disease*. L. A. Lewis, and J. J. Opplt, eds. Boca Raton, Florida: Chemical Rubber Co. Press, Inc.

114. Feldman, E. B. and Wallace, S. L. 1964. Hypertriglyceridemia in gout. *Circulation*. 29: 508.

115. Naito, H. K. and MacKenzie, A. H. 1979. Secondary hypertriglyceridemia and hyperlipoproteinemia in patients with primary asymptomatic gout. *Clin. Chem.* 25: 371.

116. Beck, P. 1973. Progress in endocrinology and metabolism—contraceptive steroids: modifications of carbohydrate and lipid metabolism. *Metabolism* 22: 841.

117. Ferreri, L. and Naito, H. K. 1978. Effect of estrogens on rat serum cholesterol concentration: consideration of dose, type of estrogen and treatment duration. *Endocrinology* 102: 1621.

118. Wallace, R. B., Hoover, J., Sandler, D., Rifkind, B. M. and Tyroler, H. A. 1977. Altered plasma-lipids associated with oral contraceptive or estrogen consumption. *Lancet* 2: 11.

119. Furman, R. H., Alaupovic, P. and Howard, R. P. 1967. Effects of androgens and estrogens in serum lipids and the composition and concentration of serum lipoproteins in normolipemic and hyperlipemic states. *Prog. Biochem. Pharmacol.* 2: 215.

120. Gustafson, A. and Svanborg, A. 1972. Gonadal steroid effects on plasma lipoproteins and individual phospholipids. *J. Clin. Endocrinol. Metal.* 35: 203.

121. Yang, M. U., and Van Stallie, T. B. 1976. Composition of weight lost during short-term weight reduction. *J. Clin. Invest.* 58: 722.

122. Crane, M. G., Harris, J. J. and Winsor, W., III. 1971. Hypertension, oral contraceptive agents and conjugated estrogens. *Ann. Intern. Med.* 74: 13.

123. Fisch, I. R. and Frank, J. 1977. Oral contraceptives and blood pressure. *JAMA* 237: 2499.

124. Mann, J. I. and Inman, W. H. W. 1976. Oral contraceptives and death from myocardial infarction. *Br. Med. J.* 2: 245.

125. Collaborative group for the study of stroke in young women. 1975. Oral contraceptives and stroke in young women—associated risk factors. *J. Amer. Med. Assoc.* 231: 718.

126. Wessler, S., Gitel, S. N., Wan, L. S. and Pasternack, B. S. 1976. Estrogen-containing oral contraceptive agents, a basis for their thrombogenicity. *J. Amer. Med. Assoc.* 236: 2179.

127. Jenkins, C. D. 1976. Recent evidence supporting psychologic and social risk factors for coronary disease. *N. Engl. J. Med.* 294: 987 and 1033.

128. Friedman, M. and Rosemann, R. 1974. In: *Type A Behavior and Your Heart*. New York: Alfred A. Knopf.

8

NUTRITION AND BEHAVIOR

————————◄•►————————

ABRAM HOFFER, M.D., PH.D.

Introduction

FROM THE BEGINNING, unicellular organisms responded to the presence or absence of food. For all species the need for food remains one of the most important factors influencing behavior; when hunger is satisfied other drives are relatively more powerful. Even man is not free of the effect of food on behavior.

Technologically advanced societies seldom suffer from hunger. They are unaware how powerful a force food remains in shaping behavior. Even less is their awareness of the deleterious impact of a national nutrition characterized by an abundance of calories combined with a deficiency of some essential nutrients. Like the atmosphere of which we are unaware unless it is perturbed, so are we unaware of what food does to us unless we are hungry, overfed or have had foods which make us sick. We live in an era of affluent malnutrition, a phenomenon so new that physicians and nutritionists have not yet recognized it.

During the gathering/hunter stage of man's evolution, hunger was a much more common problem. Food was available or not available, but it was not processed, adulterated and deprived of important nutrients. Starvation was common for various periods of time, but surplus calorie malnutrition must have been very rare.

Agriculture developed about ten thousand years ago in response to increasing population pressure. A more or less steady supply of livestock, cereal grains and vegetables created cities; first small, today enormous in size. The need to harvest, transport and store food for city populations created the conditions for deterioration of the food. Special problems such as scurvy arose

222

when man migrated to colder areas and had less available fruit. It also made man much more vulnerable to seasonal changes. Survival over the winter in colder areas became a serious problem. When industrialization developed, other diseases appeared; smoke from chimneys, industrial smoke and lack of sunlight due to working conditions created rickets, the vitamin D_3 deficiency.

The classical deficiency diseases such as beriberi, pellagra, rickets and scurvy have been controlled, at least in technologically developed nations, but they have been replaced by a more subtle pervasive group of diseases of malnutrition due to deficiencies of vitamins and minerals combined with a surplus of calories from the sugars and a scarcity of food fiber. Hunger is no longer a problem; chronic disease from affluent malnutrition is.

Hunger and the need to grow and prepare food has had a positive influence in shaping our society. The provision of food has demanded cooperation, division of labor, trade and the work ethic. Hunger in normal people seldom creates antisocial behavior even though it cannot long be tolerated, and leads to serious effects on growth and to death by starvation.

There is another form of malnutrition—cellular hunger. The body is unable to metabolize food properly because of a deficiency of nutrients even though caloric intake is adequate and often more than adequate. This type of cellular hunger creates antisocial behavior, behavior which is destructive in any society and is a major burden.

My theme in this section is that just as normal nutrition is an important ingredient in normal behavior, so is abnormal nutrition a factor in causing abnormal behavior. Affluent malnutrition is directly responsible for a major portion of behavioral abnormalities and psychiatric disease.

Orthomolecular Nutrition

If man lived solely on whole foods, foods which are alive (fruit, vegetables, nuts and seeds) or which have recently been alive (fresh fish and meat), and if this food grew on soils which contained adequate amounts of essential minerals and trace elements while free of toxic heavy metals, and if adequate quantities of this food were freely available, then the majority of people would be well; this is the kind of food to which we have adapted. Even then a substantial fraction of any society would have special nutritional needs for supplements. Orthomolecular nutrition is the newer form of clinical nutrition developed by physicians who have used nutritional treatment for large numbers of patients. They have studied the connection between nutrition and health. In their practice they have seen the importance of Roger Williams's work on biochemical individuality.[1,2] They use nutritional expertise to preserve health and to restore it even when every known standard treatment has failed.

Orthomolecular nutrition became essential because nutrition as taught in universities has been fossilized for the past forty years.[3] It has failed to understand what modern technology has done to food, how it has been stripped of much of its mineral and vitamin content. Medical schools have ignored nutrition and the role of modern nutrition (or affluent malnutrition) in the causation of a large number of chronic degenerative diseases.

The first food chemists studied foods by breaking them down into simple constituents. These fractions were obtained by applying chemical and physical procedures to these foods. They were pure and had definite physical and chemical properties. One set of procedures yields nitrogen-containing complex molecules called proteins; they in turn can be split into twenty amino acids. Of these, eight cannot be made in the body and are classified as essential. This is an unfortunate term as it suggests the remaining twelve amino acids are not essential. All are equally essential, but the twelve can be made in the body from the "essential" eight. If a person could not make any one of these nonessential from one of the essential eight, it too would be considered essential. Bessman[4,5] considers phenylketonuria an example of a condition in which a person is not able to convert phenylalanine to tyrosine. Tyrosine for these people is an essential amino acid. The enzyme which catalyzes this conversion is lacking.

Another set of chemical procedures yields fats, also called lipids. They contain molecules which are short or long, contain little oxygen and usually do not have any nitrogen. These fats are greasy, and vary in softness from liquids (oils) to harder substances (butter). A third set of procedures yields carbohydrates. These are solid materials rich in oxygen and free of nitrogen. These three major substances make up the whole bulk of any foodstuff. Carbohydrates are classified into complex carbohydrates such as potatoes, and simple carbohydrates such as glucose, fructose and sucrose. They are also known as sugars. Complex carbohydrates include fiber, found in cereals and vegetables. They are richest in leaves and in bran.

Because these three major components accounted for all the bulk or weight of any food it was natural to conclude that they only were required for nutrition. Chemists and nutritionists were convinced one needed only protein, fats and carbohydrates. This conclusion created the conditions for the development of the nutritional diseases from which we still suffer.

Primitive food technology which consisted of procedures for cooking food, or for taking some of the bran out of whole grain flour, was not as harmful as the technology of the past one hundred years which polished brown rice to white and milled the almost pure white flour from whole flour. Stripping germ and bran from rice led to beriberi. A monoculture of corn only created pellagra. For years it has been known that pellagrins are more prone to antisocial behavior. The prevalence of beriberi led to the discovery of thiamin (vitamin B_1). The study of pellagra eventually led to the recognition that the pellagra-preventing vitamin B_3 was niacin and/or niacinamide. Today about twenty vitamins are known; more will be discovered when we again begin to search for them. The importance of minerals was recognized about the same time as vitamins. The role of trace minerals in nutrition became recognized much later. More recently, enzymes are being examined, and will probably turn out to have a role. It does make sense for the body to use enzymes which helped make the food to help in digesting it. Today we understand the role of the forty essential nutrients.

Finally, in the past decade, the importance of the biological structure of foods and their fiber content has been recognized. Whole food has biological advantages not present in processed foods:

(a) The food is digested more slowly at a pace which the digestive apparatus can handle. In sharp contrast, processed food, such as syrup or the sugars, is absorbed easily and quickly, and overloads digestive mechanisms designed to deal with sugars which are normally released slowly in the body. Enzymes which are released to digest complex carbohydrates are not used; whether they remain innocuous or are harmful is not known. The rate of release of nutrients varies enormously. For example, it would be very difficult to eat five apples or five oranges in thirty seconds; this food has to be consumed more slowly. The sugar in the fruit is released slowly. On the other hand, one can consume the same amount of sugar (about five teaspoons or 20 grams) in a few seconds. Abnormally large quantities of sugar can be dumped into the stomach, absorbed into the blood, and overload the digestive apparatus designed to absorb, store and metabolize sugar. Sucrose (table sugar) under these conditions is absorbed by the liver and is shunted into the fat stores.

(b) Food contains all the fiber originally present which is very important in the digestive process. The digestive tract has adapted to a high fiber diet which assists in peristalsis, in the propulsion of food through the intestines. Fiber provides the necessary bulk. In the absence of fiber, the intestinal contents become too hard and the material moves too slowly. Constipation is a problem common for people who live on a highly processed diet too deficient in fiber and too rich in processed carbohydrates. Fiber has other uses: it provides a medium for bacteria, absorbs toxic heavy metals like mercury and lead, and absorbs organic toxic substances ingested or excreted into the intestines. By increasing the rate of movement through the bowel the toxic constituents are in contact with the bowel for shorter periods. This may account for the decreased incidence of cancer of the lower bowel and rectum in people who live on high fiber diets.

The components of food are not food. The combination of parts is not equivalent to the whole. In fact, these components do not exist free in nature; nature does not lay down pure protein, pure fat or pure carbohydrate. Their molecules are interlaced in a very complex three dimensional structure which even now has not been fully described. Intermingled are the essential nutrients such as vitamins and minerals, again not free, but usually combined in complex molecules. Since food components are not complete foods they should not be called food for this perpetuates the myth that these components comprise good food. They are food artifacts. Protein, fat, carbohydrate (i.e., fiber, starch, the sugars), vitamins and minerals are all food artifacts. It follows that when foods and artifacts are combined the whole mixture becomes food artifact. Hereafter, only food which is whole, alive, or has recently been alive will be called food. Everything else is artifact.

Food artifacts vary in quality. Some, such as vitamins, amino acids, and minerals, can be used to improve nutritional quality. Others are nutritionally useless and may be harmful, such as sugar. These useless artifacts are popularly known as junk. Any food which contains junk also becomes junk. The more junk that is present, the more difficult is it for the contaminated food to make up for the deficiencies caused by the junk.

Additives comprise a large group of artifacts. They are used to color or bleach, to stabilize, preserve, alter the taste, feel, and consistency to produce a product which resembles food or food products that populations have considered nutritious. One of the objectives of food technology is to produce a stable product, like gold, which will never deteriorate. Recently, the dairy industry was very pleased with a milk that can be stored outside a refrigerator for three months or more. These products no longer sour; they simply go bad.

Junk additives are divisible into two groups:

(a) Cosmetic additives, which are added deliberately to "improve" the product in many ways except nutritionally; none of the junk artifacts have been shown to be as nutritious as the foods from which they are made.

(b) Trace additives, which are traces of chemicals which are present in all food artifacts. The preparation of starch requires a number of chemical processes. Traces of each chemical will be present in the final product for it would be prohibitively expensive to try to remove them. Even pure table sugar, 99.99 percent pure, contains 0.01 percent of these trace additives. When these food artifacts are used in the preparation of other food artifacts (i.e., starch for making imitation caviar or pies) these trace elements are carried along. Even pure chemicals considered pure enough for human consumption contain traces of other chemicals in them. The final food processor who makes the cakes, sweets and frozen foods, is not aware of the presence of these trace additives. Surely, there must be thousands of these. Thus, food artifacts contain artifacts in varying proportions sharing this in common: they are deficient in vitamins, minerals and fiber, are too rich in sugars, and contain unknown quantities of cosmetic and trace elements.

The preparation of food artifacts reduces nutritional quality in other ways. In most processes, heat and moisture are required. When any food is heated, the destructive effect on some essential food components is accelerated. Proteins are altered chemically; anyone who has fried an egg knows what heat can do. However, people believe these changes are beneficial, whereas some changes are not. Proteins are denatured, i.e., changed from their natural state. After this, enzymes in the body, developed to digest natural protein, no longer act as efficiently. Higher temperatures destroy more of the protein. Soft boiled eggs are more nutritious than hard boiled, but fried eggs, where the protein is exposed to temperatures higher than the boiling point of water, are destroyed most of all. Another change which is potentially more serious is the reaction of amino acids with each other and with additives present in the food artifact. Some of these unnatural new compounds are carcinogenic. Nitrites in foods increase these reactions, while reducing compounds such as ascorbic acid inhibit them.

Heat has a similar destructive effect on fats (oils) and on carbohydrates. It destroys a few of the vitamins such as vitamin C and vitamin A. Heat and other processes leach out water-soluble vitamins and minerals. Thus all chemical processes used to convert food into food artifact decrease the nutritive quality of the foods. This is why commercial french fries contain a small fraction only of the original vitamin C. The quality of food artifact is so poor that any person living mostly on food artifact cannot avoid developing a variety of chronic deficiency metabolic diseases. These are responsible for a large proportion of all behavioral disturbances.

Orthomolecular nutritionists have been studying the effect of food technology on the quality of the food. One of the most important, Ross H. Hall, in *Food for Nought* describes in detail what these processes are. Orthomolecular physicians study the effect of food artifact in the production of disease, and even more, the effect of food in restoring good health and in preventing chronic disease.

But even perfect food will not be adequate for everyone, for there can be no perfect food for everyone. There can be a perfect fit between food and an individual, or at least one can aspire to this. An unknown proportion of any population has food requirements which cannot be met by the best possible diet. They have increased requirements for essential nutrients which must then be used to supplement their diet. They include vitamins, minerals, amino acids and perhaps certain fats and carbohydrates. There are many reasons for these individual differences which are genetic or which may be acquired. For example, many have inherited a need for increased quantities of vitamin B_3. These people will be the first to develop pellagra on a vitamin B_3 deficient diet, but will eventually become ill even on a diet containing quantities of this vitamin which are adequate for most people. On the other hand, people who have been subjected to severe stress combined with malnutrition remain permanently impaired. They require large amounts of vitamin B_3 for the rest of their lives. Most of the prisoners of war incarcerated in the Far East war camps who survived have remained ill and only respond when given large doses of this vitamin. When a person with average requirements for vitamin B_3 eats a diet too low in this vitamin, he will develop pellagra. This is a deficiency disease where the error is in the diet. Where the metabolic need is so great no normal diet could provide enough vitamin, the same relative deficiency is present. But since the diet is not at fault the condition is called a dependency. A dependency may then be genetic or acquired during a chronic period of malnutrition and stress.

One day we will have simple inexpensive tests which will help us decide which nutrients are required in above average quantities. Today orthomolecular physicians must depend upon their own experience in using these nutrients in above average amounts. Once a dependency has been discovered it must be treated by a diet of food only (avoidance of food artifact or junk) and by supplementation with the appropriate nutrients. Each person must determine the optimum quantity by gradually increasing amounts consumed until the best therapeutic result is obtained. Fortunately, nutrients are as safe as food and can be used in varying doses until the optimum dose is found. This will vary with time depending upon the physiological state of the body. Optimum quantities of protein, fats and carbohydrates also must be determined by each person.

Since food artifacts do not occur in nature it is wrong to equate foods with protein, fat or carbohydrate. It is accurate to describe foods as being rich or less rich in these substances. We should consider beans and meats as protein-rich foods, olives as fat-rich foods and potatoes as carbohydrate-rich foods.

If we eat only food, we no longer need to be concerned about our diet being too rich in protein, fat, carbohydrate or in other nutrients, for even consuming large quantities of any food will be reasonably safe compared to the consumption of food artifacts. People have remained well on meat diets, but not on a diet containing meat from starving animals which had no fat.

But there is probably some variation in optimum amounts of protein-rich, fat-rich, or carbohydrate-rich foods. Many people remain well on diets rich in carbohydrate foods while others do not remain well unless they consume a lot of protein-rich foods.

This then is the subject matter of orthomolecular nutrition. It is the task of the orthomolecular physician to help each patient discover that nutrition for which she or he is best suited using food and supplements. It is the duty of each orthomolecular nutritionist and scientist to make this task simpler so that patients can be helped more quickly. It is also the duty of all orthomolecular theorists and therapists to educate their clients, patients, the community, industry, the healing profession and people who control national food policy.

Links Between Nutrition and Behavior

In order to establish a theoretical link between malnutriton and malbehavior we must show that pathological behavior will result from malnutrition and that we understand how the function of the brain biochemically is influenced by nutrition so that there is a logical link from malnutrition to disordered brain chemistry, to changes in perception and thinking and other manifestations of brain function, to an interaction with the psychosocial environment which becomes pathological or abnormal behavior.

Link one: nutrition influences brain function

We are concerned only with those elements of brain activity which directly affect transmission of stimuli from one set of neurons to another. A neuron (brain cell) influences another by transmitting electrical impulses away from its body along nerves. These nerves terminate in little enlargements called terminal boutons, which are in very close proximity to, but do not actually touch, the body of the next neuron. There is a very narrow gap between bouton and nerve body called a synapse. The electrical stimulus stops at the bouton, but a set of reactions is started which results in a stimulus to the cell body to which it is closest. A number of chemicals are released in the synapse and move across to the other side. On reaching the far side they are absorbed onto special areas or receptors which have a specific electrical pattern to which these chemicals are attracted. These chemical messengers are called neurotransmitters. They include natural substances such as noradrenaline, adrenaline, acetylcholine, serotonin and several others. There is no doubt that as neuropharmacologists refine and perfect their pharmacological techniques additional neurotransmitters will be discovered.

There are other chemicals which the brain uses to control its behavior that influence glands. They are the neurohormones, and there is growing evidence that other classes of chemicals such as endorphins are used to control other functions such as modulation of pain or hunger.

Every chemical in the body has to be synthesized from a preceding natural chemical. Food is the major source of nutrients from which these essential brain chemicals are made. Acetylcholine is made by combining acetate, which is abundant in the body, and choline, which is a fat-soluble vitamin present in fats such as lecithin. If the diet is deficient in choline it will become increasingly difficult to make enough acetylcholine. Changes in acetylcholine certainly do influence electrical activity of the brain.

A number of neurotransmitters originate from the amino acid phenylalanine. This is converted into tyrosine except in patients who suffer from phenylketonuria and thus lack the enzyme essential to effect this conversion. No one doubts that the behavior of infants, children and adults with this problem is altered. Ketonuriac children may manifest psychotic behavior and adults typically schizophrenic behavior. Tyrosine is converted into noradrenaline

which is converted into adrenaline. Each one of these neurotransmitters is changed into a number of end products including
adrenochrome. Adrenochrome, which is made in the body, is
an hallucinogen.[6] This was the basis of Hoffer and Osmond's
adrenochrome hypothesis of schizophrenia which was responsible
for the initial use of vitamin B_3 and ascorbic acid in treating
schizophrenics. Thus a deficiency of phenylalanine will lead to a
variety of behavioral changes while any abnormality in the metabolism of these amines will lead to other types of behavioral changes.

Another neurotransmitter, serotonin, derives from the amino
acid tryptophan. This amino acid is converted into a variety of
intermediate compounds flowing into nicotinamide adenine dinucleotide (NAD) or into another variety of substances flowing into
serotonin. The quantity of serotonin in the brain is influenced by
the amount of tryptophan ingested. Ingestion of pure tryptophan
on an empty stomach, so that it does not have to compete with
other amino acids, will rapidly increase serotonin levels. For
some people l-tryptophan at bedtime elevates serotonin enough
to increase ability to fall asleep. Too much sugar in the diet will
also influence brain serotonin levels by interfering with transfer of
tryptophan into the brain.

Histamine, another neurotransmitter, comes from the amino
acid histidine. It is not difficult to believe that histidine levels
will influence histamine levels.

Neuropharmacologists now have ample evidence that nutrition
can influence the production and concentration of neurotransmitters
which they have always equated with the action of drugs known
to influence behavior, such as tranquilizers and antidepressants.
But two new findings have shown how vitamins can have a direct
effect on brain receptors that are independent of how they are
made or from which precursor.

Tolbert, Thomas, Middaugh and Zemp,[7] and Thomas and
Zemp[8] found that ascorbic acid is as potent a substance as Haldol ™
in blocking dopamine receptors in the brain. It is believed by
many neuropharmacologists that Haldol ™ and other tranquilizers
act by adhering to these receptors and blocking their response to
dopamine; ascorbic acid does the same. The major difference is
that ascorbic acid does not readily cross the blood/brain barrier;
only a small fraction gets into the brain. The amount which gets
in is directly related to the dose which is taken. A much larger
fraction of Haldol ™ gets across, probably because it is a foreign
molecule for which the brain has not established an effective
blood/brain barrier. Another major difference is that tranquilizers
cause a number of dangerous side effects such as tardive dyskinesia,

whereas there has not been a single case reported in people who have taken very large doses of ascorbic acid for up to several decades. The brain can control the amount of ascorbic acid that gets in; it has no way of protecting itself against tranquilizers. The price for many is very high.

Ascorbic acid is a powerful reducing substance and has a profound effect on centrally active amines such as dopamine, noradrenaline and adrenaline. It is likely ascorbic acid has an affinity with the dopamine receptors because of its electrical configuration. It has an affinity for both dopamine, with which it will combine, and the receptors. Being a natural constituent it would not be as damaging to the colony of receptors, and would be less apt to stimulate the formation of new receptors. It is believed tardive dyskinesia may be a result of an overproduction of receptors, a response of the brain to the dopamine receptor blockade by the tranquilizers.

Nicotinamide, one of the two vitamin B_3 members, also has an effect on brain receptors. A class of antianxiety drugs, the diazepines (Valium,™ Librium,™ Serax,™) are attracted to receptors called diazepine receptors; Mohler, Polc, Cumin, Pieri and Kettler[9] discovered that nicotinamide is also attracted to these receptors. They suggest nicotinamide is the natural molecule with benzodiazepine-like action. Nicotinamide crosses the blood brain barrier with difficulty, as does vitamin C; this is why large doses are required. Once it gets into the brain it is a very powerful diazepine-like substance, without any of the bad side effects such as addiction.

Link two: brain changes can distort brain function psychologically.

We can understand that changing the functioning of the brain will change behavior, but this understanding does not help us understand how undesirable behavior is produced. Why does the biochemical pathology simply not put the patient to sleep as do anesthetics, or at least decrease the level of consciousness? In fact these changes hardly ever occur. Instead there are behavioral changes in people whose memory is normal, who are fully conscious and who are not confused. But there is an important clue—this is the ubiquitous presense of perceptual changes and/or thought disorder. Any biochemical changes might then act preferentially on those synapses and neurotransmitters which control the relation of the brain to the senses which inform us about our world, internal and external. I will show later how certain well-known nutritional diseases do cause this type of brain behavioral change.

Any organism reacts to the environment if it can detect what must be reacted to. Complex animals such as man react in complex ways, depending upon a large number of factors. To simplify this description, I will use a computer analogy. This is not meant to show that humans in any way are like computers, because obviously we are not. So far no computer has created a man, but the computer analogy clarifies how we react to our environment and how our perception of our world can affect behavior.

A computer has four basic functions: an input function by which information is entered into the computer; the human input includes our senses—seeing, hearing, tasting, feeling, smelling, being aware of our orientation with respect to gravity, awareness of pain and so on. The second main function is storage of information and the ability to perform the calculating and retrieval functions which may be demanded of the machine. These are also some of the functions of the brain. The third function is to accept and to act upon orders entered into the machine, i.e., its program. A computer must be programmed to perform certain operations on the data entered therein. Humans also are programmed, but not in the same way. Ours begins before birth as soon as the developing brain becomes aware of sensations such as noise. From birth the individual is programmed (shaped) by all the many psychosocial variables we are all exposed to. This includes our culture, station in life, experiences, education and so on. The last function is the response which a computer does by sorting cards, writing on a terminal or making meaningful noises. The human response is speech, which is a particular example of behavior. It is a motor response, a response which requires muscular activity.

A computer can malfunction in many ways. These may be due to computer technicians' errors or to a breakdown in the complex apparatus. If the wrong information is put into the computer it cannot yield a sensible answer, i.e., input error will cause output error. In the same way, human input or perception can be distorted; the output will then be distorted. This will be made clear later by clinical examples. There may be errors in the computer mechanism as there may be in the brain, and there may be errors in programming as there are in the development of personality.

Perceptual changes are the easiest to relate to behavioral changes. The relation between schizophrenia, a classic disease which causes behavioral disturbances, and perception was first described in clinical detail over a century ago. Conolly [10] described insanity as a disease of perception combined with an inability to judge whether these changes were real.

Let us examine a few perceptual changes and how they can

alter behavior. All perceptual changes can be divided into illusions and hallucinations. A visual illusion is present when objects develop an unusual appearance in either form, color or shape. Those who have taken LSD or any other hallucinogens will understand these changes. There are auditory, taste, smell and other illusions which can affect every human sense. Hallucinations are objects which are seen or sounds which are heard when there is no object or sound upon which these could have been based. There is of course no sharp demarcation between them, one running into the other. The variety of illusions and hallucinations is amazing; even after thirty years I am surprised at the illusions and hallucinations my patients describe.

When a number of people witness an event they more or less see the same thing, but they do not record it in their memory as would a TV camera. The interpretation of what was seen is altered by the person's program. Presumably identical twins brought up in the same way would perceive the event the same way. Once the event has been perceived there must be a reaction. The variety of reactions to the same event is even wider than the way it was perceived. One person may respond with interest, another with fear, a third with disgust, a fourth with hysteria, while a fifth may faint. These reactions to the same event are determined by that person's program.

Certain perceptual changes lead to psychotic behavior. Assume that there is a visual hallucination, i.e., the person sees an extraterrestrial creature. As soon as this has been seen the person must decide what it means, if it is real or not, and what is behind it. If the person decides it is unreal, i.e., an hallucination, behavior will be altered, but not enough to be considered psychotic. It may cause some anxiety, some fear there is something wrong with the person. But if the person concludes the hallucination is real this will elicit a change in behavior, the form of which will be determined by that person's lifetime program. One person may see a God, and later develop a paranoid grandiose delusional psychosis. In each case, that person's program will be one of the factors which determines the response. In our book *How to Live with Schizophrenia*, we have described in detail how perceptual changes influence behavior. One example will illustrate how one's personality determines response to perceptual changes. This happened to a middle-aged woman who had had one or two afternoon cocktails for decades—she had never considered she was harming herself. However, her ability to resist alcohol slowly and insidiously weakened until she developed delirium tremens. In hospital she appeared to be in little distress as she described her vivid visual hallucinations. She told me the room was full of dogs so that it appeared as if the room was covered with a rug of dog backs. My reaction was to exclaim, "Isn't that awful!" Her response to her hallucinations was benign because of her previous experience in loving dogs and her personality; mine would have been much different.

But many reactions are not as benign. Patients have murdered because the people they were seeing took on the appearance of the devil, or of a feared enemy. Several of my patients lost the ability to distinguish faces and became very paranoid. One woman no longer recognized her husband and while still living with him treated him as a stranger—totally inappropriate behavior.

Other perceptual changes can elicit abnormal behavior, but in every case the patient believes he is behaving in a rational way, as would anyone else with the same programming and the same perceptual changes, even though to others, and even to the patient when well, this would be judged as abnormal behavior.

Perceptual changes alone are not adequate to cause serious behavioral changes. There must also be some thought disorder, i.e., the ability to judge that the changes are unreal is impaired. There may be very few perceptual changes and gross thought disorder. These are very difficult to treat. An example is a nurse who was convinced she was pregnant. She was obese, her abdomen protruded and she walked as if she were eight months pregnant. Over the years she had persuaded a succession of doctors to examine her, but she never believed them. She had become alienated from her husband and had had no intercourse for at least a year when I first saw her. She was aware that to be "pregnant" meant she must have become pregnant without spermatozoa, but was willing to accept this as a better alternative than to think she was not pregnant. I discovered that she felt movement in her abdomen, which ruled out an abdominal tumor. How else could she explain the aliveness of her abdomen? She suffered from a somatic perceptual change where her brain signaled movement, probably in response to normal peristaltic movement. Only after she lost this perceptual change did she give up her pregnancy delusion.

Brain changes not only *can* cause changes in perception and in thinking, they do. There are two main lines of evidence: (a) from diseases which are known to distort brain chemistry and cause these brain symptoms, and (b) from studies of hallucinogenic drugs. A large class of psychiatric patients are characterized by changes in perception and in thinking. These are the schizophrenias and the deliria from chronic intoxications. Similar changes are produced in normal individuals when they take adequate amounts of the hallucinogenic drugs such as LSD or mescaline or MDA, or any one of a larger number.[6] When perceptual tests are given to schizophrenics or to normal subjects under the influence of these drugs, they yield identical scores. High scores are obtained when a large number of perceptual illusions and hallucinations are present.[12]

The relation between malnutrition and perceptual changes is proven by the characteristic symptoms of one of the classic deficiency diseases, pellagra. Pellagra is a vitamin B_3 deficiency disease, with other deficiencies superimposed. It is generally caused by a diet consisting primarily of corn or other cereals low in tryptophan or vitamin B_3. Corn is a particularly bad food when it is the main source of calories since it is low in tryptophan and low in vitamin B_3, and what is present is so tightly bound it can not be released in the body. It is also too rich in leucine and too low in isoleucine. This combination increases loss of vitamin B_3 into urine. Pellagra can also come from a deficiency of pyridoxine (B_6).

Pellagra is characterized by perceptual symptoms. It can be distinguished from schizophrenia only with great difficulty. At one time when it was endemic, the only sure way to diagnose the cases was to give them vitamin B_3; if they were well in a few days, they were diagnosed pellagra.

I think it can be accepted that malnutrition can cause changes in perception by altering brain biochemistry, that the relation between the person and the psychosocial environment is disturbed by these perceptual changes, and that this is responsible for abnormal behavior.

An apparent contradiction is the observation that many adult behaviorally disturbed people, formerly called psychopathic, do not have perceptual changes. Many, if not all, of these people suffered from childhood schizophrenia with typical perceptual changes and thought disorder. A number of childhood schizophrenics diagnosed by L. Bender, using strict diagnostic criteria, were reexamined after they became adult. Every one had had visual and/or auditory hallucinations, but when they became adult one-half were typical New York street delinquents and psychopaths who denied having had any perceptual symptoms. They could not remember the ones they had suffered as children. I have seen at least twelve childhood schizophrenics become adult. Whether they had recovered or not, they could not remember the hallucinations that had been so disturbing in their childhood. Like a nightmare, the memory of hallucinations tends to disappear in time.

The other half were in mental hospitals, chronic schizophrenics. Today they will be wandering the streets of New York City, living in rundown hotels or nursing homes in slum areas, mostly under control by heavy tranquilizers. L. Bender's study has never been disproven, and it is supported by my observation of childhood schizophrenics who, for a variety of reasons, could not be treated or did not respond to treatment. They too have begun a career of criminal behavior with frequent visits to jails, mental hospitals, and psychiatric wards. Their referral centers are the courts, and the police act as their social workers. Their behavior was shaped by their early prolonged experience with schizophrenia; they have been unable to develop normal social relationships or the ability to empathize with other people. Their own needs are paramount and must be consummated immediately. Any person in their way must be removed like any inanimate object.

Behavioral Diseases Due to Malnutrition

Any kind of brain disorder will lead to behavioral abnormalities. Life is so complex that it requires a fully efficient, normal, stable brain for normal relationships to be established and maintained. When the brain becomes disordered, it becomes almost impossible to remain normal. Since there are four major brain functions, it is possible to divide all behavioral disorders under these four categories.

Behavioral disorders due primarily to perceptual changes

These include the schizophrenias; a proportion of children with learning and/or behavioral disorders; intoxications with alcohol, the hallucinogens, marihuana, and other street drugs; and deliria.

Behavioral disorders due primarily to thought disorder

These include chronic patients whose perceptual changes have gone or receded, but the thought disorder and personality pattern generated by the illness has remained. I would include in this category many of the criminals who become members of terrorist groups, and have no compunction in using and destroying any humans in order to achieve their aims. Among a society of normal people they would not be acceptable, among terrorists and other criminals they find themselves useful and needed.

The diseases due to perceptual and thought disorder are caused by a number of biochemical changes. I will not discuss conditions such as hypothyroidism, general paresis of the insane, or the hallucinogens which cause the schizophrenic syndrome. Orthomolecular physicians have added three new classes of syndrome: the

238 Nutrition

cerebral allergies, the vitamin dependencies, and the heavy metal toxicities. And we are beginning to study the amino acid dependencies.

The Cerebral Allergies: Every tissue and organ in the body can react to molecules pathologically; some of these reactions are called allergic reactions. The skin responds with itching and swelling— general or local such as hives; joints become swollen and painful; the respiratory system develops asthma, hayfever, coughing or sneezing. The reaction between allergen and cell releases histamine; edema and swelling with itching result, the affected tissues weep or secrete. Milk commonly causes secretion in the sinuses and throat often described as mucus. Some foods are so often involved they have become popularly known as mucous-producing foods, but of course, only people who are allergic are so affected.

Some tissues react in an obvious way. It is simple to spot and feel hives or to feel the effects of mucus, but certain organs can respond with results not easily recognized. If the liver responds how could one relate the symptoms to an allergic reaction of the liver? The brain also is hidden; it can not be seen to swell and does not develop an itch or a rash.

Usually when an organ is disturbed by an allergic reaction its function is disturbed. One can then judge that the organ is disturbed by recognizing this relationship. The brain or central nervous system is the organ of perception, thinking, feeling, and it orders behavior. When the brain is disturbed by an allergic reaction, any one of these functions will be altered in the same way that the hallucinogens alter brain function, as has already been described. The idea that milk can produce hallucinations is still so new it is unacceptable to most psychiatrists, but this concept must be accepted since the data which establish it are very large and persuasive.

The data relating allergies to cerebral function are at least eighty years old if one accepts medical reports in current medical journals as evidence, but the knowledge that certain foods make people mentally ill certainly was known thousands of years ago. A few allergists and internists, such as Walter Alvarez, described how allergic reactions caused tension, irritability and depression. Every sufferer of allergies is aware of this. I have seen no asthmatics cheerful, happy and relaxed when suffering from an attack. The importance of this relationship between mood and allergic reaction was neutralized by psychosomatic explanations which began around 1945. Psychosomatic theorists suggested that personality and/or psychosocial factors caused the allergic reaction and that the discomfort of the reaction caused the mood changes. They failed to recognize that both mood and allergic somatic reactions were the result of a brain reaction or cerebral allergy. These theories suppressed any further examination of the causes of mood and allergic reactions by forcing attention on psychological and subconscious matters.

The evidence relating allergies to brain function changes (to behavioral disorders) is divisible into the following findings:

1. Abnormal behavior is present as long as the offending allergen is in the body, and (a) removal of the allergen results in recovery, (b) reintroducing the allergen causes relapse.

2. Neutralizing the reaction results in a recovery.

3. Preventing the organ from reacting also prevents the abnormal behavior.

Abnormal behavior present as long as allergen is present— Every physician who has seen the effect of a four-day fast on the behavior of some patients is surprised and most are excited. A patient came to see me several years ago. Several months before, she had fasted, become normal and subsequently identified, by adding one food to each meal, what had been making her sick. With some excitement and enthusiasm she reported this to her family physician. He became very angry with her, they had a bitter argument, and she demanded a referral to see me which he did. But she had at the same time decided never to see the doctor again. This doctor had not suggested the fast. He must have thought that the biggest sin a patient could commit was to get well for the wrong reason.

Clinical ecologists have been using deprivation diets for many years to discover what their patients were allergic to. Fasting has been used for centuries to make people feel better. I have no doubt that our ancestors many thousands of years ago had to fast pretty often and that some of them would have noted that after each fast or after some fasts they were better. Perhaps this is why fasting and religion are so intimately related. Fasting therapy is not new. What is new is its application to behavioral diseases, to psychiatry.

Marshall Mandell[13] was the first clinical ecologist who forced orthomolecular psychiatrists to pay attention. Before him E. Rees[14] had reported the importance of certain diets in curing children with learning and behavioral disorders. But these reports did not have the same impact as those by Mandell and by W. Philpott, his collaborator. There is nothing as dramatic as seeing a chronic psychotic become normal after a four-day fast. The following case illustrates such a response in a patient who was too sophisticated a patient to respond by any placebo reaction. He was, in fact, what I call a professional schizophrenic, i.e., he had been ill too long and had become accustomed to a life in and out of hospital, continuously on welfare, and free of any need to make any decision.

I first saw this patient in 1952, about ten years after he had been discharged from a tuberculosis sanitorium where he had been a patient for a couple of years. The treatment then demanded that patients be well fed and if possible slightly overweight. This was achieved by forcing milk and its derivatives. After discharge he was well until in 1952 he developed anuria; he could not urinate. After a complete urological examination with no evidence of physical disease he was transferred to the psychiatric ward and became my patient. He was clearly schizophrenic with visual and auditory hallucinations, severe thought disorder and anxiety with depression. As I was then testing vitamin B_3 I started him on niacin up to 6 grams per day. He began to respond slowly and after several admissions was able to remain relatively well and to work. In 1957 he had a minor relapse; he had stopped taking his vitamins, placed himself under the care of a Winnipeg psychiatrist who started him on the then new tranquilizers. He returned to Saskatchewan and came back to me again around 1960. He was and had been psychotic from his recurrence in 1957; he no longer responded to any treatment including drugs, vitamins and ECT. Eventually not even a very good home with a tremendous understanding of schizophrenia was able to keep him and he was sent to a mental hospital. About ten years later, he was transferred from the mental hospital to City Hospital in Saskatoon because of anuria; again there was no physical reason and I was asked to take over. Again, I saw him exactly as he had been from 1957 even though he had been thoroughly tranquilized throughout.

I had just started fasting a number of chronic patients who had not responded to vitamin treatment. The patient agreed to do a four-day water fast. On the fifth day, to my surprise, he was normal, he was free of hallucinations, was no longer paranoid, was not depressed or tense. I then began to test foods giving him first a glass of milk. Within one hour he was sick mentally and physically, all his psychotic symptoms reappeared and he also suffered nausea, abdominal cramps and diarrhea. The next day he was better. I told him he was allergic to milk and would have to eliminate all milk products. He replied he had known all along milk made him sick. He added that he would not discontinue milk, that he was not prepared to live on his own, seek work or take on the responsibilities of a normal person. He demanded another psychiatrist. As soon as he was given dairy products he regained the psychotic symptoms that had been his companion for nearly twenty years and returned to the mental hospital where he died several years later of leukemia.

Over a two-year period I supervised a four- to nine-day fast (usually four days) on about 160 patients who had not responded or had responded poorly to treatment. By the end of the fast about 100 were well. The majority of these remained well; the remainder relapsed because they could not or would not follow the new dietary program. This sudden improvement in a large number of my chronic patients had an unforeseen effect on my practice. Before I had treated these patients using the allergy approach, I had a number of patients on my waiting list for admission to hospital. Most would be given ECT in combination with orthomolecular treatment. After the two-year period, this waiting list vanished and I had to use ECT very infrequently. This has remained the case for the past eight years.

The use of elimination diets and recovery at the end of the fast with the resurgence of the psychosis when certain foods were reintroduced establishes the first main line of evidence. The only exception occurs in patients who have been off the offending foods for a long time. When the food is introduced they may have no reaction, but if the food is used more frequently, approaching the use before the fast, the psychosis will emerge. Another apparent exception occurs in patients who use rotation diets and eat foods they are allergic to every four or five days.

Neutralizing allergic reactions—When the allergic reaction is neutralized the psychosis will not reappear. This has been described by a number of clinical allergists who have used desensitization techniques ranging from injections of food extracts or extracts of any offending material, sublingual administration of the same or similar extracts. Urine injections have also been used taking samples from patients who are suffering allergic reactions at the time.

Decreasing or preventing reactions—Decreasing the intensity of the reaction also reduces the intensity of the psychosis. This may be done using chromoglycate, found useful in treating children, and antihistamines. Tranquilizers and antidepressants have antihistaminic properties although this aspect of their biological activity has been more or less ignored for the past twenty years. Pharmacologists have been more interested in their effect on substances such as serotonin or noradrenaline. One antidepressant, Mianserin,™ has no effect on these latter two neurotransmitters and is an effective antidepressant; it also has good antihistamine properties. Elsewhere I have suggested [15,16] that most patients with depression respond to antidepressants because they are really examples of cerebral allergies with depression as the main symptom.

Behavioral disorder arising from depression and irritability

Depression is not considered a cause of antisocial behavior. Suicide is a major risk in seriously depressed patients, but laws against suicide are not enforced and would-be suicides are not charged; murder-suicide is a rare complication of depression.

Depression and irritability often co-exist. When the main symptom is irritability, especially in children and adolescents, a good deal of antisocial behavior can be generated. These patients develop almost explosive behavior and may become involved in antisocial behavior. Their irritability is increased by street drugs, by junk food including alcohol, and by other equally irritable youths. Our modern diet of food artifact has created a large number of adolescent boys and girls who have perceptual illusions so they can not or do not enjoy reading, who have short attention span, who are restless and irritable, who seldom laugh or feel happy, and who excite each other to similar states of hyperactivity, sometimes frenzy. They are temporarily calmed by pot or alcohol and other street drugs. The street is their drugstore, while pushers are their therapists. Modern advertisers have recognized this increased level of irritability and have equated it with energy and good life. This can be seen on many modern TV commercials advertising food artifacts. These are hyperactive ads with children, young men and women jumping about in a frenzy of activity. Many believe that hyperactivity and feeling good are synonymous.

The connection between food artifacts and abnormal behavior

Two types of food artifacts are most often associated with abnormal behavior: (a) the consumption of food artifacts rich in the sugars and processed starches and (b) food additives present in food artifacts, including cosmetic and trace additives. In practice both factors should be considered together since most processed foods contain both.

The current interest in the effect of additives followed B. Feingold's publications[17] dealing with the effect of certain cosmetic additives on children's behavior. He studied the effect of common food dyes and foods which naturally contain similar substances. His work has been received with scorn and hostility by most of the experts in pediatrics and child psychology. Parents of hyperactive children have become convinced he is correct as are physicians and all the professional people who have followed his diet and seen its calming effect on children. At last corroboration has been published and more will follow once the critics become more humble and more willing to try his diet rather than to simply criticize it.

I have seen children who had been on additive-free diets become very hyperactive after eating one chocolate bar; over the next four days they engaged in stealing and lying and became very aggressive. Adults, too, have reacted in the same way. Over the past ten years I have treated around 800 children. I estimate that about half respond well to a junk-free diet. The main problem is persuading these children to keep away from junk.

Even whole foods which ought to be good and nutritious may contain additives which create hyperactivity. Parents of one of my hyperactive patients noted that one commercial egg would make their child much worse whereas an egg from a neighbor's hens did not. Commercial eggs contain additives from the feed given these birds which may include antibiotics and growth stimulants as well as other substances. This six-year-old child could not have had a placebo reaction; how could he know eggs can be so different?

The relation between certain vitamin dependencies and abnormal behavior

A vitamin dependency exists when a person requires large doses of any vitamin in order to remain well. These doses are so large that even the best diet could not possibly provide enough. Dependencies are congenital or acquired; most of them are acquired. They occur during periods of severe malnutrition combined with great stress. The best modern example occurred in Japanese war camps nearly forty years ago, but they may also occur in modern hospitals. I have seen a number of patients who had to be in hospital several weeks following gastrointestinal surgery. Recently such a patient had to be on intravenous feeding following the stress of a second operation for a recurrent condition. The psychological stress was severe. When she could eat she was offered gelatin, ginger ale and a thin soup made from boullion cubes. This "diet" made her sick and she refused to eat it, preferring intravenous feeding. Six weeks after discharge she became much worse, depressed and tense. Generally, long periods of malnutrition and stress are much more apt to produce vitamin dependencies. Very few of the ex-prisoners of war, who spent forty-four months in war camps in the Far East, have remained well. Most ex-POW's suffer from a variety of physical and mental changes which respond to high doses of vitamin B_3. I have estimated that one year in such a camp aged each prisoner about 5 years.

The following vitamins are involved.

Thiamin (B_1): A dependency for thiamin is most apt to occur in people who consume large amounts of simple carbohydrates, especially alcohol. Alcoholics may develop Wernicke-Korsakov syndrome, a disease recognized to require large doses of thiamin. I would expect that some ex-POW's are also thiamin-dependent since many of them suffered beriberi.

Niacinamide/niacin (B_3): Vitamin B_3 dependency is apt to develop after severe stress and malnutrition such as occurred in the ex-POW. Chronic pellagrins, when this disease was more common, also developed a vitamin B_3 dependency.

Pyridoxine (B_6): I suspect that children who consume large quantities of milk will develop a pyridoxine dependency. The large intake of protein increases the requirement for pyridoxine. These children develop behavioral changes.

Orthomolecular Treatment

The first step in solving any problem is in understanding some of its roots, otherwise there would be no point in reciting the many reasons why behavior is disturbed. Nor do we understand all the factors, but we have enough information to start remedial treatment. We can not wait for another hundred years when we will understand much more. Scientists are under no pressure and can leisurely pursue their studies until they are certain. We physicians and all the people in agencies which must deal with the problem do not have this luxury of time. We must act now. This last section of this chapter outlines a treatment proposal which in my opinion will sharply reduce the incidence and prevalence of antisocial behavior.

General principles or ethics

Orthomolecular psychiatry uses the medical model as described by Siegler and Osmond.[18] This statement had to be made to contrast our practice with the flight from the medical model of most American psychiatrists. There is strong evidence they have realized their error and leaders of American psychiatry are encouraging a return to the medical model. Within the medical model both patient and physician have rights and responsibilities. The patient has the right to be told the diagnosis, to have it explained and to be given the best possible treatment, whether or not it is a popular or accepted treatment. The patient has a responsibility to be truthful and to cooperate with treatment.

Each patient is different and each treatment program must be individually tailored much as a dress fitter fits a dress. The physician must be skillful in use of all treatments including drugs, provided they will not harm the patient. The amount of supplements must be varied to work out an optimum dose.

Nutrition

For patients free of food allergy: The best diet is the diet of food only, free of food artifact. This allows meats, fish, vegetables, nuts, fruit, grains, raw where possible, lightly cooked when cooking is essential. Each person must discover the best distribution of foods from those available. Some will be healthier on greater quantities of protein-rich foods; others will do better with less. Some may be vegetarian; others heavy meat and fish consumers. The best rule is to totally eliminate all junk. If this restores health, no further modification is necessary. If there is only a partial recovery one, can experiment with various programs until the best one is found. If no nutritional variation is successful, supplements will be required.

For food allergic patients: The presence of cerebral allergies is diagnosed by means of a careful history beginning with infancy. The presence of allergies in children is suggested by gastrointestinal problems, by colic, by any physical manifestation of allergy. Special attention should be given to the dietary history and the relationship of food to symptoms. Many people have been aware that they felt worse after eating certain foods, but the idea that foods could make anyone suffer depression, anxiety or fatigue is so novel few people consider the relationship valid.

The final diagnostic test consists of various forms of testing, often after food deprivation. One of the most accurate is a fast, usually four to nine days, followed by individual food tests. Other tests are being used which are quicker but may be less accurate. Of these the best are the sublingual food tests. The least accurate are the intradermal tests probably because foods seldom interact with skin as it does with the mucosa of the gastrointestinal system. They are much more accurate for contact allergens. Once the offending foods are identified, they are not consumed. They may have to be avoided forever, but in most cases after a prolonged abstinence it may be possible to eat these foods sparingly and occasionally. If the patient is allergic to a large number of foods special rotation diets may be required.[13] It is also essential to search for factors which may decrease the resistance to allergies. There is evidence that conditions such as chronic monilia infection,[19] and hypothyroidism may be responsible for multiple food allergies which clear when these conditions are corrected.

Supplements

Vitamins: Two groups of vitamins have been used most frequently: vitamin B_3, vitamin B_6, vitamin B_{12}, folic acid and ascorbic acid for psychiatric conditions; and vitamins A, D_3 and vitamin E for physical conditions. There is no sharp division nor can other vitamins be ignored. The body requires adequate amounts of all the vitamins. For each vitamin, optimum quantities per day should be determined, usually by using several dose ranges. Fortunately, vitamins are safe when used at an optimum dose defined as an effective-therapeutic dose which does not cause side effects.

The psychiatric vitamins are used in treating schizophrenias, children with learning and behavioral disorders, and, in fact, for most psychiatric conditions. With the mood disorders, they are used in much lower dosages. They are especially helpful in treating the addictions.

The physical vitamins A and D_3 are used for treating some allergies, especially asthma,[20] and arthritis. Vitamin E is used in treating cardiovascular diseases and in slowing down the ravages of age.[21]

For all vitamins, once the illness has subsided, it is possible to discover maintenance doses which are lower than the curative doses, but many will have to use maintenance—for health—for ever.

Minerals: All essential minerals are required in optimum doses. A few are water soluble and easily lost from the body, such as zinc and manganese. Zinc salts are especially important since zinc is so easily lost under any stress, physical and psychological, and is present in diminished amounts in our food artifacts. With adequate intake of zinc, copper levels are reduced. It is even being used with success to treat Wilson's disease, a condition where copper levels build up in the body, and it may be more effective than copper-chelating substances such as penicillamine.

Other treatments: The use of nutrition with supplements does not mean that other treatment is to be avoided; each patient requires the best possible treatment program which will alleviate suffering and cause a recovery. Such a program may require any drug available today, but it must be used skillfully. We use tranquilizers, antidepressants, antibiotics, any special drug available, and, for a very small number of psychotic patients, we may have to use electroconvulsive treatment (ECT).

When drugs are used, in most cases smaller doses can be used compared to use of drugs without nutritional therapy. This decreases the chance of side effects. In my own series of schizophrenics treated over twenty-five years, I have not seen tardive dyskinesia develop. Those I have treated have come to me with this condition already fully developed. D. Hawkins [22] reports that he has seen no cases in over 15,000 patients treated over fifteen years. Patients on tranquilizer therapy alone show a 10 to 20 percent incidence. When smaller doses of tranquilizers are used, less manganese is chelated from the body.[23] When tardive dyskinesia does develop, it is easily treated by giving manganese and vitamin B$_3$.

Once the patient has recovered or is close to recovery, the dose of any drug is reduced very slowly; a sharp reduction may cause a sharp rebound reaction and precipitate a relapse. It is important to get the dose down as quickly as possible without precipitating a relapse, for a tranquilized person is unable to function normally in society.

Diseases treated

Although the general principles of treatment and the use of nutrition, supplements and drugs applies to all diseases, there are certain specific treatments unique to each class of diseases.

The Schizophrenias: The particular syndrome, whether an allergy, a vitamin dependency or a mineral problem, must be determined as well as finding out which particular biochemical subtype it is.[24,25,26,27]

Vitamin B$_3$, either form, is one of the primary vitamins. For adults the minimum dose is 1 gram three times per day, but much larger quantities may be required. For each patient the maximum dose is the dose which is just below that dose which causes nausea and, if not discontinued, vomiting. It is seldom possible to go higher than 6 to 9 grams per day for nicotinamide. Many patients can take much more nicotinic acid, but doses higher than 3 grams per day are only used if there is not a satisfactory response. Higher doses are needed during the recovery phase of the treatment, but during convalescence these doses may be reduced. One always aims at the optimum dose, which is equivalent to the minimum effective dose. Three grams per day is preferable to 6 grams, if it works as well.

Pyridoxine (vitamin B_6) is especially indicated for the sub-group of the schizophrenic syndrome, pyroluria.[25] This group excretes large quantities of kryptopyrrole (KP), a toxic substance first discovered by Irwin, Bayne and Miyashita.[28,29] KP binds pyridoxine and zinc, and this may be responsible for the double deficiency. The symptoms are the schizophrenic syndrome and certain physical changes including changes in skin (white areas under nails, stretch marks), changes in hair, impotence, premenstrual tension, impaired growth in adolescents, and changes in sensation of smell and taste. The amount of KP can be measured in the urine. The dose of B_6 varies between 100 to 3,000 milligrams per day, but is usually between 250 and 500 milligrams.

Ascorbic acid is used as an antistress and anti-infective substance. It thus decreases the probability of relapse. Schizophrenics are most susceptible to relapse during these physical stresses. In a few cases, very large doses of ascorbic acid have been more effective than tranquilizers in relieving severe anxiety in schizophrenic patients.

Children with learning and behavior disorders: There are many different diagnostic terms for disturbed children, but they have low reliability and validity. When children are seen by a number of therapists, they usually receive different diagnoses. Nor does the diagnosis suggest which treatment should be used. For this reason I no longer use any of these terms. I find it much more important to determine why these children are sick so that definitive treatment can be offered.

Orthomolecular therapists have recognized three broad classes of causes, each of which requires its own specific treatment. The broad outlines of treatment already described are used with modification for each child. Drugs are seldom required. In nearly a decade of practice I have started fewer than five children on Ritalin,™ (out of about 800 seen). I do use one of the tricyclic antidepressants, Imipramine,™ 25 milligrams per day, very rarely 50 milligrams, at bedtime usually. This is for children who respond slowly to treatment, who are depressed or who wet the bed, but in each case it is important to get them off this drug as soon as possible. I hardly ever use tranquilizers.

Vitamin doses are smaller than for adults; with children the usual starting dose is 500 milligrams three times per day for B_3 and ascorbic acid, and for pyridoxine, it is about 250 milligrams per day. These are then increased to optimum levels. Nicotinamide is preferable as children do not tolerate the nicotinic acid flush well, but when the nicotinamide causes serious side effects the other form is used. When both cause side effects I use inositol niacinate (Linodil™) which is not available in the U.S.A. but can be obtained over the counter in Canada. It is an excellent nicotinic acid derivative which releases the nicotinic acid slowly in the body. Inositol also has useful centrally active relaxing properties.

Children generally have fewer allergies than adults. They have not been exposed for as long. They may be divided into several groups:

A. Reactive to additives and to certain foods rich in substances similar to salicylates.[17] Dr. Feingold considered these toxic reactions rather than true allergies, which is probably correct.

B. Reactive to foods and food artifacts. The common ones are sugar and all products containing added sugar, milk products, and cereal grains—especially wheat and corn. But they may be allergic to any food. Diagnosis is established by elimination diets and provocative food tests.

Summary

In this review I have outlined the thesis that malnutrition can lead to malbehavior, and have shown the links between nutrition and disturbed behavior. I have not discussed a large number of psychosocial factors which are involved. Psychosocial factors have been examined seriously for centuries. We do understand how important they are in shaping behavior, but the vast majority of studies and nearly every social scientist has ignored nutritional factors. The attempts to modify behavior have not included nutritional modification; is this why our criminal justice system has had to face so much difficulty? I believe it is.

When we accept the role played by malnutrition in causing antisocial behavior in the context of a psychosocial system which influences it, when we ensure that all persons involved in antisocial behavior are adequately nourished as well as adequately treated, we will find that the problems will become more soluble. If we persist in ignoring nutrition and biochemistry, none of the psychosocial factors will be adequate. We need good nutrition and good psychosocial factors, not just one or the other. If only one can be used, then I suggest that it should be good nutrition as it will be more effective, more economical and more feasible. For an excellent general review see Hippchen.[30]

REFERENCES

1. Williams, R. J. 1969. *Biochemical Individuality*. Austin, Tx.: University of Texas Press.
2. Williams, R. J. 1973. *Nutrition Against Disease*. New York: Bantam Books.

3. Hall, R. H. 1974. *Food for Nought. The Decline in Nutrition*. New York: Harper & Row.
4. Bessman, S. P. 1972. Genetic failure of fetal amino acid "justification": a common basis for many forms of metabolic nutritional and "nonspecific" mental retardation. *J. Pediatrics* 8:834.
5. Bessman, S. P. 1979. The justification theory: the essential nature of the nonessential amino acids. *Nutrition Reviews* 37:209.
6. Hoffer, A. and Osmond, H. 1967. *The Hallucinogens*. New York: Academic Press.
7. Tolbert, L. C., Thomas, T. N., Middaugh, L. D. and Zemp, J. W. 1979. Ascorbate blocks amphetamine-induced turning behavior in rats with unilateral nigrostriated lesions. *Brain Research Bulletin* 4:43.
8. Thomas, T. N. and Zemp, J. W. 1977. Inhibition of dopamine sensitive adenylate cyclase from rat brain striatal homogenates by ascorbic acid. *J. Neurochemistry* 28:663.
9. Mohler, H., Polc, P., Cumin, R., Pieri, L. and Kettler, R. 1979. Nicotinamide is a brain constituent with benzodiazepine-like actions. *Nature* 278:563.
10. Conolly, J. 1964. *An Enquiry Concerning the Indications of Insanity, 1830*. London, England: Reprinted Dawsons of Pall Mall.
11. Hoffer, A. and Osmond, H. 1978. *How to Live With Schizophrenia*. New York: Citadel Press.
12. Hoffer, A., Kelm, H. and Osmond, H. 1975. *The Hoffer-Osmond Diagnostic Test*. Huntington: R. A. Krieger Pub. Co.
13. Mandell, M. and Scanlon, L. W. 1979. *Dr. Mandell's 5-Day Allergy Relief System*. New York: Thomas Y. Crowell.
14. Rees, E. L. 1973. Clinical observations on the treatment of schizophrenic and hyperactive children with megavitamins. *J. Orthomolecular Psychiatry* 2:93.
15. Hoffer, A. 1979. Obsessions and depressions. *J. Orthomolecular Psychiatry* 8:78.
16. Hoffer, A. 1980. Allergy, depression and tricyclic antidepressants. *J. Orthomolecular Psychiatry* 9:164.
17. Feingold, B. F. 1974. *Why Your Child Is Hyperactive*. New York: Random House.
18. Siegler, M. and Osmond, H. 1974. *Models of Madness, Models of Medicine*. New York: Macmillan Pub. Co., Inc.
19. Truss, C. O. 1978. Tissue injury induced by Candida albicans: mental and neurologic manifestations. *J. Orthomolecular Psychiatry* 7:17.
20. Reich, C. J. 1971. The vitamin therapy of chronic asthma. *J. of Asthma Research* 9: 99.
21. Shute, W. E. and Taub, H. J. 1969. *Vitamin E for Ailing and Healthy Hearts*. New York: Pyramid Publications.

22. Hawkins, D. R. 1980. From a private communication with A. Hoffer.
23. Kunin, R. A. 1976. Manganese and niacin in the treatment of drug-induced dyskinesias. *J. Orthomolecular Psychiatry* 5:4.
24. Hawkins, D. R. and Pauling, L. 1973. *Orthomolecular Psychiatry*. San Francisco: W. H. Freeman & Co.
25. Pfeiffer, C. C. 1975. *Mental and Elemental Nutrients*. New Canaan, Ct.: Keats Publishing, Inc.
26. Pfeiffer, C. C. 1978. *Zinc and Other Micro Nutrients*. New Canaan, Ct.: Keats Publishing, Inc.
27. Pfeiffer, C.C., Sohler, A., Jenney, M. S. And Iliev, V. 1974. Treatment of pyroluric schizophrenia (malvaria) with large doses of pyridoxine and a dietary supplement of zinc. *J. Applied Nutrition 26:21*.
28. Irvine, D., Bayne, W. and Miyashita, H. 1969. Identification of kryptopyrrole in human urine and its relation to psychosis. *Nature* 224:811.
29. Hoffer, A. and Osmond, H. 1963. Malvaria: a new psychiatric disease. *Acta Psychiatric Scand*. 39:335.
30. Hippchen, L. J. 1978. *Ecologic Biochemical Approach to Treatment of Delinquents and Criminals*. New York: Van Nostrand Reinhold Co.

9

IMPLICATIONS OF
CHRONIC VITAMIN UNDERNUTRITION

———————◄●►———————

RAYMOND J. SHAMBERGER, PH.D.

Introduction

MAJOR vitamin deficiencies in people with poor nutrition have been recognized for a number of years. However, chronic or marginal vitamin deficiencies resulting in clinical symptoms in humans are largely unrecognized. The increasing awareness and interest in these problems by the medical community have come about through problems of caring for patients on parenteral nutrition, aged patients and cancer patients. Advances in the clinical technology of laboratory measurement of vitamins and metabolites have resulted in increasing quantitation of chronic or marginal vitamin deficiencies. The objective of this chapter is to summarize knowledge in regard to chronic or marginal vitamin deficiency.

Stages of Vitamin Deficiency

Listed in Figure 9.1 are the events that occur if the vitamin supply is less than minimum requirement during a short period of time or in some cases if a suboptimal amount of vitamin is supplied during a longer period of time.[1] All stages are passed through with the first type of vitamin deficiency, but with the second kind, an equilibrium is reached at one of the indicated stages.

The first stage is characterized by a diminution of the body reserves as evidenced by lowering of the body vitamin content or by lowering the vitamin concentration in certain tissues or blood. These decreases can be identified by measuring the amount of

Figure 9.1
Stages of Vitamin Deficiency*

Stage		*Biochemical disturbances*	*Morphological changes*	*Functional disturbances*
1	Duration of severity of deficiency	Lowering of body vitamin content or Lowering of vitamin concentration in certain tissues or blood ↓		
2		Lowering of metabolite concentrations ↓		
3		Lowering of activity of vitamin-dependent enzymes or hormones ↓		
4		Early signs of metabolic disturbances ↓	Early signs of morphological changes ↓	Early signs of functional disturbances ↓
5		↓ Severe metabolic disturbances ↓	↓ Severe morphological changes	↓ Severe functional disturbances ↓
6			Irreversible morphological changes	Irreversible functional disturbances

*Permission granted from S. Karger AG, Base I

vitamin decrease in the plasma or a decrease of the vitamin in the urinary content. Lowering of metabolite concentrations is observed in the second stage, but the metabolism of the host is not disturbed. In stage three, the activity of vitamin-dependent enzymes or hormones is reduced. Erythrocyte transketolase is decreased when there is a reduced supply of vitamin B_1. The activity of this enzyme is measured with and without the addition of thiamine pyrophosphate. The ratio of these two measurements can be used as a measure of vitamin B_1 status.[2] In the fourth stage, initial signs of metabolic, morphological or functional disturbances are observed. Examples are: the increased clotting time of vitamin K deficiency; fatigue which occurs as one of the first signs of vitamin C deficiency; and slow calcification of bones in vitamin D deficiency seen as morphological change on roentgenogram. For many vitamins, the borderline or chronic deficiency states are often unspecific and not easy to diagnose. Finally, in the last two stages are the well-known symptoms of vitamin deficiency, which result in irreversible damage to the tissues. Each individual vitamin and its possible physiological defect are listed.

Vitamin A

The recommended daily intake for normal males is 1,000 μg or retinal equivalents (RE) of retinal, females 800 μg, and children and infants 400 to 700 μg.[3] One RE equals 3.33 International Unit (IU). Severe vitamin A deficiency can cause many lesions. One early symptom is a failure of the retina to obtain retinal for rhodopsin formation resulting in night blindness. Night blindness is reversible, but may be followed by structural changes in the retina which may result in xerosis of the cornea, followed by corneal distortion if deficiency continues. In untreated cases, the corneal structure melts into a gelatinous mass resulting in changes known as keratomalacia. Xerosis can occur throughout the body and mainly replaces columnar epithelia in many sites by thick layers of horny stratified epithelium. The early process is metaplasia, but later the epithelia becomes horny or keratinized. Numerous anatomic deformities can occur in the fetus from vitamin A deficiency of the maternal diet. Because vitamin A is transported on protein, in particular retinal binding protein, protein deficiency accentuates retinal deficiency. Hypovitaminosis A can occur in conjunction with fat absorption diseases: celiac disease, obstructive jaundice, infectious hepatitis and cystic fibrosis of the pancreas. Vitamin A absorption is dependent on the presence of bile acids in the intestinal tract which may explain why vitamin A deficiency is associated with biliary obstruction disorders.

Russell et al[4] have observed a subclinical vitamin A deficiency in thirteen patients with regional enteritis, celiac sprue and jejunal diverticulosis.[5] Although they were without overt evidence of a nutritional defect, the patients were found to have abnormal dark-adaptation tests. Reversal with 3,500 to 10,000 IU units was found in half of the patients. The rest required larger doses of vitamin A indicating that routine vitamin supplementation cannot always be relied upon. The frequency with which defective vitamin A dependent dark-adaptation was found in patients with small intestine disease suggests that subclinical disease in these and other chronic diseases is more frequent than has heretofore been recognized. Mahalanabis et al[5] have observed that 70 percent of their Indian patients infected with *Ascaris lumbricoides* had vitamin A malabsorption. The results of their study indicate that *ascariasis* in populations on marginal intakes of vitamin A and its precursors is an important contributing factor in producing clinical vitamin A deficiency in India where it ranks as one of the major causes of preventable blindness.

The elderly are particularly vulnerable to vitamin deficiencies because of their high incidence of illness and disability in the later years of life and because of other common problems, such as low income, poor appetite and social isolation. Davidson et al[6] in a study of 104 elderly Bostonians found less than adequate blood levels of vitamin A in 7 percent of the people studied. Steinkamp et al[7] studied a group of 229 elderly subjects in Berkeley, California. One-fourth had intakes of vitamin A that were less than two-thirds of the recommended amounts. Levine[8] has demonstrated a reversible depression of the vitamin A concentration in serum in seven healthy volunteers receiving 2 g of neomycin daily for one week. Cholestyramine [9] also reduces the concentration of vitamin A in the serum. Mineral oil acts as a solvent for fat soluble vitamins, especially β-carotene, and will interfere with the absorption.[10]

Vitamin D

The recommended daily intake of vitamin D^3 from infants to age nineteen in males and females is 10 μg cholecalciferol (10 μg = 400 IU vitamins D).

Males and females, age nineteen to twenty-two should take in 7.5 μg per day. Vitamin D brings about normal mineralization of bone and endochondral calcification, thus preventing the disease rickets in the young and osteomalacia in the adult. Vitamin D also prevents hypocalcemic tetany, a function it shares with the parathyroid hormone.

In chronic renal disease 1, $25\text{-}(OH)_2D_3$ is not made in sufficient amounts and thus vitamin D deficient intestine and, ultimately, bone result. Malabsorption and steatorrhea result in a diminished absorption of ingested vitamin D. Chronic pancreatitis, celiac disease and biliary obstruction were found to malabsorb vitamin D. Absorption occurs in the jejunum and/or ileum. Bile is essential with most of the vitamin D present in the chylomicrons of the lymphatic system. Vitamin D is then concentrated in the liver and transferred to an α_1-globulin with a molecular weight of

52,000 and acts as a carrier for the vitamin and its metabolites. Marginal vitamin D deficiency can be followed by observing the slow calcification of bones, determinable as a morphological change seen by roentgenogram. Simple chemical methods to monitor vitamin D in blood are not yet available. Brin et al[11] have summarized elderly populations who have an inadequate or marginal intake of vitamin D.

Subclinical vitamin deficiency has been reported in slow-growing Indian children of puberty and adolescent age.[12] The incidence of this type of deficiency may be greater than previously anticipated in the adolescent group. Ford et al[13] have examined the prevalence of vitamin D deficiency among older children in the Bradford Asian community, the largest in the United Kingdom and compared these results to children of white or West Indian parents living in the Bradford area. Biochemical evidence of rickets was present in 45 percent of the Asians; whereas no rickets were detected in the white sample and some minor biochemical abnormalities were present in nine of the forty West Indian children.

Children on a macrobiotic vegetarian diet had only marginal vitamin D, calcium and phosphorus intakes.[14] Vitamin D supplements were rarely given. Thirty-two children on a macrobiotic vegetarian diet showed prior physical and roentgenographic evidence of rickets. Two children had evidence of rickets. Seventeen other vegetarian children showed no present or prior evidence of rickets.

Subclinical vitamin D deficiency has been observed following gastric surgery.[15] Eleven patients, all of whom had previously undergone gastric surgery had bone biopsy specimens taken before and after an intravenous dose of vitamin D. The osteoid volume was found to be normal in all cases. In three patients with a raised serum-alkaline-phosphatase, there was an increase in the osteoid-surface area and a decrease in the proportion of osteoid with a calcification front. Administration of vitamin D resulted within eight days in a marked increase in the proportion of osteoid with a calcification front. The data suggest that vitamin D is necessary for the proper formation of the calcification front, but that a decrease in the proportion of osteoid with a calcification front is an early indication of vitamin D deficiency.

Ovesen[16] has summarized several situations where drug intake has led to a concomitant vitamin D deficiency. Abuse of irritant cathartics which may act through damage to the intestinal wall or through increased peristalis has resulted in symptoms of vitamin D deficiency. Mineral oil taken for a long period may result in osteomalacia or rickets. One patient had symptoms of vitamin D deficiency after receiving cholestyramine for two years. About 15–30 percent of patients receiving long-term chronic intakes of anticonvulsant drugs had radiologic evidence of vitamin D deficiency accompanied by reduced serum calcium and increased alkaline phosphatase concentration. Most of these patients had received phenytoin, phenobarbital, primidone or pheneturide for more than five years. Osteomalacia developed in one woman who had been taking 500 mg of glutethimide for ten years for insomnia. The structure of glutethimide resembles phenobarbital, and the mechanism of action is probably the same as with anticonvulsants.

Vitamin K

The recommended daily intake for vitamin K for adults is 70–140 μg.[3] Other recommended intakes are: infants to 6 months, 12 μg; infants 6 months to 1 year, 10–20 μg; children 1 to 3 years, 15–30 μg; children 4 to 6 years, 20 to 40 μg; adolescents 7 to 10, 30 to 60 μg; adolescents over 11, 50 to 100 μg. A normal mixed diet in the United States will contain from 300 to 500 μg of vitamin K per day, an amount more than adequate to supply the dietary requirement. The anticoagulant effect of vitamin K deficiency is caused by a reduction in the content of plasma prothrombin. Three other coagulation proteins—Factor VII, Factor IX and Factor X—are also regulated by vitamin K.

Primary vitamin K deficiency is uncommon in man because of the widespread distribution of vitamin K in plant and animal tissues. In addition, the microbiologic flora of the normal gut synthesize the menaquinones in amounts that may supply the bulk of the requirement for vitamin K. Healthy adult subjects fed diets low in vitamin K (less than 20 μg per day) for several weeks show minimal signs of vitamin K deficiency as evidenced by prothrombin values of 60 to 90 percent, unless they were given bowel-sterilizing antibiotics such as neomycin. In one study neomycin was required to lower the vitamin K-dependent clotting factors to below 20 percent of normal in four weeks. The microorganisms synthesizing vitamin K must reside in the gut because up to 500 mg per day instilled into the cecum did not elevate depressed coagulation factors in anticoagulated patients.

Any disorder that hinders the delivery of bile from the small bowel, such as obstructive jaundice or bile fistula, reduces the absorption of vitamin K from the bowel and causes a reduction of plasma concentration of the vitamin K-dependent factors. Malabsorption syndromes associated with sprue, pellagra, bowel shunts, regional ileitis and ulcerative colitis also cause a secondary vitamin K deficiency. In chronic liver disease, hypoprothrombinemia with bleeding may occur because of lack of functional hepatic ribosomes to respond to vitamin K.

Marginal vitamin K deficiency could result in patients with the above bowel diseases or patients with a sterile intestine from taking antibiotics or sulfa drugs. Mineral oil[10] and cholestyramine may reduce the absorption of vitamin K. In a study of sixteen neonates born to mothers treated with anticonvulsant drugs for two or more years, Mountain et al[17] demonstrated a severe coagulation defect in seven and a mild defect in one of the neonates. The authors recommend that the vitamin should be given to the mother intravenously during labor. Coumarins are vitamin K antagonists, finding widespread application in the prophylaxis of thrombosis. Salicylates in doses of 4 to 6 g daily and cinchona alkaloids in conventional doses act synergistically with coumarin anticoagulants resulting in serious bleeding manifestations.

Vitamin E

The recommended daily intake of vitamin E[3] is 10 mg in adult males, and 8 mg in adult females. In children ages 1 to 10, 5 to 7 mg are recommended, whereas infants up to 1 year should take in 3 to 4 mg/day. The average intakes of α-tocopherols by adults is 15 mg/day, but the variation could be quite large, since individuals fed diets high in protein and low in plant fat would consume less than 10 mg/day, whereas diets high in polyunsaturated oils might contain 60 mg/day. More vitamin E is thought to be required in individuals on high polyunsaturated fat diet especially when the fats are oxidized or contain large amounts of fish oil. Fish oils have a high peroxidative potential and low levels of tocopherol.

Although mammals on vitamin E-deficient diets can show a wide spectrum of pathologic conditions, there is no good evidence to indicate that man is susceptible to vitamin E deficiency when he consumes an average American diet. The anemia of prematurity and its relationship to inadequate absorption of α-tocopherol by the premature infant has been observed. Some pediatricians supplement vitamin E from the tenth day in premature infants. Immature infants have been shown to have a lower incidence of retrolental fibroplasia when supplemented with vitamin E. In addition, vitamin E administration during the acute phase of therapy for the respiratory distress syndrome in premature neonates may favorably modify the development of bronchopulmonary dysplasia.

Oski et al[18] have described a hemolytic anemia in premature infants associated with reticulocytosis, thrombocytosis, schistocytes and peripheral edema. These changes resolve with treatment. Malabsorption also may contribute to vitamin E deficiency. Improvement in cystic fibrosis patients is observed with added vitamin E. A seven-year-old boy with severe malabsorption developed proximal muscle weakness and peripheral neuropathy.[19] After treatment with water-soluble vitamin E clinical improvement was observed. Marginal vitamin E deficiencies have been observed in the elderly.[12]

Thiamin

The recommended daily requirement for infants up to 1 year is 0.3–0.5 mg; children age 1 to 3, 0.7 mg; age 4 to 6, 0.9 mg; age 7 to 10, 1.2 mg; males 11 to 51, 1.2 to 1.5 mg; females 11 to 51, 1.0 to 1.1 mg.[3] Thiamin in the form of pyrophosphate participates as a coenzyme in the oxidative decarboxylation of alpha keto acids to aldehydes. The major known deficiency disease of humans is beriberi. Clinically, beriberi presents a spectrum of manifestations. Early symptoms are a peripheral neuropathy. Initially, the deep tendon reflexes are increased; later they may be absent. The muscles are often tender and may atrophy. Fatigue, decreased attention span and impaired capacity to work may occur. This type of beriberi is so-called dry or atrophic beriberi. If even less thiamin is taken in, cardiovascular signs and symptoms become apparent. The heart is often enlarged and edema may be present. Tachycardia occurs with the slightest effort in the so-called subacute or wet beriberi. The most acute of thiamin deficiencies is Wernicke's encephalopathy, which occurs primarily in alcoholics, or vomiting associated with pregnancy, or surgery on the gastrointestinal tract. High morbidity and mortality are associated with Wernicke's encephalopathy. Infantile beriberi may appear as acute cardiac failure in a previously healthy appearing child. Marginal thiamin deficiencies have been observed in a small percentage of children and adults studied in Denmark.[20] Elderly subjects frequently have inadequate intakes of thiamin[11] and marginal thiamin deficiency. About 40 percent of 112 elderly patients in a medical ward had inadequate thiamin intake and marginal deficiency.[21] Lonsdale et al[22] have studied twenty patients who consumed large amounts of "junk" foods, carbonated or sweet beverages and candy. The patients presented symptoms similar to early beriberi and were improved by the administration of thiamin.

Riboflavin

The recommended daily intake[3] for infants is 0.4 to 0.6 mg; children 1 to 10 years, 0.8 to 1.4 mg; adult females 1.2 to 1.3 mg;

and adult males 1.4 to 1.7 mg. Riboflavin deficiency manifests itself as a corneal vascularization. Angular stomatitis, glossitis and seborrheic dermatitis about the nose and scrotum also occur. Erythrocyte glutathione reductase, which is decreased when the consumption of riboflavin is deficient, has been used to evaluate population groups. Marginal riboflavin levels were observed in about 8 percent of elderly patients in a medical ward.[21] Riboflavin deficiency is known to be endemic in Trinidad[23] and it manifests in particular in the second trimester of pregnant women.

An adolescent population ranging in age from 13 to 19 years, and of a low socioeconomic status in New York City, had an overall deficiency in 26.6 percent of those studied.[24] Ahmed et al[25] studied twenty-three apparently healthy Indian women of the middle and low income group before they started taking estrogen-containing hormonal contraceptives. Reduced levels of erythrocyte glutathione reductase activity were observed. Some of the subjects developed glossitis. Newman et al[26] found twenty-four of fifty-six women of low socioeconomic status who were on birth control pills to have reduced erythrocyte glutathione reductase activity. Eng et al.[27] have observed subclinical riboflavin deficiency leading to a low glutathione reductase activity present in almost 50 percent of the adult and newborn Malaysians, especially among Malays and Indians.

Niacin

The recommended daily intake for infants is 6 to 8 mg; children age 1 to 10, 9 to 16 mg; adult males, 16 to 19 mg; adult females, 13 to 15 mg.[3] Although pellagra has been endemic in corn-eating areas of the world for over 200 years, it was not until 1908 that the diagnostic symptoms were recognized. The early symptoms are weakness, lassitude, anorexia and indigestion. These are followed by the classic "three D's," dermatitis, diarrhea and dementia. The mental symptoms that often accompany the early stages of pellagra are irritability, headaches, sleeplessness, loss of memory and emotional instability. Toxic confusional psychosis, acute delirium and catatonia have been observed in advanced cases of niacin deficiency. The deficiency of dietary intake of nicotinic acid, or tryptophan-containing proteins, can be obtained by analyzing the urine for its N'-methylnicotinamide content. Niacin is reduced in Parkinson patients treated with l-dopa, benserazide and carbidopa.[28] Griffiths[29] has described two cases who developed pellagra while on isonizid therapy for seven and nine months respectively.

Pantothenic Acid

The recommended daily intake of pantothenic acid is 2 to 3 mg for infants up to one year of age; children age 1 to 11, 3 to 7 mg per day; and adults 4 to 7 mg per day.[3] Pantothenic acid is so widely distributed in foods that a deficiency of the vitamin is extremely rare. Significant amounts of pantothenic acid are lost when foods are canned, cooked, frozen or processed. In malnutrition, multiple deficiencies often occur and a pantothenic acid deficiency may not be apparent. Serum contains free pantothenic acid and no coenzyme A, while most of the vitamin is present in the erythrocytes as coenzyme A. The symptoms of a pantothenic acid deficiency have been observed in human volunteers on a diet deficient in pantothenic acid and on a pantothenic acid antagonist, omega methyl pantothenic acid. Subjects on the pantothenic acid deficient diet developed vomiting, malaise, abdominal distress and burning cramps. Later the volunteers developed tenderness in the heels, fatigue and insomnia. The symptoms developed earlier in the group who received both the omega methyl pantothenic acid and the deficient diet. Marginal deficiencies of pantothenic acid are not known, but might exist in populations with general chronic vitamin deficiencies, which could mask symptoms from a pantothenic acid deficiency.

Pyridoxine

The recommended daily intake of pyridoxine in infants is 0.3 to 0.6 mg; children age 1 to 10, 0.9 to 1.6 mg; adult males 1.8 to 2.2 mg; and adult females 1.8 to 2.0 mg.[3] Patients on deficient diets were observed to be characterized by weakness, irritability, nervousness, insomnia and difficulty in walking. Convulsive seizures and nervous irritability were observed in infants fed a commercial liquid milk formula low in B_6. Clinical improvement on supplementation was confirmed by return of the abnormal electroencephalographic patterns to normal. Vitamin B_6 deficiency has been induced in human adults with the pyridoxine antagonist, 4-deoxypyridoxine. Subclinical vitamin B_6 deficiency using a tryptophan loading test has been observed in 30 Polish children who were treated with isoniazid.[30] In other studies isoniazid, hydralazine, D-penicillamine, and levodopa, as well as oral estrogen-containing contraceptives, have caused subclinical pyridoxine deficiency.[16] Diet surveys have indicated that elderly subjects have inadequate intakes of B_6.[11] Age per se influences the blood levels (and presumably nutritional adequacy) of vitamin B_6. Hamfelt[31] has shown that vitamin B_6 levels are measured both by tryptophan tolerance tests and by pyridoxal phosphate determination decrease strikingly with age. A familial case of pyridoxine deficiency has been reported in a Japanese family.[32]

However, this type of deficiency is probably very rare.

Folic Acid

The recommended daily intake for folic acid is 30 to 45 μg for infants; children 1 to 11, 100 to 300 μg; and adult males and females 400 μg. Folic acid as well as vitamin B_{12} is required for the synthesis of thymidylate, and therefore of DNA. Lack of adequate DNA synthesis causes many hematopoietic cells to die in the bone marrow, very possibly without ever completing the S phase of cell replication (a form of ineffective erythropoiesis). Megaloblastosis (the presence of giant germ cells) is the endproduct of deranged DNA synthesis. The underlying biochemical defect which translates poor thymidylate synthesis into morphologic megaloblastosis may be failure to elongate DNA chains in the presence of a relatively normal capacity to initiate DNA synthesis. Progressive dietary folic acid deprivation in man results in a series of biochemical and hematologic sequence of events. Low serum folate will result in hypersegmentation of blood cells in about six to eleven weeks; at about thirteen weeks a high urinary formiminoglutamate is evident; at seventeen weeks low folate is seen in the red blood cells; macroovalocytosis is seen at eighteen weeks; and at nineteen weeks megaloblastic marrow followed by anemia can result from the low serum folate. Folate coenzymes involve transfer of a 1-carbon unit. These reactions include: (1) *de novo* purine synthesis; (2) pyrimidine nucleotide biosynthesis; (3) amino acid conversions, serine to glycine, histidine to glutamic acid and homocysteine to methionine; (4) generation of formate into the formate pool; and (5) methylation of small amounts of transfer RNA.

In addition to a poor intake, other clinical conditions can result in low serum folate: inadequate absorption from the upper one-third of the small intestine due to malabsorption or drugs such as Dilantin,[™] alcohol and barbiturates; inadequate utilization due to metabolic blocks due to folic acid antagonists such as methotrexate; increased requirement due to parasitization, hyperthyroidism and the Lesch-Nyhan syndrome; increased excretion due to B_{12} deficiency; and increased destruction due to scurvy. Folate is usually determined by radioimmunoassay, the results of which are quite precise and able to determine marginal folate deficiencies. Subnormal red cell folate values were encountered in twenty of sixty-three thalassemic subjects in a population with a low incidence of megaloblastosis.[33] Some drugs such as cholestyramine, oral contraceptives, anticonvulsants such as phenobarbital, phenytoin and Primidone,[™] sulphasalazine, aspirin, methotrexate, pyrimethamine, trimethoprim and triamterene lower folate in the body.[16] Dietary surveys and biochemical investigations of elderly subjects have indicated inadequate intakes of folate.[11]

Vitamin B_{12}

The recommended daily intake for B_{12} is 0.5 to 1.5 μg for infants up to one year; children 1 to 10 years, 2.0 to 3.0 μg; and adult males and females 3.0 μg. Both B_{12} and folic acid are required for synthesis of thymidylate, and therefore of DNA. A vitamin B_{12}-containing enzyme removes a methyl group from methyl folate and transfers it to homocysteine, thereby converting homocysteine to methionine and regenerating tetrahydrofolic acid from which the 5,10-methylene-tetrahydrofolic acid is synthesized. In addition to the methyl transfer from methylfolate, vitamin B_{12} deficiency results in neurologic damage to the myelin, and the neuropathies and cerebral manifestations that arise from myelin disorders. Since B_{12} is required for the hydrogen transfer and isomerization whereby methylmalonate is converted to succinate, B_{12} is involved in both fat and carbohydrate metabolism. Vitamin B_{12} is also involved in protein synthesis through its role in the synthesis of the amino acid methionine and B_{12} appears concerned in maintenance of sulfhydryl groups in the reduced form necessary for the function of many SH-activated enzyme systems. Low serum B_{12} can result from inadequate intake, inadequate absorption due to stomach lesions, inadequate utilization due to antagonists and other factors, increased requirement due to hyperthyroidism, increased excretion, and increased destruction possibly due to excessive vitamin C intake. Deficiency results in megaloblastic anemia accompanied by leukopenia and thrombopenia. Vitamin B_{12} is measured accurately by radioimmunoassay. Therefore, marginal serum values can be easily recognized. Drugs affecting B_{12} requirements are cholestyramine, neomycin, potassium chloride (slow release), bioguanides, para-aminosalicylic acid, colchicine and oral contraceptives.[16] Dietary surveys and biochemical investigations of elderly subjects have indicated inadequate intakes of B_{12}.[11] There is also evidence[34] that many people in developing countries have subclinical intestinal malabsorption due to structural changes in their small intestines which in developed countries would be associated with overt gastrointestinal disease. This has been documented in Australia (in aboriginals), Bangladesh, the Dominican Republic, Egypt, Guatemala, Haiti, India, Iran, Nigeria, Pakistan, Puerto Rico, Singapore, Thailand and Uganda.

Ascorbic Acid

The recommended daily allowance for vitamin C for infants is 35 mg; children 1 to 10, 45 mg; and adult males and females, 50 to 60 mg.[3] The onset of scurvy can be detected between 60 and 90 days after beginning a diet that contains no ascorbic acid. The earliest manifestations consist of a few petechial spots and small ecchymoses which later become larger. At the same time follicular hyperkeratosis develops, especially on the buttocks, thighs and calves. Many hyperkeratotic lesions contain fragmented or coiled hairs, but some demonstrate the classical lesion of scurvy: the hyperkeratotic follicle with a red hemorrhagic halo. Later the gums become swollen and bleed easily. A unique symptom of scurvy is the development of Sjogren's syndrome, dryness of the mouth and eyes, hair loss, itchy dry skin and loosening of teeth and dental fillings. Scurvy may produce weakness and lethargy, aching legs and joint effusions. Psychologic changes are common and have been characterized by hysteria, depression and hypochondriasis. Ascorbic acid is a powerful water-soluble antioxidant which may protect other antioxidants even though they may be lipid-soluble. Ascorbic acid facilitates gastrointestinal absorption of iron and may help convert folic acid to its active form, folinic acid. Ascorbic acid may be an important factor in hydroxylation reactions which help detoxify poisonous substances. Ascorbic acid is necessary for the hydroxylation of proline for the synthesis of collagen. This reaction may be important in wound healing. Ascorbic acid is important in other hydroxylation reactions and is thought to be essential for conversion of hydroxyphenylpyruvate to homogentisic acid in the formation of tyrosine. Drugs such as aspirin, tetracycline and oral contraceptives can increase the requirement of vitamin C.[16] Dietary surveys and biochemical investigations of elderly subjects have indicated inadequate intakes of vitamin C.[11] Twelve of thirty-five elderly Australian men who were living alone had intakes of vitamin C which were in the range of asymptomatic scurvy.[35] Subclinical hypovitaminosis C has been outlined in a case report of two patients.[36] Subclinical vitamin C deficiency frequently occurs in South African black mineworkers who are individuals subjected to a variety of stresses. Stress hastens use of ascorbic acid by the adrenals thereby increasing the requirement for vitamin C.[37] There seems to be a relationship between body stores and vitamin C plasma levels. Renal turnover rises steeply above 0.8 mg/100 ml. Hodges et al[38] carried out investigations with volunteers and showed that the first sign of scurvy can be observed at plasma vitamin C levels between 0.2 and 0.3 mg/100 ml. Ginter has reviewed the effects of chronic marginal vitamin C deficiency on the biochemistry and pathophysiology of man and animals.[39]

Biotin

The recommended daily requirement for biotin is 35 to 50 μg for infants up to one year; children ages 1 to 10, 65 to 120 μg and male and female adults 100 to 200 μg per day. Biotin is an essential cofactor for the enzymes acetyl CoA carboxylase, propionyl CoA carboxylase, pyruvate carboxylase, β-methylcrotonyl carboxylase, geranoyl CoA carboxylase and methyl-malonyl CoA transcarboxylase. In animals biotin deficiency decreases the incorporation of ^{14}C-labeled acetate into the phospholipids of liver tissue and also decreases gluconeogenesis, probably resulting from the inhibition of pyruvate metabolism. Decreased utilization of glucose for protein synthesis may be due to an interference with protein synthesis at the level of RNA metabolism.

An experimental biotin deficiency in human subjects has been induced by feeding raw egg-white diets. A scaly dermatitis, graying of mucous membranes, increasing skin dryness, depression, lassitude, muscle pains, anorexia, nausea, hypercholesteremia and finally electrocardiogram abnormalities were found during a ten-week course of deficiency. Administration of large doses of antibiotics or sulfa drugs has been used to produce a biotin deficiency in experimental animals. However, in humans the commonly used doses of antibiotics for limited periods, probably have little effect on biotin synthesis. Administration of biotin has been beneficial in alleviating symptoms of seborrheic dermatitis and Leiner's disease in some infants. Treatment of the mothers of breast-fed infants with seborrheic dermatitis by injection of biotin has been reported to be beneficial. In humans, rare inborn errors of metabolism involving the activity of propionyl CoA carboxylase and β-methylcrotonyl carboxylase respond sometimes to doses of biotin.

Choline

The need for choline is dependent to some extent on methionine availability, and the vitamin B_{12} and folacin content of the diet. Because of the interaction of choline with these and other dietary components, the requirement for choline by human beings is not known. In animals, the most common signs of choline deficiency are fatty infiltration of the liver and hemorrhagic kidney damage. Poultry suffer from perosis, a tendon defect resulting in permanently deformed legs. Choline participates in transmethylation reactions. Choline donates a labile methyl group to homocystine to form methionine which in turn reacts with guanidoacetic acid to form creatinine. Transmethylation allows the replacement of choline with methionine or homocystine, betaine and ethanolamine in diets without incurring a specific choline deficiency.

In humans the use of choline in the treatment of the fatty liver of alcoholism and kwashiorkor has proven to be ineffective. Administration of choline may alleviate symptoms of tardive dyskinesia and Huntington disease, but the effect appears to go beyond specific dietary needs for choline in normal people.

Other factors

Under normal conditions it has not been demonstrated that there is a human requirement for bioflavonoids, carnitine and inositol.

REFERENCES

1. Brubacher, G. 1979. Relevance of a borderline vitamin deficiency in relation to the question of vitamin requirement. *Biblio. Nutrit. et Dieta* 28:176.
2. Brin, M. 1964. Erythrocytes as a biopsy tissue in the functional evaluation of nutritional status. *J. Am. Med. Assoc.* 187:762.
3. Food and Nutrition Board. 1980. *Recommended Dietary Allowances.* Ninth Revised Edition. Washington, D.C.: National Academy of Sciences, National Research Council.
4. Russell, R. M., Smith, V. C., Multack, R., Krill, A. E. and Rosenberg, I. H. 1973. Dark-adaptation testing for diagnosis of subclinical vitamin-A deficiency and evaluation of a therapy. *Lancet* 2:1161.
5. Mahalanabis, D., Jalan, K. N., Maitra, T. K. and Agarwal, S. K. 1976. Vitamin A absorption in ascariasis. *Amer. J. Clin. Nutr.* 29:1372.
6. Davidson, C. S., Livermore, J. and Andersen, P. 1962. The nutrition of a group of healthy aging persons. *Amer. J. Clin. Nutr.* 10:181
7. Steinkamp, R. C., Cohen, N. L. and Walsh, H. E. 1965. Resurvey of an aging population: fourteen year follow-up. *J. Am. Diet. Assoc.* 46:103.
8. Levine, R. A. 1967. Effect of dietary gluten upon neomycin-induced malabsorption. *Gastroenterology* 52:685.
9. West, J. and Lloyd, J. K. 1975. The effect of cholestyramine on intestinal absorption. *Gut.* 16:93.
10. Fingl, E. 1975. In: *The Pharmacological Basis of Therapeutics.* Goodman and Gilman, eds. New York: MacMillan Publishing Co.
11. Brin, M. and Bauernfeind, J. C. 1978. Vitamin needs of the elderly. *Postgraduate Med.* 63:155.
12. Teotia, S. P. S., Teotia, M., Singh, R. K., Teotia, N. P. S. and Malhotra, V. 1976. Subclinical D-deficiency in adolescents. *Indian J. Physiol. Pharmacol.* 20:261.

13. Ford, J. A., McIntosh, W. B., Butterfield, R., Preece, M. A., Pietrek, J., Arrow-Smith, W. A., Arthurton, M. W., Turner, W., O'Riordan, J. L. H. and Dunnigan, M. G. 1976. Clinical and subclinical vitamin D deficiency in Bradford children. *Arch. Dis. Child.* 51:939.

14. Dwyer, Johanna T., Dietz, William, H., Hass, Gerald and Suskind, R. 1979. Risk of nutritional rickets among vegetarian children. *Am. J. Dis. Child.* 133:134.

15. Bordier, P. H., Matrajt, H., Hioco, D., Hepner, G. W., Thompson, G. R. and Booth, C. C. 1968. Subclinical vitamin-D deficiency following gastric surgery. *Lancet* 1:437.

16. Ovensen, L. 1979. Drugs and vitamin deficiency. *Drugs.* 18: 278.

17. Mountain, K. R., Hirsh, J. and Gallus, A. S. 1970. Neonatal coagulation defect due to anticonvulsant drug treatment in pregnancy. *Lancet* 1: 265.

18. Oski, F. A. and Barnes, L. A. 1967. Vitamin E deficiency: a previously unrecognized cause of hemolytic anemia in the premature infant. *J. Pediatr.* 70: 211.

19. Tomasi, L. G. 1979. Reversibility of human myopathy caused by vitamin E deficiency. *Neurology* 29: 1182.

20. Reinken, L., Stolley, H. and Droese, W. 1979. Biochemical assessment of thiamin nutrition in childhood. *Eur. J. Pediatrics* 131: 229.

21. Wenger, Von R., Ziegler, B., Kruspi, W., Syre, B., Brubacher, G. and Pillat, B. 1979. Relationship between vitamin status (A, B1, B2, B6, and C), clinical features and nutritional habits in a population of old people. *Wein. Klin. Wochenschr.* 91: 557.

22. Lonsdale, D. and Shamberger, R. J. 1980. Red cell transketolase as an indicator of nutritional deficiency. *Am. J. Clin. Nutr.* 33: 205.

23. Clarke, H. C. 1976. In Trinidad: angular stomatitis and pregnancy. *Internat. J. Vit. Res.* 46: 366.

24. Lopez, R., Schwartz, J. V. and Cooperman, J. M. 1980. Riboflavin deficiency in an adolescent population in New York City. *Am. J. Clin. Nutr.* 33: 1283.

25. Ahmed, F., Bamji, M. S. and Iyengar, L. 1975. Effect of oral contraceptive agents on vitamin nutrition status. *Am. J. Clin. Nutr.* 28: 606.

26. Newman, L. J., Lopez, R., Cole, H. S., Boria, M. C. and Cooperman, J. M. 1978. Riboflavin deficiency in women taking oral contraceptive agents. *Am. J. Clin. Nutr.* 31: 247.

27. Eng, L. L., Ng, T., Wan, W. P. and Ganesan, J. 1975. Stimulation of erythrocyte glutathione reductase activity by Flavin Adenine Dinucleotide (FAD) in Malaysian adults and newborns and their parents. *Brit. J. Haematol.* 31: 337.

28. Bender, D. A., Earl, C. J. and Lees, A. J. 1979. Niacin depletion in Parkinsonian patients treated with L-dopa, benserazide, and carbidopa. *Clinical Science* 56: 89.

29. Griffiths, W. A. D. 1976. Isoniazid-induced pellagra. *Proc. Royal Soc. Med.* 69: 313.

30. Lewenfisz-Wojnarowska, T., Kubicka, K. and Wroblewska-Kaluzewska. 1967. Studies in subclinical vitamin B6 deficiency in children treated with isoniazid. *Pediatria Polska* 42: 775.

31. Hamfelt, A. 1964. Age variation of vitamin B6 metabolism in man. *Clin. Chim. Acta* 10: 48.

32. Miyasaki, K., Matsumoto, J., Murao, S., Nakamura, K., Yokoyama, S., Hayano, M. and Nakamura, H. 1978. Infantile convulsion suspected by pyridoxine responsive seizures. *Acta Path. Jap.* 28: 741.
33. Tso, S. C. 1976. Significance of subnormal red-cell polate in thalassemia. *J. Clin. Path.* 29: 140.
34. Baker, J. 1976. Subclinical intestinal malabsorption in developing countries. *Bull. World Health Organ.* 54: 485.
35. McClean, H. E., Dodds, P. M., Stewart, A. W., Beaven, D. W. and Riley, C. G. 1976. Nutrition of elderly men living alone, Part 2, vitamin C and thiamin status. *N. Z. Med. J.* 84:345.
36. Booth, J. B. and Todd, G. B. 1972. Subclinical scurvy hypovitaminosis C. *Geriatrics* 27: 130.
37. Visagie, M. E., DuPlessis, J. P. and Laubscher, N. F. 1975. Effect of vitamin C supplementation on black mineworkers. *So. Afr. Med. J.* 49: 889.
38. Hodges, R. E., Hood, J., Canham, J. E., Sauberlich, H. E. and Baker, E. M. 1971. Clinical manifestations of ascorbic acid deficiency in man. *Am. J. Clin. Nutr.* 24: 432.
39. Ginter, E. 1979. Chronic marginal vitamin C deficiency: biochemistry and pathophysiology. *Wld. Rev. Nutr. Diet.* 33: 104.

10

DIETARY FIBER

──◄●►──

DENIS BURKITT, M.D.

Historical Aspects

ALTHOUGH nothing was known about dietary fiber at the time, Hippocrates recognized the laxative effect of unprocessed wheat and wrote, "To the human body it makes a great difference whether the bread be made of fine flour or coarse, whether of wheat with bran or without the bran." He went on to describe the laxative effects of coarse bread. A Persian physician, Hakim, made a similar observation in the ninth century A.D. and stated: "Wheat is a beneficial cereal. Chupatties are made from wheat flour. The chupatties, containing more bran come out of the digestive tract quicker, but are less nutritious. Chupatties containing little bran take a long time to be excreted."

In the last quarter of the nineteenth century, John Harvey Kellogg in the U.S. and T. R. Allinson in England were extolling the benefits of bran, the outer layers of grains of wheat, as being beneficial to health. The name of the former was commemorated in the Kellogg breakfast cereals and the name of the latter was removed from the medical register because his practice of not only prescribing but also of manufacturing and selling whole-meal bread was deemed to be unethical. The name on the plate outside his London consulting rooms thence bore the words, "Dr. T. R. Allinson, Ex. L.R.C.P." However, his name lives on in Britain in Allinson's whole-meal bread.

One of Allinson's treatises on bread was printed in the *Weekly Times* in 1890 in which he stated: "The innutritious bran . . . by bulk . . . helps to fill the stomach and keep us from eating too much. It also aides in filling up the small intestine, and stimulates the unvoluntary muscle of the bowel, thus causing daily laxation.

269

One great curse of this country is constipation of the bowels, which is caused in great measure by white bread. From this constipation come piles, varicose veins, headaches, miserable feelings, dullness and other ailments." He must have been the first physician to link over-nutrition, hemorrhoids and varicose veins with a deficiency of dietary fiber.

Later in the last century, a London surgeon, Albuthnot Lane, became so absorbed with the notion that much disease was caused by stagnation of colon content and absorption of poisons that he recommended removal of the colon, a terrible insult in the light of what we now know of the important functions fulfilled by that organ. Fortunately, he later changed his approach and recommended high fiber diets to aid the elimination of noxious bowel content.

In the 1930s, Cowgill and Anderson,[1] Williams and Olmstead,[2] and Fantus et al[3] in the U.S. were among the first to make definitive studies on the effect of fiber on bowel behavior and content. A few years later, a young British physician, Ted Dimmock, recognized the relationship between constipation and health, and spent much time weighing and examining stools under different dietary regimes. His thesis for the London M.D. examination was entitled, "The treatment of habitual constipation by the bran method."[4]

The current, almost explosive, wave of renewed interest in the importance of fiber in food springs largely from the work of a British naval physician, Thomas Latimer Cleave, although many others made major contributions which were, like Cleave's, largely unrecognized at the time.

A. R. P. Walker in South Africa has been emphasizing the importance of fiber in the diet ever since his dietary studies on prison inmates during the Second World War. He has made many major contributions to this field of study.

Cleave's contribution must rank among the major advances in medical knowledge. With quite remarkable insight he recognized not only that there were a number of major diseases that were characteristic of modern western culture, but also that a factor common to all of them was the refining of carbohydrate foods. He was among the first to appreciate that this process had two complementary results, the removal of fiber on the one hand and an increased consumption of fiber-depleted carbohydrate, sugar in particular, on the other. His emphasis initially was much more on the detrimental effects of sugar rather than on the beneficial effects of fiber, but he recognized the significance of both. Regrettably, he first published his revolutionary concept in a little-read publication, the *Journal of the Royal Naval Medical Service*.[5] It was revolutionary in suggesting that many totally different diseases might share a common causative factor. The significance to medicine of this concept was not recognized at the time. Later he summarized his beliefs and the results of his prodigiously painstaking correspondence with doctors throughout the world in his book, *Coronary Thrombosis and the Saccharine Disease*,[6] in which he was assisted by a man with wide experience of diabetes, G. D. Campbell. Later this work was revised with a section on diverticular disease by N. S. Painter, and then was again revised under the name *The Saccharine Disease*.[7]

Hugh Trowell, renowned for his pioneer work on kwashiokor[8] wrote his book *Non-infective Disease in Africa*,[9] after thirty years teaching medicine in that continent. In this, his list of diseases characteristic of modern western culture closely approximated that made by Cleave. Trowell had also hinted that roughage in the diet might play a protective role against these diseases. After being introduced to Cleave's work, he was to make many major contributions to the understanding of fiber and was responsible for the use of the current term "dietary fiber" to replace the now obsolete concept of "crude fiber."[10]

Neil Painter, a British surgeon, had, in 1964[11] presented evidence strongly suggesting that diverticular disease of the colon was actually caused by a deficiency of fiber in the diet. His work reversed the treatment of this disease which previously had consisted of actually prescribing low-residue diets. Among others who played key roles in the current understanding of the concept are Martin Eastwood and Ken Heaton, both British workers. The outstanding contributors to the understanding of the chemical nature of fiber have been Pater Van Soest of Cornell University in the U.S. and David Southgate of the Dunn Laboratory, Cambridge, in England.

The major reasons for the neglect of fiber in both medical and nutritional science was a misunderstanding of its nature. It had been thought to be synonymous with cellulose, which was a grave error, and because it contributed little to nutrition it was viewed as a useless component of food that could be discarded with impunity. In food tables it was listed as "crude fiber," which denoted merely that fraction of plant food that survived heating first in acid and then in alkali, a test that measured merely the lignin and part of the cellulose. The all-important hemicelluloses, or to use the more modern term, the non-cellulosic polysaccharides, which are destroyed by this test, were completely ignored.

The enormous interest in the importance of fiber that has over the last decade increased annual publications on the subject from under ten to over 400 owes much to increased knowledge of the geography of disease. It is now well recognized that many of the major diseases in more affluent western societies are rare in traditionally living communities, and dietary changes, including a fall in fiber intake, are believed to play a dominant role.

The recent report of the Royal College of Physicians in England on *Medical aspects of dietary fiber*[12] has raised the subject out of the realm of food quackery to which it was once believed to belong.

Epidemiological Features

There is now a well-recognized list of diseases that are related to modern western culture.[13] Many but not all of these have been definitively related to changes in diet.[14] The concept is that man throughout his long history has been adapted to the environment, including the dietetic environment, in which he has lived. During something like two million years or approximately 80,000 generations, he was a hunter-gatherer, and by extrapolation from what is known of the diets of the few hunter-gatherer populations still surviving an estimate of the composition of his diet can be made. Then for some 10,000 years, or 400 generations, he lived, as the majority of people in the Third World still live today, as a peasant farmer. During the last 200 years, only a mere eight generations, which is a moment in time compared to man's existence on earth, western man has drastically changed his dietetic environment to one to which he has not been evolutionarily adapted. (I am using the word "man" in an anthropological rather than a theological sense, recognizing that the Biblical concept of man is that he is more than a merely biological creature.)

The diseases that have their maximal prevalences in economically developed western countries and their minimal in rural communities in the Third World include the following:

Gastrointestinal diseases—dental caries, constipation, diverticular disease, appendicitis, large bowel cancer, hemorrhoids and hiatus hernia.

Cardiovascular diseases—ischemic heart disease (IHD) and varicose veins.

Metabolic diseases—gallstones, diabetes and obesity.

All of these diseases have, as will be indicated below, been related to changes in diet. The etiology of other characteristically western diseases, including multiple sclerosis, Crohn's disease, ulcerative colitis and thyrotoxicosis, remain obscure.

There is no evidence that any of the diseases listed above were other than relatively rare even in western communities prior to the present century, and all available data suggest that diseases like IHD, and diverticular disease were uncommon until after the Second World War.

These diseases have comparable prevalences in black and in white Americans today. Two generations ago, those for which information is available were much less frequent in black than in white Americans. When the forebears of American blacks arrived in the western world their prevalences of these diseases cannot have been greater than they are at the present time in village Africans.

The diseases listed were comparatively rare in Japan until after the Second World War, but have been increasing since.[15] In second and subsequent generations of Japanese who have emigrated to Hawaii and California, prevalences are comparable to those in other ethnic groups.[16,17] The same applies to Polynesians who have become New Zealand Maoris.[18] Urban and otherwise more westernized communities in Africa and Asia are more prone to these diseases than are rural communities.[19] This and much other evidence indicates that they must be predominantly the result of environmental rather than of genetic factors.

Incrimination of Diet

Since all of these diseases have been shown to be directly or indirectly related to the gastrointestinal tract it would seem reasonable to examine changes in diet before considering other associated environmental changes inherent in increased mechanization and technological change, though diminished exercise must be considered a contributory factor.

More profound changes in diet have been made by modern western man during the last two centuries, and particularly during this one, then have been made in the whole of man's previous history.[20] The major dietary changes are illustrated in Figure 10.1. It will be observed that total protein intake has not altered greatly, although its source has largely changed from vegetable to animal, as those who were formerly peasant agriculturists have become westernized. Hunter-gatherers, however, ate as much animal protein as we do today. As the contribution made by starch has fallen, that of fat has been greatly increased. Sugar has been a relatively recent innovation and it now supplies some 20 percent of the total energy requirements of modern western man. His fiber intake of around 20 g/d is only a third of that of peasant agriculturalists, in addition to which the source of fiber has changed. Constant availability of fruit and green vegetables has resulted in the fiber from those sources replacing that of starch staples, and of cereals in particular, which from a health standpoint has been a poor exchange. Salt intake has drastically increased and this has been incriminated in the pathogenesis of hypertension.[21]

Figure 10.1
Changes in Food

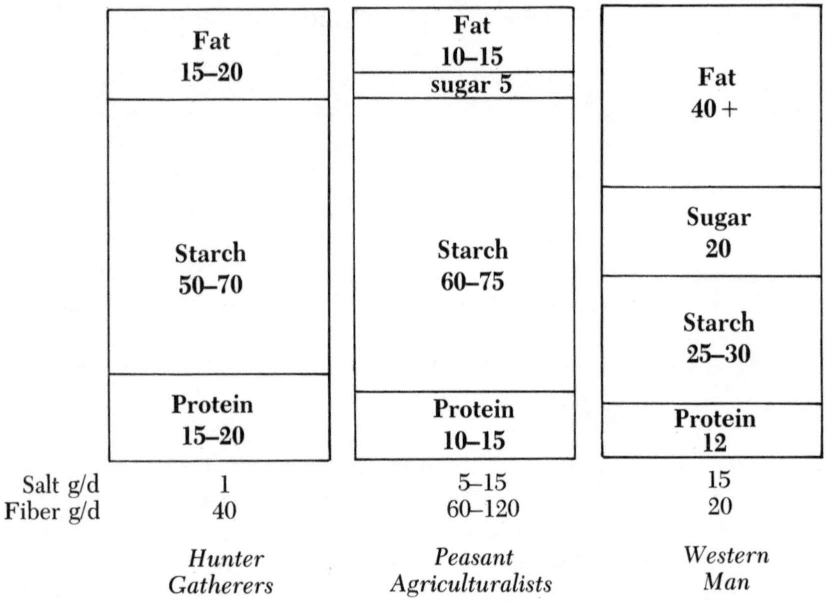

Hunter Gatherers	Peasant Agriculturalists	Western Man
Fat 15–20	Fat 10–15 / sugar 5	Fat 40+
Starch 50–70	Starch 60–75	Sugar 20 / Starch 25–30
Protein 15–20	Protein 10–15	Protein 12

	Hunter Gatherers	Peasant Agriculturalists	Western Man
Salt g/d	1	5–15	15
Fiber g/d	40	60–120	20

In addition to these changes in the proportions of energy provided by different dietary components, total energy intake has increased. As will be discussed below, the removal of fiber from plant foods has been incriminated in the cause of all the diseases listed. Sugar which is the prime example of fiber-depleted carbohydrate can only be made available by the removal of the fibrous skeleton in which it was originally resident. White flour is the next most obvious example of refined carbohydrate. Over-ingestion of fat has been incriminated in some of these diseases, notably IHD, and large bowel cancer.

Nature of Dietary Fiber

The carbohydrate content of food can be divided into mono- and disaccharides (sugars) on the one hand, and polysaccharides on the other. Polysaccharides can then be subdivided into the absorbable fraction, starch, and the fraction largely undigested in the small intestine, fiber. The latter can again be divided into cellulose and non-cellulosic polysaccharides. But in addition to these polysaccharides, fiber also contains lignin which is not a polysaccharide.[22] Perhaps the simplest, but not totally accurate definition of dietary fiber is that part of plant food that passes through the small intestine undigested.

As an understanding of the nature of fiber has increased it has become evident that it can no longer be viewed as a single substance, but as a group of entirely different entities having characteristic chemical compositions and physiological actions. The situation is somewhat analogous to the manner in which what was formerly known as vitamin B was subsequently subdivided into the whole group of B vitamins. Not only does the nature and content of fiber differ from one plant to another, but it varies in individual species according to the age of the plant. It is also modified by cooking.

Of the different components of fiber, the pentoses, predominant in cereals, have the greatest action in increasing the bulk and softness of stools.[23] Lignin binds bile acids,[24] pectins have been shown to reduce blood lipids,[24] and gums appear to be most effective in reducing postprandial blood glucose levels.[25,26] These particular actions will be referred to when dealing with the different diseases in the pathogenicity of which fiber-deficiency has been implicated.

Dental Caries

Dental caries and periodontal disease are the most prevalent of all diseases in western communities. At the age of three to four years, no less than 25 percent of London children had dental caries.[27] An estimated 15 percent of the population in Scotland are edentulous by the age of thirty.[28]

Dental caries were rare in ancient Britain and most children were free of this disease. It was found to be seven times commoner in the British in 1957 than it had been in Anglo-Saxons.[29] This disease today is much less prevalent in rural Third World communities than it is in western nations.

Dental plaque plays a major role in the pathogenesis of dental caries. Not only does the consumption of refined and soft carbohydrate foods play a prominent role in the formation of this plaque, but the chewing of more abrasive fiber-rich foods helps to remove it.[30] Genetic and other factors also play a major role.

Bowel Content and Behavior

The consistency, bulk and speed of transit of intestinal content is now believed to profoundly influence the development of a number of the diseases associated with western culture.[31] The concept of constipation is usually a subjective assessment. It has relatively little meaning, at least in an epidemiological content, unless average daily stool output and intestinal transit time can be measured. Consistency of stool is very relevant, but no reliable and simple method has yet been devised to measure stool viscosity. The frequency of defecation is not necessarily related to the amount of feces voided. Although there are wide variations in bowel behavior in the same individuals on different occasions and between individuals consuming comparable diets, overall patterns of bowel behavior are characteristic of different communities. Diet is the dominant factor influencing the volume, consistency, and speed of transit through the gut of intestinal content, and the dietetic influence is mediated almost entirely through the fiber content of food.[23]

The average stool output in western countries is in the region of 80–120 g/d and that in Third World communities, 300–500 g. Intestinal transit times in the former are usually over seventy-two hours and in the latter under forty.[31]

Effects of Raised Intraluminal Pressures

Diverticular disease: Diverticular disease consists of the presence of pouches of colonic mucosa that have been forced out through weak spots in the overlying muscle coat by raised intracolonic pressures. The additional pressures required to propel small and viscid, in place of large and soft, fecal masses along the colon lead to hypertrophy of the muscle coat. This results in narrowing of the lumen, which in turn results in further increases in intraluminal pressure. Contraction of circular muscle can divide the pelvic colon into segments between areas where the lumen has been totally occluded by muscular contraction. It is in these closed segments that maximal pressures are generated with consequent blowing out of diverticula. The mechanism can be compared to squeezing clay in a clenched fist. Its extrusion between the fingers corresponds to the extrusion of bowel content with the bowel mucosa between bundles of circular muscle.[33] When these pouches become infected, they constitute diverticulitis. It is thus easy to appreciate why dietary fiber, by maintaining normal volume and softness of colon content is protective against the development of diverticular disease.

It is tragic that fiber should ever have been designated "roughage" in the mistaken concept that fibrous foods might be abrasive in the colon. The reverse is, of course, the case, and much suffering could have been avoided if the more appropriate term "softage" had been used instead. As might be expected, diverticular disease has been shown to be much less common in vegetarians who consumed approximately twice as much fiber as did carnivorous controls, the main difference in their respective diets being the content of cereal fiber.[33] The need for surgical intervention can be greatly reduced by prescribing high-fiber diets for all patients suffering from diverticular disease.[34]

Appendicitis: Appendicitis is usually a generalized lesion of the appendix mucosa distal to a more or less distinct line of demarcation between normal and diseased tissue. Any proportion of the appendix from the tip proximally may be involved. In view of the pathological features, together with the clinical aspects, commencing with epigastric colic, it is now generally agreed that the initial lesion is obstruction to the appendix lumen and that the inflammatory changes supervene when pressures generated distal to the obstruction jeopardize the blood supply of the mucosa.[35] Although by no means proved, there is reason to suspect that the presence of firm fecal particles in the appendix lumen may contribute to its obstruction in a manner analogous to that by which firm fecal masses can lead, through excessive muscular activity, to closure of the very much larger lumen of the pelvic colon. The higher frequency of appendicitis in young people could be explained by the narrower appendix lumen before progressive atrophy of the lymphoid tissue in its wall takes place. High-fiber diets, by reducing the presence of firm fecal particles in the appendix, might be expected to be protective against appendicitis.

Effects of Raised Intraabdominal Pressures

Hiatus hernia: The most frequent type of hiatus hernia consists of an upward protrusion of the gastroesophageal junction, together with the adjacent portion of the fundus of the stomach through the esophageal hiatus in the diaphragm and into the thoracic cavity. This must be due to a push from below, a pull from above or a combination of both. The contrast between the frequency with which this lesion is observed in western communities and its rarity in Third-World countries is consistent with the hypothesis that increased pressures below the diaphragm are predominantly responsible. The valsalva maneuver, comparable to straining at stool, raises intraabdominal pressures to a greater extent than does weight-lifting. When sitting on a raised toilet seat intraabdominal pressures during this maneuver have been shown to be around 200 cm H_2O while those above the diaphragm were under 70 cm, making a differential of about 130 cm H_2O.[36] It is easy to appreciate how these pressures frequently exerted could force the gastroesophageal junction upwards. The concept is comparable to the manner in which contained water can be expressed out through a hole in the wall of a ball when it is squeezed. When squatting at stool in the traditional manner rather than sitting on a raised western type toilet seat, intra-abdominal pressures are much lower[36] and this may well be an additional factor protecting Third-World communities against the development of hiatus hernia.[37] The fact that radiologists instruct patients to perform a valsalva maneuver in order to demonstrate a hiatus hernia is consistent with this concept, as is the rarity of the disease in all communities in which people normally evacuate a large daily stool volume.

Varicose veins: Whatever the factors responsible for develop-ment of varicose veins, such conventional concepts as man's erect posture, pregnancy, constrictive clothing or corsets or genetic defects can now be discounted as primary causative factors in the light of current epidemiological evidence.

Raised intraabdominal pressures have been shown to be readily transmitted to the major venous trunks at the back of the abdo-men that drain the blood from the legs. These pressures, transmit-ted retrogradely down the unsupported superficial veins, are initially arrested by the uppermost vein valves. In time, often repeated rises in pressure within the veins are believed to lead to their dilatation and the stretching of the ring to which the valve cusps are attached. This prevents the cusps from meeting one another and renders the valve incompetent so that the raised pressures are then transmitted to the next valve below, where the process of stretching and resultant incompetence are repeated.[38]

Raised intraabdominal pressures are almost certainly not the only factors responsible for the occurrence of varicose veins, and straining at stool is not the only cause of raised intraabdominal pressures. Varicose veins have been observed to occur more frequently than usual in tri-shaw riders in Southeast Asia and in porters carrying loads up the Himalayas.

In the epidemiological studies of Beaglehole et al[39] in Polyne-sians living in islands with different extents of contact with west-ern culture and in Maoris and Caucasians in New Zealand, the only factor found to relate consistently to the prevalence of vari-cose veins was the adoption of western customs. Two studies showed that patients with radiologically demonstrable colonic diverticula had a significantly higher than expected risk of also having varicose veins, which is consistent with the hypothesis that both disorders may share some common causative factor. [40,41] In our present state of knowledge, dietary fiber can be expected to be to some extent, protective against the development of varicose veins.

Other Effects of Increased Viscosity and Reduced Volume of Feces

Hemorrhoids: The conventionally accepted concept that hemorrhoids are varicosities of the veins in the superior hemorrhoidal venus plexus, and analogous to varicose veins in the legs, seems no longer to be tenable. Thomson[42] injected the vessels of the anal region in 100 babies who died near birth, with suitable substances for radiological and other examination. He demonstrated the well-developed presence of three vascular sub-mucosal cushions presumably present for the purpose of maintaining fecal continence. Not only does the presence of firm fecal masses in the rectum necessitate straining, which results in engorgement of these cushions, but the passage of these fecal masses through the anal canal acts like a ramrod forced down the barrel of a rifle, and in time ruptures the attachment of the cushions to the sphincter muscles and allows their prolapse towards the external anal orifice. As with varicose veins, there will be other factors contributing to the development of complications in hemorrhoids, but it is being increasingly accepted that a fundamental aspect of treatment in every case must be the provision of a fiber-rich diet.[34,43] This has been shown to greatly reduce the requirement of surgery.

Large-bowel cancer: It is now generally accepted that frequency of cancer of the large bowel is predominantly determined by dietary factors.[44,45] There is considerable evidence to suggest that fat in the diet may play a causative role and that the responsible fecal carcinogens are bacterial metabolites.[46] The various hypotheses that have been postulated have been discussed elsewhere.[47,48]

It has recently become generally agreed that whatever the factors responsible for the formation of carcinogens in the feces, dietary fiber exerts a protective role against this characteristically western form of cancer. There are many mechanisms which probably operate in supportive combination with one another. They may be listed as follows:

1. When fecal volume is large, all contained carcinogens or pre-carcinogens will be diluted, and vice versa. This will certainly influence their effectiveness.

2. The more rapid transit of large-volume feces will reduce time of contact between carcinogens and bowel mucosa.

3. Bowel cancer risk appears to be directly related to fecal pH[49] and this in turn is directly related to the content of fiber in the diet.

4. In vitro studies have shown that a small reduction in pH can greatly increase the bacterial conversion of primary into secondary bile acids, the latter being potentially carcinogenic.[50]

5. High-fiber diets are protective against overnutrition and obesity and these per se have been shown to predispose to development of cancer in general.

6. The amount of mutagens in the stools can be greatly reduced, either by reducing the fat or increasing the fiber content of the diet.[51]

For these and other reasons, fiber, and the fiber of starch staples in particular, can be expected to offer protection against large-bowel cancer.

Fiber and Gallstones

Either excessive cholesterol excretion in the liver or inadequate secretion of bile acid and phospholipid renders the bile supersaturated with cholesterol with the consequent tendency for the formation of gallstones.

The bile-acid content of the bile is related to the size of the bile-acid pool, and a reduced pool size is thought by many to be the result of suppressed bile-acid synthesis in the liver. Patients with gallstones usually have both excessive secretion of cholesterol and a small bile-acid pool.[52] Several studies have shown that adding wheat bran to western diets reduces the saturation of bile.[53]

Although gallstones are very rare in wild animals they have been produced experimentally in a wide variety of species. The carbohydrate component of the diets used in these experiments has in all instances been largely depleted of its fiber.[52] When fiber has been added, the diets have lost their lithogenic effect.

In addition to the epidemiological and experimental evidence that is consistent with the hypothesis that fiber provides protection against gallstones is the observation that the formation of stones is associated both with overnutrition and with obesity. Fiber-rich foods exert some protection against both of these states.

Fiber and Obesity

Fiber gives bulk to food without providing energy. Fiber-rich foods are consequently of low energy density, and have a low energy-satiety ratio, meaning that they make you feel full before excessive energy is consumed. The reverse is the case with foods with a high energy density, and consequently they encourage overnutrition and predispose to obesity.[54]

In addition, the fibrous structure of plant foods necessitates chewing. This both reduces the rate of food ingestion and increases the amount of saliva swallowed. For these and other reasons, such as the palatability of sugar, refined fiber-depleted carbohydrate foods predispose to the development of obesity in those genetically vulnerable in this respect.[55]

In addition to these dietetic factors, certain individuals are much more prone than are others to put on weight irrespective of the amount they eat. There is now strong evidence that this tendency to obesity is related to the amount of brown fat in the body. Brown fat has been shown to convert excessive energy intake into heat and thus prevent its conversion into adipose tissue.[56]

It would thus appear that in the case of both diabetes and obesity, individuals have differing genetically determined tendencies to these diseases but that the disorder to which they are prone is only expressed in a certain dietetic environment, and that in both instances fiber-rich foods are at least to some extent protective.

Fiber and Diabetes

The traditional practice of reducing carbohydrate intake in the treatment of maturity-onset diabetes would appear unreasonable in the light of the geographical distribution of the disease. Lowest prevalences are found in communities with the highest proportion of their energy provided by plant foods. It is now recognized that whereas mono- and disaccharides (sugars) are detrimental to diabetics, polysaccharides (starches) containing their natural complement of fiber are beneficial. Certain components of fiber, and particularly gums, found predominantly in certain legumes, increase the viscosity of upper intestinal content so that energy is released much more slowly than in the case of diets rich in refined carbohydrate foods.

Fiber has thus been shown to have a strongly beneficial effect on glucose-tolerance curves.[57,58]

Fiber and Ischemic Heart Disease

Opinions vary as to the role of fiber in IHD.[24] Communities consuming fiber-rich diets have low rates of IHD, but their food is reciprocally low in fat. Adding fiber to diets in the form of miller's bran doesn't appear to alter serum lipid levels, but putting people with high levels on a diet high in starch and fiber and low in fat and sugar does.

Morris et al[59] found in a twenty-year study of men in London that smoking was the major risk factor for IHD in this group and that cereal fiber, but not that of fruit and vegetables, was the strongest protective factor in those investigated.

It may be that as in the case of bowel cancer, high-fat diets are detrimental and high-fiber diets protective.

The hypotheses that have been postulated to explain a possible protective role of dietary fiber against development of IHD, can be summarized as follows:

1. Epidemiologically excessive energy intake is associated with IHD, and fiber-depleted carbohydrate foods predispose to overnutrition.

2. Atherosclerosis is linked with excessive production of insulin and with obesity. Both of these diseases are in turn associated with fiber-depleted diets.

3. Under certain circumstances, dietary fiber increases fecal excretion of bile acids and the employment of cholesterol to replace this loss may lower serum cholesterol concentrations.

4. There is some evidence that fiber alters blood clotting mechanisms. Venous thrombosis is much less common in Third-World than in western communities[60] and Latto et al[34] have shown that adding wheat bran pre- and postoperatively to patients' diets reduces the prevalence of postoperative deep-vein thrombosis and pulmonary embolism.

Practical Considerations

Merely adding fiber to an otherwise fiber depleted diet will combat constipation and in consequence may be expected to provide protection against diseases known, or postulated to be, directly caused by constipation.

The simplest and most cost-effective way to add fiber is in the form of miller's bran. This will not combat diseases due to metabolic and other effects of fiber-depleted diets, and it is vastly preferable to consume fiber-rich foods. From the standpoint of bowel behavior, bread made from high-extraction flour, brown or preferably whole-meal, and fiber-rich breakfast cereals are the best source of fiber. Legumes are also rich in fiber. It must be emphasized that potatoes are not fattening, provided they are neither cooked nor eaten with fat.

It is surprising to many that fruits and green vegetables, includ-

ing salads, are a relatively poor source of fiber, though a good source of food from other standpoints.
Important though it is, fiber must not be considered in isolation from other components of food. Western diets are too high in fat, sugar and salt, and too low in fiber and starch. A reasonable and practical approach would be to at least double our starch and fiber, halve our sugar and salt, and reduce our fat by a third. This does not present any great difficulties.

REFERENCES

1. Cowgill, G. R. and Anderson, W. E. 1932. Laxative effects of bran and washed bran in healthy men. Comparative studies. *J. Am. Med. Assoc.* 98:1866.
2. Williams, R. D. and Olmsted, W. H. 1936. The effect of cellulose, hemicellulose and lignin on the weight of the stool: contribution to the study of laxation in man. *J. Nutr.* 11:433.
3. Fantus, B., Kopstein, G. and Smidt, H. R. 1940. Roentgen study of intestinal motility as influenced by bran. *J. Am. Med. Assoc.* 144:404.
4. Dimmock, E. M. 1936. The treatment of habitual constipation by the bran method. M. D. Thesis, University of Cambridge.
5. Cleave, T. L. 1956. The neglected natural principles in current medical practive. *J. R. Nav. Med. Serv.* 42:55.
6. Cleave, T. L. and Campbell, G. D. 1966. *Diabetes, Coronary Thrombosis and the Saccharine Diseases.* Bristol, England: Wright & Sons, Ltd.
7. Cleave, T. L.: *The Saccharine Disease.* 1975. New Canaan, CT: Keats Publishing, Inc.
8. Trowell, H. C., Davies, J. N. P. and Dean, R. 1952. *Kwashiokor.* London: Edward Arnold.
9. Trowell, H. C. 1960. *Non-Infective Disease in Africa.* London: Edward Arnold.
10. Trowell, H. 1972. Ischemic heart disease and dietary fiber. *S. J. Clin. Nutr.* 25:926.
11. Painter, N. S. 1964. The etiology of diverticulosis of the colon with special reference to the action of certain drugs on the behavior of the colon. *Ann. Roy. Coll. Surg. Eng.* 34:98.
12. *Medical Aspects of Dietary Fiber.* A report of the Royal College of Physicians. 1980. London: Pitman Medical.
13. *Western Diseases—Their Emergence and Prevention.* 1981 H. C. Trowell and D. P. Burkitt, eds. London: Edward Arnold. *Also:* Cambridge, MA: Harvard University Press.
14. *Refined Carbohydrates Foods and Disease—Some Implications of Dietary Fiber.* 1975. D. P. Burkitt and H. C. Trowell, eds. London, New York: Academic Press.
15. Yamamoto, S. 1981. *Western Diseases. Their Emergence and Prevention.* H. C. Trowell and D. P. Burkitt, eds. London: Edward Arnold.
16. Stemmermann, G. N. 1970. Patterns of disease among Japanese living in Hawaii. *Arch. Env. Health* 20:266.
17. Wynder, E. L. and Shigematsu, T. 1967. Environmental factors of cancer of the colon and rectum. *Cancer* 20:1520.

18. Prior, I. and Tasman-Jones, C. 1981. New Zealand Maori and Pacific Polynesians. In: *Western Diseases, Their Emergence and Prevention.* H. C. Trowell and D. P. Burkitt, eds. London: Edward Arnold.
19. Burkitt, D. P. 1973. Some diseases characteristic of modern western civilization. *Brit. Med. J.* 1:274.
20. Trowell, H. C. 1975. In: *Refined Carbohydrate Foods and Disease.* D. P. Burkitt and H. C. Trowell, eds. London: Edward Arnold, p. 43.
21. Trowell, H. C. 1980. Salt and hypertension. *Lancet* 2:88.
22. *Medical Aspects of Dietary Fiber.* London: Pitman Medical, pp. 12–25.
23. Eastwood, M. A., Brydon, W. G. and Tadesse, K. 1980. Effects of fiber on colon continence. In: *Medical Aspects of Dietary Fiber.* G. A. Spiller and R. McP. Kay, eds. New York and London: Plenum Medical Books.
24. Story, J. A. 1980. Dietary fiber and lipid metabolism: an update. In: *Medical Aspects of Dietary Fiber.* G. A. Spiller and R. McP. Kay, eds. New York and London: Plenum Medical Books, p. 137.
25. Jenkins, J. A. 1980. Dietary fiber and carbohydrate metabolism. In: *Medical Aspects of Dietary Fiber.* G. A. Spiller and R. McP. Kay, eds. New York and London: Plenum Medical Books. p. 175.
26. Jenkins, J. A., Wolever, T. M. S., Leeds, A. R., et al. 1978. Dietary fiber, fiber analogues and glucose tolerance: the importance of viscosity. *Brit. Med. J.* 1:1392.
27. Wynter, G. D., Rule, D. C., Mailer, G. P., James, P. N. C. and Gordon, P. H. 1978. The prevalence of dental caries in pre-school children age 1–4 years. *Br. Dent. J.* 130:271.
28. Todd, J. E. and Whitworth, A. 1974. *Adult Dental Health in Scotland.* H.M.S.O. London.
29. Hardwick, J. L. 1960. The incidence and distribution of caries throughout the ages in relation to the Englishman's diet. *Br. Dent. J.* 108:99.
30. Carlsson, J. and Egelberg, J. Effect of diets on early plaque formation.
31. Burkitt, D. P., Walker, A. R. P. and Painter, N. S. 1974. Dietary fiber and disease. *J. Am. Med. Assoc.* 229:1068.
32. Painter, N. S. 1975. *Diverticular Disease of the Colon.* New Canaan, CT: Keats Publishing, Inc., p. 111.
33. Gear, J. S., Ware, A., Furdson, P., Mann, J. I., Nolan, E. J., Broadribb, A. J. M. and Vessey, M. P. 1979. Symptomless diverticular disease and intake of dietary fiber. *Lancet* 1:551.
34. Latto, C. 1978. Practical experience. In: *Dietary Fiber: Current Developments of Improvement to Health.* K. W. Heaton, ed. London: Newman Publishing, p. 151.
35. Burkitt, D. P. 1975. Appendicitis. In: *Refined Carbohydrate Foods and Disease.* D. P. Burkitt and H. C. Trowell, eds. London and New York: Academic Press, p. 87.
36. Fedails, S., Harvey, F. F. and Burns-Cox, F. J. 1979. Abdominal and thoracic pressures during defecataion. *Brit. Med. J.* 1:91.
37. Burkitt, D. P. 1981. Hiatus hernia. Is it preventable? *Am. J. Clin. Nut.* 34:428–431, and Almay, Thomas P. 1981. Editorial, *Am. J. Clin. Nut.* 34:432–433.
38. Burkitt, D. P. 1976. Varicose veins, facts and fantasy. *Arch. Surg.* 111:1327.
39. Beaglehole, R., Prior, I. H. M., Salmand, C. E. and Davidson, F. 1975. Varicose veins in the South Pacific. *Int. J. Epidem.* 44:295.
40. Latto, C., Wilkinson, R. W. and Gilmore, O. J. A. 1973. Diverticular disease and varicose veins. *Lancet* 1:1089.

41. Broadribb, A. J. M. and Humphreys, D. M. 1976. Diverticular disease, Part I. Relation to other disorders and fiber intake. *Brit. Med. J.* 1:424.
42. Thomson, W. H. F. 1975. The nature of hemorrhoids. *Br. J. Surg.* 62:542.
43. Huibregtse, K. 1979. Non-surgical therapeutic possibilities in hemorrhoidal disease. In: *Hemorrhoids: Current Concepts in Causation and Management.* London: Academic Press.
44. Modin, B. and Lebin, F. 1980. Epidemiology of colon cancer: fiber, fats fallacies and facts. In: *Medical Aspects of Dietary Fiber.* C. A. Spiller and R. McP. Kay, eds. New York and London: Plenum Medical Books, p. 119.
45. Weisburger, J. H., Reddy, B. S., Spingarn, N. E. and Wynder, E. J. 1980. Current views of the mechanisms involved in the etiology of colo-rectal cancer. In: *Colorectal cancer: Prevention Epidemiology and Screening.* S. J. Winawer, D. Schottenfeld and P. Sherlock, eds. New York: Raven Press.
46. Wynder, E. L. and Reddy, V. S. 1975. Dietary fat and colon cancer. *J. Natl. Cancer Inst.* 54:7.
47. Walker, A. R. P. and Burkitt, D. P. 1976. Colonic cancer: hypotheses of causation, dietary prophylaxis and future research. *Am. J. Clin. Nutr.* 31:910 (1978).
48. Burkitt, D. P. 1980. Fiber in the etiology of colorectal cancer. In: *Colorectal Cancer: Prevention Epidemiology and Screening.* S. J. Winawer, D. Schottenfeld and P. Sherlock, eds. New York: Raven Press.
49. MacDonald, I. A., Webb, G. R. and Mahoney, D. E. 1978. Fecal hydroxysteroid dehydrogenase activities in vegetarians, Seventh-Day Adventists controlled subjects and bowel cancer patients. *Am. J. Clin. Nutr.* 31:223.
50. MacDonald, I. A., Singh, G., Mahoney, D. E. and Mier, C. G. 1978. Effect of pH on bile salt degradation by mixed fecal cultures. *Steroids* 32:245.
51. Land, P. C. and Bruce, W. R. 1976. *Origins of Human Cancer.* Coldspring Harbor, New York: Coldspring Harbor Laboratory.
52. Heaton, K. W. 1975. Gallstones and cholecystitis. In: *Refined Carbohydrate Foods and Disease.* D. P. Burkitt and H. C. Trowell, eds. London, New York: Academic Press, p. 173.
53. Pomare, E. W. and Heaton, K. W. 1973. Alteration of bile salt metabolism by dietary fiber (bran). *Brit. Med. J.* 4:262
54. Heaton, K. W. 1975. The effects of carbohydrate refining on food ingestion, digestion and absorption. In: *Refined Carbohydrate Foods and Disease.* D. P. Burkitt and H. C. Trowell, eds. London, New York: Academic Press, p. 60.
55. Haber, J. B., Heaton, K. W., Murphy, D. and Burroughs, L. F. 1977. Depletion and disruption of dietary fiber: effect on satiety, plasma, glucose and serum insulin. *Lancet.* 2:679.
56. Jung, R. T., Shetty, P. S., James, W. P. T., Barrand, M. A. and Callighan, B. A. 1979. Reduced thermogenesis in obesity. *Nature* 279:322
57. Jenkins, D. J. A. 1980. Dietary fiber and carbohydrate metabolism. In: *Medical Aspects of Dietary Fiber.* G. A. Spiller and R. McP. Kay, eds. New York: Plenum Medical Books, p. 175.

58. Anderson, J. 1981. Diabetes mellitus. In: *Western Diseases—Their Emergence and Prevention*. H. C. Trowell, and D. P. Burkitt, eds. London: Edward Arnold.
59. Morris, J. N., Marr, J. W. and Clayton, D. G. 1977. Diet and heart: a postscript. *Brit. Med. J.* 2:1307.
60. Burkitt, D. P. Deep vein thrombosis and hemorrhoids. In: *Refined Carbohydrate Foods and Disease*. D. P. Burkitt and H. C. Trowell, eds. London, New York: Academic Press, p. 143.

Those wanting a comprehensive list of articles on dietary fiber, until and including 1977, are referred to *Dietary Fiber in Human Nutrition: A Bibliography*. H. C. Trowell. Published by John Libbey: London for Kellogg Company of Great Britain.

11

IMPLEMENTING
NUTRITIONAL EDUCATION
IN A GENERAL MEDICAL PRACTICE

SCOTT RIGDEN, M.D.

THE CHALLENGE of teaching proper nutritional habits to patients in a general practice of medicine is an extremely difficult, but rewarding, proposition. Patients generally are slow to accept that nutrition plays any role in the prevention or course of their illnesses. Even if they do accept this premise, often they are unwilling to change, because of the comfort they have achieved with their diet. In addition, there are also resistances related to ethnic preferences, ease of procurement of certain foods and convenience of fast-food living, which may prevent them from integrating effective preventive nutritional concepts into their own and their families' lives.

Physicians wishing to integrate a comprehensive approach within a family practice, including nutrition, exercise, stress reduction, patient education and preventive medicine, must constantly be teaching and motivating in their attempts to help the patients change constructively.

This comprehensive preventive nutritional approach towards health care is based upon four basic premises:

1. The physician is a teacher and health adviser; the goal of every physician/patient interaction is the imparting of some information to patients which will help them to be more independent and to understand their problems better. The ability to evaluate patients in terms of their responsiveness to education and to motivate them to change their lives can be taken as an index of the sucesss of a physician.

287

2. Comprehensive care in a general medical practice optimally stresses preventive medicine and continuity of care: as Dr. Kenneth Cooper has stated, ". . . We are not dying, but killing ourselves."[1] He cites mortality statistics on males in their forties that show five of the leading six killers are heart disease, lung cancer, auto accidents, cirrhosis of the liver and strokes, and maintains that these could be significantly modified with appropriate changes in life-style and preventive health-care orientation.

3. The patient must become activated. It is no longer acceptable for patients to come passively to the office and unload all of their problems on the physician and expect that the physician is doing his or her part by delivering palliative medication. Patients must accept personal responsibility for their health and work with the physician in attaining high levels of it.

4. Comprehensive care, particularly as it relates to implementing nutrition via patient education, must emphasize the team concept with the patient being part of the team. Physicians must delegate responsibilities to other staff members within the office to monitor and impart patient education.

Medical Literature Supporting Patient Education

A frequently heard objection by many physicians to a commitment regarding patient education and nutrition is that research has not proven the value or efficacy of nutritional therapies. Several recent studies have indicated that the success of these nutrition approaches to a great degree depends upon physicians' attitude about the implementation of nutrition education in their practices. Talkington found that patient compliance could be improved if the physician-patient interaction emphasized building a partnership with the patient.[2] The patients repeatedly seemed to react favorably to feeling they were valued enough that the health professional took the time to care for them beyond conventional expectations. Ley et al documented that anxious and depressed patients significantly reduced medication errors when they were presented with an easily comprehensible leaflet explaining how and why they should take their medication.[3] Significantly, they also showed that similar leaflets with sophisticated terminology were not helpful.

Physicians working at the general medical clinic of the Johns Hopkins University Hospital entered into tutorials to improve their effectiveness as educators of patients with essential hypertension.[4] They subsequently allowed more time for patient education and achieved increased patient knowledge. The patients were more compliant with drug regimes and had better control of blood pressure than patients of untutored physicians. The authors conclude, ". . . The personal physician, if he is provided with strategies identifying the noncompliant patient and for intervening in that behavior, can apply a stimulus to his patients that results in improved compliance and better control of hypertension."

Newkirk et al documented that a self-instructional health educational program could be educationally effective in the ambulatory clinical setting.[5] Specifically, they developed an audio-visual program dealing with infant and child nutrition that was played in the waiting room of the University Hospital pediatric clinic. Mothers, primarily in their late twenties, significantly improved their knowledge in this important area. It has been found that preventive medical behavior of large groups can be altered with patient education coupled with multiphasic screening. Rodnick and Bubb combined the use of a health hazard appraisal multiphasic screening in patient education to achieve a reduction in cardiac and other risk factors in a group of 292 patients.[6]

Singman et al documented that 1,113 males over a fifteen-year period in their "anti-coronary club" in New York City were able to utilize the teaching of a "prudent diet" to lower coronary heart disease incidence rates, serum cholesterol and weight.[7] A similar but smaller study in Chicago featuring 519 males over a fifteen-year period led to weight loss, slowing of pulse rate, reduction of serum cholesterol levels and sustained decreases of blood pressure.[8]

The Stanford Three Community Study by Fortmann et al[9] suggests that mass media health education can achieve lasting changes in diet, obesity and plasma cholesterol on a community level.

In summary, physician advocates of patient education need no longer apologize if their cohorts demand references from the literature for supporting the importance of nutritional education. It must be acknowledged that not all studies show such salutary effects, but this could easily be due to suboptimal motivation of the health professionals or their patients, suboptimal ability of the health professional to teach, motivate and communicate, or a suboptimal setting which was not conducive to patient education.

Written Patient Aids

Written patient aids form a keystone of the patient education efforts on nutrition. There are increasing opportunities for the interested physician to obtain excellent materials. Sources include drug company pamphlets, features in medical or lay journals, *Instruction for Patients* by Griffith,[10] and *Patient Education for* the Family[11] recently written by Brunworth and Rigden. The latter two books contain numerous one-page handouts that can be easily photocopied and given to the patient. Table 11.1 lists the written nutrition patient aids that many offices commonly use with their patients.

TABLE 11.1

Written Nutrition Patient Aids

ADA Diets 1000 Calories	How to Live with Hypoglycemia
ADA Diets 1200 Calories	Hypoglycemia Diet
ADA Diets 1500 Calories	Infant Feeding
ADA Diets 1800 Calories	Ironing Out Your Diet
ADA Diets 2200 Calories	Lactose Free Diet
ADA Diets 2600 Calories	Low Salt Diet
ADA Food Exchange Lists	Nutritional Analysis Form
A Bran New You	Nutritious Snacks
Coping with Stress and Stress Eating	Substitutions for any Recipe
Foods High in Potassium	Tips for Weight Loss
Glucose Tolerance Test Prep Diet	Whole Grain Recipes

It should be emphasized that written handouts are not used instead of verbal communication, but rather to complement instructions. Written materials are kept in a centrally located nurse's station, alphabetized and color-coded, as seen in Figure 11.1 This facilitates giving the materials to the patient after the physician has concluded his or her evaluation. For example, the physician may note on a fee slip which is attached to the chart that the patient needs patient education on "irritable colon" and the use of bran. The nurse or medical assistant then retrieves the appropriate written patient aid and reviews it with the patient. The materials may also be used by a staff member during an individual nutrition appointment or as a part of special information packets given to the prenatal or neonatal patients, and as supplementary handouts to various nutrition classes and groups.

Physicians may wish to write their own nutrition patient education aids. This will enable them to develop handouts that reflect their own individual style and approach and to individualize education according to their own patient population. It has been found that much of the content of these materials evolves from often-repeated discussions with patients. Most primary care physicians are literally teaching and educating all day long, but may not be consciously aware of this. A reflection on their patients' most common questions and problems will help them in the

Figure 11.1
Infant Feeding Recommendations

General: infant nutrition is a rapidly expanding and dynamic topic. New research and ideas are being published weekly, so talk with your doctor about your infant's nutrition.

Currently, it is our recommendation and the recommendation of the American Academy of Pediatrics that mother's milk fed on a demand schedule is the feeding method of choice. It is also advised that whether mother's milk or formula is used, that they be continued for 1 year before the introduction of regular cow's milk.

Additionally, recent studies strongly point to the early introduction of solid foods as the leading cause of childhood obesity and possibly many adult illnesses such as obesity, high blood pressure and diabetes. For these reasons, we suggest no solid foods until 4 months of age.

For breast fed infants, see our handouts on breast feeding techniques.

For formula fed infants, the following table may be helpful in judging average amounts of formula taken per twenty-four hours.

1 month: 20–24 oz. in 6 bottles.
2 months: 24–30 oz. in 5 bottles.
3 months: 30–32 oz. in 4–5 bottles.
4 months: 26–32 oz. in 4–5 bottles.
6 months: 16–24 oz. in 3–4 bottles or cups
9–12 months: discontinue bedtime bottle, try and establish schedule of 3 meals/day.

SOLID FOODS:
At about 4 months of age the baby will develop signs that he/she is ready for solid foods. Such signs include A) the appearance of teeth, B) excessive salivation or C) inadequate filling with milk alone.

Although there is no proven scientific rationale as to which foods to begin in any given order, a program found satisfactory by many parents follows:

A) Begin only one new food every 5–7 days so that any allergic reaction such as rash or diarrhea may be specifically isolated to that newly introduced food.

B) Home made infant foods are probably fresher and more nutritious and definitely less expensive. Simply make or grind regular table food into a consistency which is easily swallowed by the child.

C) Do not add salt, sugar or honey to the foods—this prevents developing dependence on these substances for the taste which is naturally present in whole foods.

D) If commercial baby foods are used—avoid the ones with added sugar, salt or modified food starches for the above reason.

E) Begin first with cereals such as rice, oat, barley or wheat working up to 1–2 tablespoonful per serving.

F) After the infant has successfully enjoyed the cereals, he/she will be ready for vegetables. Introduce all the vegetables at least once. Obviously, there will be some infants enjoy more than others, but try most of them so that a wide range of taste preferences can be learned.

G) Following vegetables, introduce the meats/fishes, A 2:1 ratio of white: red meat/day is preferred because of its lower cholesterol count. Gradually advance up to 2 oz. of meat twice daily.

H) By this time the infant is ready to begin fresh fruits—raw or cooked with no sweetener added. Banana, applesauce, pears, peaches are good to begin with. Citrus fruits may be given at nine months.

I) Egg yolks up to four per week may be begun at approximately six months.

J) Whole eggs at nine months.

formulation of specific education materials. The content of the nutrition patient education materials must be up-to-date, accurate, and agree with what the patient is told verbally. A periodic routine review of all materials should be integrated into the program for potential updating where necessary.

The format of these aids should be to effectively transmit information to the patient in clear, concise, brief language. The language should vary depending upon whether the physician is treating a rural, college town or intercity practice, but it should not contain "buzz" words. Illustrations and diagrams may enhance communication. If the physician has a talented artist in the practice, they may be able to collaborate in the formulation of such materials.

Assessing the Patient

There are several methods that can be conveniently used in a family practice to assess the patients' nutritional status. Questionnaires can be used for different age groups which concern the intake of alcohol, caffeine, sugar and standard foods. Many of these assessment tools can also be important as education devices

TABLE 11.2

What Do You Know About Sugar?

1. Government figures show that we as a nation consume _____ pounds of sugar per year per person.
   a) 10 pounds   b) 75 pounds   c) 110 pounds
2. What percentage of our total sugar intake is from processed foods?
   a) 15%   b) 45%   c) 70%
3. Refined sugar contains essential nutrients such as vitamins and minerals. True or False.
4. Obesity, cavities, hyperactivity,and constipation can be problems related to high sugar consumption. True or False.
5. Sugar is present in most cereals, crackers, salad dressings and bologna. True or False.
6. Pre-sweetened cereals have_____percentages of sugar.
   a) 5%   b) 15%   c) 40–60%
7. Sugar is the #1 food additive. True or False.
8. Refined sugar is a needed nutrient by the body. It should be consumed daily. True or False.
9. Honey and molasses and sorghum are sweeteners that can be used to replace sugar in most recipes. True or False.
10. Honey tastes sweeter to the tongue than sugar. Therefore only half as much is needed for sweetening. True or False.

10	Correct	Very good. Wonderful. You are aware.
5–9	Correct	You know the problem.
1–5	Correct	Not bad. You're beginning to realize the problem.
0	Correct	Glad you came! You're given 4 points just for being here and wanting to learn. Go on to 1–5 correct.

for the patient, in that they bring to mind for the first time certain
nutrition relationships of which the patient has been unaware.
Such is the impact of the questionnaire entitled "What Do You
Know about Sugar?" as seen in Table 11.2 which serves to raise
the consciousness of patients concerning their refined sugar intake.
A three- to seven-day diet is very important in assessing the
nutrition intake of a patient. A comprehensive blood screen and
other detailed biochemical analyses may be useful in establishing
a patient's nutritional status, depending upon the degree of sophis-
tication of nutritional assessment employed within the office. At
minimum, a physician should be requesting dietary information
concerning the patient, looking for signs or symptoms of nutritional inadequacy and establishing a relationship with the patient
in terms of nutrition education.

Prenatal and Neonatal

The nutritional management of pregnancy and lactation[12,13] is
an important part of the efforts that a general practitioner can
provide during these times with a family. Once pregnancy has
been established in a patient, the physician may then have the
woman spend half an hour with a staff member in a teaching
session concerning nutrition and pregnancy. At this time, the risk
of alcohol, nicotine and caffeine may be discussed. In addition,
written patient aids on breast feeding may be given to the patient
to facilitate decision-making on this important area. An excellent
citation that may be used is *As You Eat, So Your Baby Grows* by
Goldbeck, which might be given to all prenatal patients. It is a
small pamphlet available from the Ceres Press, Old Witchtree
Road, Woodstock, New York, 12498.

Similarly, all new mothers and fathers may be involved in a
teaching session with the office staff about one week after discharge from the hospital concerning infant feeding and the avoidance of premature use of cow's milk.

Use of Books

Books are a very central part of nutrition education and can be
used in the following ways:

1. Books of general information may be dispalyed in the patient
   education room, so that patients may see them and become
   familiar with them;
2. Specialized books may be made available for various classes;
3. Recommended reading lists should be given to each patient;
4. Selected books should be made available for purchase, loan
   or as gifts in the office;

5. A cookbook which stresses improved diets and nutrition may be given to a family as an incentive for reinforcing improved nutrition;

6. Innovative concepts such as providing a patient a booklet entitled *A Bran New You,* along with recipes featuring bran and a one-pound package of unprocessed bran may help reinforce the patient to adopt an integrated approach toward diet and health.

Obesity

One of the most common nutrition problems[14,15] seen in a general practice of medicine is that of obesity. Problems as they relate to weight management may be divided into two categories: those who are less than forty pounds overweight, and those who are in excess of forty pounds above the ideal lean body mass.

Individual diet-nutrition counseling to identify the offender foods and putting a person on a 1,000 calorie-a-day mixed food diet may be effective for the moderately obese patient, whereas the morbidly obese patient may need more comprehensive management, including exercise, life-style, nutrition and behavior modification education.[16,17,18] These patients may attend a patient education class given during the evenings which includes positive mental attitude, reduction of stress eating, improvement of exercise, when and how to eat out, self-hypnosis, relaxation therapy and other behavior modification tools. Seeing the patients weekly during this phase is very important to developing a relationship with them and identifying psychological aspects of overeating and food preference habits. Even after completing the diet, it may necessitate another six months to a year of return visits every month to continue the established relationship the physician has with the patients, so that they continue to comply with their improved dietary habits. Patients may have developed a very important relationship with the practitioner and he or she may serve as their psychological "crutch" until they can turn the corner psychologically and be able to self-control their dietary habits, which may take more than a year after the weight loss has been achieved.

Figure 11.2
Tips for Weight Loss

1. Recognize obesity as a lifelong, incurable, but controllable disease.
2. Adopt a long-range plan:
   - • try shedding five to fifteen pounds at a time, in one to three months
   - attempt to lose one pound per week by eating less and exercising more (achieving a net loss of 500 calories per day).
3. Increase the level of physical activity:
   - walk at least an extra mile a day; don't ride short distances; park your car two blocks from your destination and walk the rest of the way
   - exercise according to physical and emotional ability; walking may be more suitable than jogging or swimming.
4. Try to avoid sampling foods while preparing meals. Keep a "free" food (like celery stalks) handy in case you get the urge for a "sneak preview."
5. To control eating habits at the table, try the following:
   - try changing to a new table setting—different design of plates and silverware
   - put food on a smaller (7" rather than 9" for example) plate, and eat with a dessert or salad fork
   - don't keep extra portions on the table; avoid serving food "family style," and no second helpings
   - put down the fork between bites; make it a point to chew each mouthful of food ten times
   - count every mouthful
   - interrupt the meal with two minute breaks—leave the table for that long
   - leave a little food on your plate at the end of each meal, then destroy this food or feed it to the dog . . . don't be a human disposal
   - meals should last *at least* twenty minutes; it takes that long to *feel* like you've eaten

- have family members scrape their own plates.

General Suggestions:
- avoid having ready-to-eat or snack foods around the house
- do your grocery shopping from a list, and avoid shopping on an empty stomach
- do all your eating in one room and in one chair, and avoid reading, watching TV or listening to the radio while eating
- keep refrigerated foods in *covered* containers and turn *off* the light bulb in the refrigerator
- try to increase your intake of the following foods: asparagus, broccoli, brussels sprouts, cabbage, cauliflower, lettuce, mushrooms, okra, peppers, radishes, sauerkraut, string beans, tomatoes, watercress. These are the lowest in calorie (often called "free foods") and good filler foods.
- make a special bank for money saved from cutting down on your eating habits. For instance, reward yourself 25 cents or 50 cents for every pound lost. It also helps to identify an item you would like (one of modest expense) and write that item on the bank. Don't buy that item until there is sufficient money saved. Sometimes a beautiful picture of something works better. You may prefer a scale of money saved (possibly in the form of a thermometer) on the bank.

Figure 11.2 (Continued)
Tips for Weight Loss

WEIGHT REDUCTION

Obesity may well be the leading health problem in this country. Over half of all adults older than thirty are at least slightly to moderately overweight. Moreover, obesity is rapidly becoming more prominent in infant, pre-school and school-age children. It is a key factor in causing heart disease, adult onset diabetes, and hypertension and aggravates arthritic conditions. In addition, it is often the key factor in causing fatigue and preventing the average person from functioning to full capacity. Obviously no one has all the answers regarding obesity. The numerous fad diets and lack of uniform success by any one method speak to that. Our feeling is that obesity is a lifelong, incurable but controllable problem. Therefore, we approach a successful weight reduction program as one which is a long-range plan, losing weight at a rate of four to six pounds per month, and in so doing maintaining excellent health. In addition, it is important that your weight reduction program becomes a practical part of your life, helping you to maintain your new weight once you have reduced. Our function as physicians will be to advise you on the four essential aspects of a weight reduction program, diet, exercise, reprogramming the subconscious mind, and behavior modification. At first, we usually see the patient frequently to help make needed adjustments with his program and overcome the initial difficulties of a new lifestyle. Gradually office visits become more infrequent and are devoted to a weigh-in and brief discussion-analysis of your progress.

DIET

Our goal is to choose an appropriate diet for you that is *practical* and that will insure your body of *good nutrition*. The choice depends on multiple factors such as your weight, frame, exercise level and general life-style. Some people respond better to general guidelines, while others need a very specific detailed diet. To help us choose the best possible program for you, we sometimes ask you to fill out a nutrition questionnaire, noting carefully everything you have eaten in a twenty-four hour period. It is our goal to make you an active partner in choosing your type of diet. In addition, whenever possible we would like to have *couples* and *whole families* involved.

EXERCISE

In order to achieve a net loss of calories per day, it is very important to increase exercise at the same time you decrease eating. This also helps to "firm up" physiques. If a person walked one mile more than his usual activity every day of the year, this could lead to a twenty to twenty-two pound weight loss. We will help you decide on forms of exercise according to your physical and emotional ability. Walking at least an extra mile a day is certainly a reasonable level for most people to start. If weather prohibits outdoor exercise, walking at a mall, indoor bicycling or jogging in place indoors are good alternatives. In your daily life deliberately park your car two blocks from your destination and walk the rest of the way. Most of you will be asked to keep an exercise log and bring it with you at each appointment.

REPROGRAMMING YOUR SUBCONSCIOUS MIND

Research has indicated one's self image is a very important part of changing one's life and habitual weight. Willpower and good intentions are not enough. If deep down in your subconscious mind you still *do not* really *believe* you can be the healthy, thin person you want to be, your chances for lasting success are small. Often, years of habitual negative programming and negative thinking undermine the two

Figure 11.2 (Continued)
Tips for Weight Loss

necessary conditions for self-improve-ment: the *desire* and the *belief* that one can change. Many have been "brain-washed" with beliefs such as "I'll al-ways be fat," "I have no self-control," "I always eat when I'm nervous," "It's not my fault that I'm fat." In addition, many people erroneously approach weight reduction with a passive atti-tude, insisting that the doctor must cause them to lose weight with various "water" and "diet pills." To become thin and healthy, you must constantly work on reprogramming your subcon-scious mind, e.g., brainwash yourself with positive throughts. See yourself looking thin and healthy, the way you want to be. Make these mental images even more real with your old pictures when you were thin, clipping pictures of clothes or styles you would like to see yourself in, etc. Pick a slogan that you can write on little signs or cards and see many times during the day. Put those in obvious view in the bath-room, kitchen, automobile, wallet, purse, etc. By *repeating* this slogan *many times* you can rid yourself of old, defeated, negative, failure images and replace them with the positive and suc-cessful images. Example of slogans that others have found useful include:

I have control over my appetite and life.
I see myself as thin, healthy and in control of my life.

BEHAVIOR MODIFICATION
The branch of behavioral science called behavior modification approaches the behavior of over-eating as a habit. Its goal is to help you modify or improve poor or self-defeating eating habits with habits that will reinforce your efforts to lose. An obvious example is the per-son who habitually comes home after work and goes to the refrigerator and eats a snack. Behavior modification would perhaps advise this person to come home and go through another door and route himself in a way that avoids the kitchen and refrigerator. Obviously, behavior modification has to be individualized. Your physician will discuss your eating habits with you and prescribe behavior modifiers for you to try. Some examples of basic behavior modification that would bene-fit most of us include: (1) avoid having ready-to-eat or snack foods around the house; (2) interrupt the meal with two minute breaks—leave the table for that long; (3) meals should last *at least* twenty minutes; it takes that long to as though like you've eaten.

Establishing a Nutrition Consciousness

It is vital that practitioners and their staff reflect an office atmosphere that nutrition is important. This starts with the practitioner him- or herself. The practitioner must teach, lead and motivate by example. A practitioner who is committed to im-proved nutrition in his or her own life sets an example for the whole staff and patients, as it relates to the importance of nutri-tion and health. Bulletin boards can be inexpensively placed in each examining room, waiting room and around the office, to exemplify the commitment to nutrition and exercise. These bulle-tin boards can contain little reminders regarding weight loss tips, recipes, pictures of the staff exercising or pictures of the commu-nity showing people vitally involved with their lives. The patient often is a captive audience awaiting the doctor, so this can be an ideal time to provide subtle psychological input.

A patient newsletter can do much to create an expanded nutritional awareness in the practice and develop a different relationship with the doctor. Nutrition classes every three or four months in the evenings may be of help in bringing patients to a higher level of nutritional awareness.

Many times rural town newspapers are clamoring for information regarding health. Topics related to nutrition are now popular and well received by these periodicals. A physician may then cite certain exemplary case studies or examples within the practice to the newspaper to help motivate the community.

Similarly, speaking in the community to various civic groups is an excellent forum for nutrition education. These presentations may include written handouts as well as visual aids.

A physician should recognize that integration of the nutritional concept into the kitchen may be another stumbling block, and that possibly cooking classes done by a local nutritionist who is sympathetic to the same spirit and philosophy of the office may be very helpful in training patients how to implement improved nutrition. Simple concepts such as learning how to bake bread with whole wheat flour may be an important first step for many patients in improving their nutritional status.

The use of audio-visual presentations in the office as either slide shows or video cassettes may also be excellent attention-getters. An audio-visual cassette presentation produced by Ross Hume Hall of McMaster University, entitled *Whole Nourishment,* has been used effectively in many offices to educate patients on the importance of the complete diet, outlining the principles of variety, minimal processing and native diets, and considers seven food categories for insuring a high quality diet.

Patients can become much more active and responsible for their own maintenance by the use of Patient Flow Sheets, as seen in Figures 11.3 and 11.4. These Flow Sheets allow the patients to chart their own progress towards a higher level of health and fitness. Patients may respond enthusiastically to being able to see a quantifiable demonstration of their improvement by looking at such things as serum cholesterol, hemoglobin and hematocrit, cholesterol to HDL ratio, potassium and serum glucose. These Flow Sheets are secured in a folder in the patient's chart to insure their use during each visit, with a copy going to the patients so that they can monitor their own improvement. The response of the patients to their dietary modification and life-style improvement should be quantified in their charts for referral, since many patients will forget how much improvement they have undergone over a period of several years.

Lastly, the use of a computerized health hazard appraisal form may be of benefit to motivate patients by utilizing the concept of biological versus chronological age. This concept is easily understood by patients and can be used as a springboard to discuss risk towards disease and how to minimize risk by integrating improved nutrition and life-style.

Nutritional Help for Common Health Problems

There are many opportunities in the course of a day for a family practitioner to integrate nutrition into a treatment regime. Two common problems (irritable colon and glucose intolerance) may illustrate how this may be done. After the diagnosis of the irritable colon has been made, the patient receives patient education and the contributing role of stress is explained. Dietary instructions may then be given, including the following:

1. Elimination or great reduction of coffee, tea and cola drinks.
2. Examination of the consumption of dairy products, alcohol and spicy foods, if they seem to correlate with symptoms.
3. The consumption of two helpings of fresh fruit and two helpings of fresh vegetables daily.
4. The consumption of two to four slices of whole grain bread daily.
5. Elimination or considerable reduction of white flour and white sugar products.
6. The consumption of a whole grain, high fiber, low sugar cereal daily with one tablespoon of unprocessed bran added.

This type of simple approach embodies recent information by authorities in the field,[19,20,21,22] is well tolerated by most patients, and has led to considerable clinical improvement in these problems.

Patients with glucose intolerance, including diabetes, may also respond very favorable to dietary revision when it is put in the proper education and behavior modification setting in the office. Instructions in this area, supported by recent research,[23,24,25,26,27,28,29,30,31,32] are also kept simple and may include the following:

1. Point out to the patients that it is important to eat three or four well balanced smaller meals a day to manifest proper blood sugar control. Encourage the patients not to skip meals, but not to oversnack and eat foods of low quality.

Figure 11.3
Cholesterol Flow Sheet

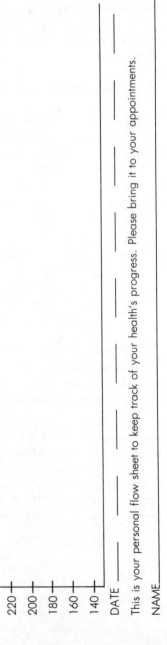

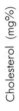

Figure 11.4
Cholesterol Ratio Flow Sheet HDL

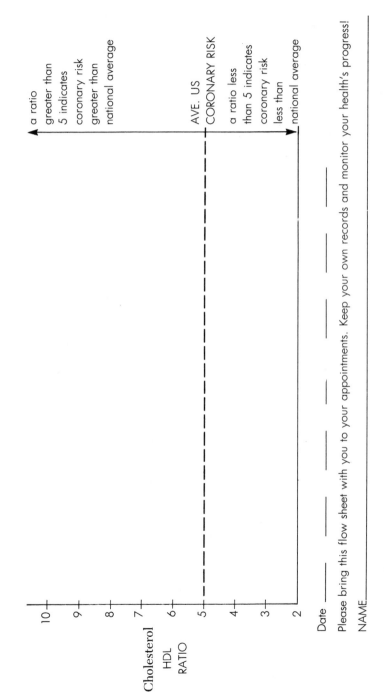

2. Sugar and other sweeteners are eliminated from the diet with the exception of a small amount of natural sugars found in fruits and vegetables. The concept of label reading is brought to the attention of the patient. It is pointed out that anything ending in -ose is a sugar, such as sucrose, dextrose or maltose.
3. Limiting coffee, tea, nicotine or alcohol is suggested because they stimulate difficulties in normalizing blood sugar.
4. The use of a reasonable high complex carbohydrate, moderate protein, low fat diet is utilized with recipes given out exemplifying this approach. The diet should be 65 to 70 percent complex carbohydrates, 20 percent fat, and 10 to 12 percent protein.
5. Whole fruits, frozen or fresh, not fruit juices, are recommended.
6. Regular exercise is suggested to normalize the body's ability to be sensitized to insulin.
7. Unprocessed bran is used, generally increasing from one teaspoon in the morning to one tablespoon each morning.

These two examples exemplify a simplistic approach towards nutritional improvement which can be used for many patients in the treatment of specific health dysfunctions which have relationship to nutrition. It is important to recall that almost all of the major chronic degenerative diseases have nutritional relationships, and therefore improvement of the average patient's diet will not only serve to reduce the risk to degenerative disease, but may also be an important part of the therapy chosen by the physician for a diagnosed degenerative disease. The successful implementation and integration of these concepts within the practice of medicine depends to a great extent on how well organized the physician and his or her staff are in educating the patient.[33,34] The concept that "patients will not change even if they know what's good for them" is only self-fulfilling when the physician and the staff do not commit themselves significantly to the importance of this particular topic. It is truly significant to see the types of patient compliance that can be achieved when the whole staff emphasizes life-style intervention and nutritional alteration as a major theme in the practice, and provides a proper support to work with the physician as a team in the improvement of that patient's health.[35,36]

The first step in the appropriate integration of these concepts within the practice of health care is for the physicians themselves to secure enough education in the area of nutrition so that they feel comfortable with delivering these concepts to their patients. Secondarily, the physicians must commit themselves to an improved nutritional base in their own lives, and then excite the staff towards the ultimate goal of patient education in this important area. As the practitioner moves forward in these areas, the more successful implementation of nutrition education in the general practice of medicine will result.

REFERENCES

1. Cooper, K. H. 1978. *The New Aerobics*. New York: Bantam Books.
2. Dugdale, A. E. and Chandler, D. 1979. Knowledge and belief in nutrition. *Amer. J. Clin. Nutr. 31*, 441.
3. Ley, P. and Anderson, S. 1977. Patient education and medication errors. *J. Medical Education 52*, 147.
4. Fineberg, H. V. and Hiatt, H. H. 1979. Evaluation of medical practices. *New Engl. J. Medicine 298*, 1086.
5. Newkirk, B., Osterhaus, K. and Huntington, B. November 14, 1978. Patient education in an ambulatory care clinic. *Patient Care*, p. 26.
6. Rodnick, P. and Bubb, T. 1978. Health hazard appraisal in cardiac risk factor reduction. *Amer. J. Epidemiology 101*, 177.
7. Levy, R. 1981. The decline in cardiovascular disease mortality. *Annual Reviews of Public Health*, vol. 2. Palo Alto: Annual Reviews, Inc.
8. Farquhar, J. W., Maccoby, N. and Wood, P. D. 1977. Community education for cardiovascular health. *Lancet*, p. 1192.
9. Griffith, D. 1980. *Instruction for Patients*. Chicago: Medical Science Publishers.
10. Brunworth, D. and Rigden, S. 1979. *Patient Education for the Family*. New York: Harper and Row.
11. Brunworth and Rigden. 1979. *Patient Education for the Family*. New York: Harper and Row.
12. Rulin, Marvin. 1973. Office Gynecology and Obstetrics. Chapter 35 in *Family Practice*. Conn, Rakel and Johnson, eds. Philadelphia: W. B. Saunders.
13. Price, Weston. 1975. *Nutrition and Physical Degeneration*. Pasadena, California: Price-Pottenger Nutrition Foundation.
14. George Bray, ed. November, 1979. *Obesity in America*. PHEW. Public Health Service. NIH Publication No. 79–359.
15. R. B. Stuart and Barbara Davis. 1976. *Slim Chance in a Fat World*. Champaign, Ill.: Research Press.
16. Peter Lindner, M.D. 1963. *Mind Over Platter*. N. Hollywood, Calif.: Wilshire Book Co.
17. Malcolm, Robert. February, 1976. Current views on the management of obesity. *South Med. J.* 69:135–140.
18. Currey, Hal, et al. June 27, 1977. Behavioral treatment of obesity: limitations and results with the chronically obese. JAMA 237:2829–2831.
19. Burkitt, Denis. 1980. *Eat Right—to Stay Healthy and Enjoy Life More*. New York: Area publishing, Inc.

20. Grimes, Davis S. February 21, 1976. Refined carbohydrate, smooth muscle spasm and disease of the colon. *Lancet* 1:395–397.
21. *Nutrition and the MD.* vol. VII, no. 7. July 1981.
22. Heaton, K. W. August 1979. The real value of fiber. *Consultant*, pp. 23–30.
23. Anderson, J. W. April, 1981. High-fiber diets in diabetes. *Cont. Educ. for the Family Physician*, vol. 14, no. 4, pp. 22–27.
24. Anderson, J. W. and Seiling, Beverly. 1979. *HCF Diets. A Professional Guide.* University of Kentucky.
25. Anderson, J. W. May, 1980. High-fiber diet. *Medical Times*, pp. 41–44.
26. Anderson, J. W. and Ward, K. 1978. Long term effects of high carbohydrate, high fiber diets on glucose and lipid metabolism. *Diabetes care* 1:77.
27. Hallfrisch, J., et al. April, 1979. Insulin and glucose responses in rats fed sucrose or starch. *American Journal Clin. Nutrition.* 32: pp. 787–793.
28. Kiehm, Y., et al. August, 1976. Beneficial effects of a high carbohydrate, high fiber diet on hyperglycemic diabetic men. *Amer. Journal Clin. Nutrition.* 29: pp. 893–899.
29. Crapo, Phyllis A., et al. February, 1981. Comparison of serum glucose, insulin, and glucagon responses to different types of complex carbohydrate in noninsulin dependent diabetic patients. *Amer. Journal Clin. Nutrition* 43: pp. 184–190.
30. Bolton, Robin P., et al. February, 1980. The role of dietary fiber in satiety, glucose, and insulin: studies with fruit and fruit juice. *Amer. Journal Clin. Nutrition* 34: pp. 211–217.
31. Albrink, M. J., et al. July, 1979. Effect of high and low fiber diets on plasma lipids and insulin. *Amer. Journal Clin. Nutrition* 32: pp. 1486–1491.
32. Riales, R., Albrank, M. J. December, 1981. Effect of chromium chloride supplementation on glucose tolerance and serum lipids including high-density lipoprotein of adult men. *Amer. Journal Clin. Nutrition* 34: pp. 2670–2678.
33. Rigden, S. Patient education in a small town family practice. Proceedings no. 2-1978 from *Patient Education in the Primary Care Setting.* Madison, Wisconsin, pp. 95–98.
34. Rigden, S. Holistic care in rural practice. Proceedings no. 3-1979 from *Patient Education in the Primary Care Setting.* Minneapolis, Minnesota, pp. 93–97.
35. Rigden, S. April, 1980. Patient education—it's good for patient and doctor. *Physician's Patient Education Newsletter*, vol. 3, no. 2, pp. 1–2.
36. Rigden, S. November, 1980. My experience with patient education. *Colloquy*, pp. 3–6.

INDEX

305